Contents

The following units are available on our website www.heinemann.co.uk/vocational:

BT30 Provide UV tanning treatments
BT31 Provide self tanning treatments

Acknowledgments

Most writers would say that writing is a particularly solitary pastime, but this has definitely not been my experience in putting together a book of this size! There are so many wonderful people to thank for their support and encouragement, without which I could not have contemplated tackling such a volume of work.

My darling husband Stephen was a tower of strength both with moral support and on the practical domestic front. He provided both the time and freedom to allow this book to develop. Thank you for the TLC and the endless cups of tea, and sherry, when required!

The team at Heinemann once again offered endless support and vision to this book. Thank you Pen Gresford for your continued guiding light, Camilla Thomas for your outstanding editing skills and copy-editor Susan Ross and proofreader Jan Doorly for never missing a thing!

Thank you to my co-authors, both experts in their field: firstly, Jeanine Connor, Beauty Therapy lecturer at the London School of Fashion, for her anatomy and physiology contribution, and my good friend Elaine Stoddart, for her epilation and business chapters. Both your inputs have enhanced this book immeasurably, giving a commercial and very professional edge, which I am sure the students will also appreciate.

Elaine also deserves a huge thank you for her commercial contacts, as many of the contributors were through her industrial links, which provided a current, commercial feeling to all the chapters. The companies were amazing, and their contribution to the photo shoot was over and above my expectations. So, my thanks to:

- Bellitas – Penny Turvey for product provisions.
- The Carlton Group – Angela Barbegelata – and Fabes & Trudy Sawyer for both equipment photos and answers to my endless technical clarification demands!
- Dale Saunas – Stephen Hipps for photographs and technical information.
- Espa International – Charlie Harmsworth for photographs.
- Face & Body Perfector – David Greenway, MD – and Emma Holmes, the therapist in the photographs for the non-surgical face and body lifting.
- Fake Bake – Jackie Howard and Julie Kelly for body exfoliation and fake tan application.
- Finders International for Dead Sea product shots.
- Floataway – Colin Stanwell-Smith for his contributions in flotation theory.
- Gareth Boden and Tony Poole for the excellent photographs and their outstanding patience with the more technical shots of epilation and the electrical equipment.
- The Guinot UK Training and Development Manager, Marie Caudwell, and Clare Boxey, the therapist in the photographs for galvanic facials.
- HABIA – Tiffany Tarrant for her support with the NVQ level 3 standards and my endless queries.
- Salon Solutions – Tracey Stephens for her contributions with spray tanning.
- SOTHYS – Jon Mills for photographs.
- Sterex Electrolysis International Ltd – Philip Woods.
- The Sunbed Association – Cathy Banks.
- Susan Molyneux – Susannah Bingham and Karen Gold for the body wrapping photos.
- Jane Holmes and her staff at Salisbury College, and the Tidworth site, for all their help with the photo shoot and excellent catering arrangements. Thank you Jane for being so helpful with models during the shoot, and thanks you to the staff and all the models for their help. Thank you also for being another professional pair of eyes for all the photos and for being a true friend.
- City Computers who fixed my computer as it crashed with the entire book stored upon it!

Jane Hiscock

The use of HABIA unit titles and element headings by kind permission of HABIA, Fraser House, Nether Hall Road, Doncaster, South Yorkshire DN1 2PH, Tel: 01302 380000, Fax: 01302 380028, Email: enquiries@habia.org.uk, Website: www.habia.org.uk.

We are pleased that this book has been approved by the Federation of Holistic Therapists, www.fht.org.uk.

The authors and publisher would like to thank the following for permission to reproduce photographs:

Harcourt Education/Gareth Boden 8, 11, 17, 23 (bottom), 24, 27, 67, 84, 97, 104, 213, 220, 228 (top, bottom two), 236 (bottom), 240, 243, 248, 252, 256, 257, 260, 261, 270, 270, 272, 278, 279, 280, 281, 285 (centre), 286 (top and bottom), 307, 319 (3rd from top), 320–23, 333, 335–342, 344, 345, 346 (top). 349, 350, 352–67, 370–79, 384–88, 391, 392, 395 (right), 396, 402, 410, 411, 415, 419, 427, 430, 431, 445–47, 449, 450, web pages 1 (left and right), 25, 26, 28–31; Carlton Professional 7, 39, 50, 51, 52,

S/NVQ Level 3

Beauty Therapy

Jane Hiscock

Elaine Stoddart

Jeanine Connor

www.heinemann.co.uk
✓ Free online support
✓ Useful weblinks
✓ 24 hour online ordering

01865 888058

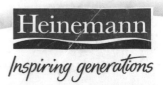

Heinemann
Inspiring generations

Heinemann Educational Publishers
Halley Court, Jordan Hill, Oxford OX2 8EJ
Part of Harcourt Education

Heinemann is a registered trademark of
Harcourt Education Limited

Text © Jeanine Connor, Jane Hiscock and Elaine Stoddart, 2004

First published 2004

2009 2008 2007

10 9 8 7 6 5 4

British Library Cataloguing in Publication Data is available
from the British Library on request.

ISBN 978 0 435 45640 5

Copyright notice

Page layout and Illustrations by Hardlines.

Original illustrations © Harcourt Education Limited, 2004

Cover design by Wooden Ark

Cover photo: © Zefa

Printed in China by South China Printing Company

54, 55, 57, 93, 95, 219 (left), 227 (first three from top), 228 (2nd and 3rd from top), 229, 237, 241, 245, 251, 263, 285 (left), 320 (bottom), 328, 330, 346 (bottom), 389, 390, 425, 464, 478; Dale Sauna 318 (bottom three), 319 (top), 461 (top), 467, 468, 480; Elemis 23 (top), 119; Daniel Lee 82; Finders International 443, 444, 475, 477; Floataway 453, 456; Guinot 125, 135 (centre), 171, 187 (centre), 187 (left), 188, 194, 197 (left and centre), 219 (centre), 227 (bottom), 234, 235, 236 (top), 250 (top), 261 (bottom right); Oxyspa 461 (bottom); Perfector 83 (left),131, 205, 219 (right), 262 (left), 272; Science photo Library 15, 42, 43, 44, 135 (left), 135 (right), 137, 139, 149, 150, 153, 154, 421; Sothys 50, 106, 114, 196, 209, 215 (bottom), 250 (bottom), 285 (right), 318 (top), 319 (2nd from top), 334

Every effort has been made to contact copyright holders of material reproduced in this book. Any omissions will be rectified in subsequent printings if notice is given to the publishers.

Introduction

Welcome to your S/NVQ level 3 in Beauty Therapy. This professional handbook has been written in an accessible format to provide all the underpinning knowledge and practical skills you need to succeed in your S/NVQ level 3 course. The book is designed to guide you through the 2004 level 3 National Occupational Standards (NOS) and is tailor-made for the level 3 general beauty therapy route, including body massage and spa treatments.

The key features used in this book to support your learning are:

Remember – highlighting specific areas that you need to pay particular attention to and to remind you of the important legal and professional issues within the industry.

Check it out – activities involving self-learning through research and investigation into products, services or treatments.

Keys to good practice – tips and suggestions to promote good practice in the salon and in your working methods.

In the salon – includes case studies based on real-life events that you may face in the salon. They are written to allow you to consider how you would respond in situations as they arise.

There are also:

- **Step-by-step photographs** to guide you through the practical application of equipment for face and body treatments.
- **Clear diagrams and tables** to support your required underpinning knowledge.
- **Knowledge checks** at the end of every section.

Each of the practical units of the qualification contains the same essentials – the **Professional basics**. This has been presented as a separate section that should be worked through and adapted to the unit you are taking at the time. The anatomy required for each unit has also been presented separately, in the **Related anatomy and physiology** section, which can be referred to easily. Anatomy is a constant theme through each unit, but remember that you only need to learn it once and apply the knowledge to the practical area you are working through. The same applies to knowledge of the skin, which is dealt with in the section **You and the skin.**

The treatments and specific skills that you will learn during this level 3 course build on the knowledge and techniques you learnt and practised in your level 2, or equivalent, course. By enhancing your expertise, this level 3 course extends your career options: you can work in a salon, for international companies, such as Virgin and Guinot, or even start your own mobile business. You could also develop your skills to work within the commercial sector, working with companies selling to salons or demonstrating to and training other therapists. Health farms, cruise ships and spa resorts all demand a high level of expertise which this qualification prepares you for. With an NVQ level 3 qualification the world is literally your oyster and your career will take off in all sorts of directions – so consider this book a good investment for your future!

Level 3 is by no means an easy option and some areas of the underpinning knowledge may seem more difficult than others. Like all areas of life, there is no substitute for hard work and revision. For example, the muscles of the body may seem like a lot to learn, but with revision, repetition, games and continuous use, you will find that remembering the names eventually become second nature.

The same can be said for the application of equipment during treatments – the practical skills. Level 3 requires practitioners to work at a very high level of skill and this demands practice and effort. Learning massage movements, for example, can be frustrating at first, with so much to remember: feet; hand direction; your posture, however practice will reap rewards, and most family members or friends are usually delighted to act as a model to help!

If you have taken an NVQ level 2 qualification you will find that the level 3 assessment is very similar to your level 2 portfolio file. The assessment books are the same format, with ranges to be covered and performance criteria to be checked against by the assessor. Level 3 assessments, however, do require more thought to coordinate and are not always done strictly per unit – you may have a client treating him or herself to a full morning of treatments, including a sauna, jacuzzi, back massage and a galvanic facial, which means you are crossing over several units and ranges. The key is to be organised: recording your treatment plan and being able to provide evidence to support your assessment. You may wish to take some treatments under assessment conditions and not others; at the start of the practical session let your tutor know that you would like to be assessed. Each training establishment may have slightly differing methods of recording assessment outcomes: student diaries, evidence sheets etc. Whichever method is used it is vital to fill out the assessment book as thoroughly as possible, to avoid missing any valuable evidence.

An essential tip to keep in mind during both the electrical and body massage assessments is to be very aware of safety, especially using electrical equipment, making sure that your treatments do not run over the commercially acceptable times required for the NOS assessment requirements. That too is quite a skill to master: preparing, carrying out a consultation, and giving a full treatment with aftercare, all within the time parameters.

Remember that the hard work will be worth it and your diverse set of skills will be a great asset to any salon owner or manager. A level 3 qualification gives you the knowledge to meet client demands and trends for most commercial salons as well as providing you with the flexibility and choices to pick your own career path.

Good luck and enjoy the book!

Jane Hiscock, Elaine Stoddart and Jeanine Connor

professional
BASICS

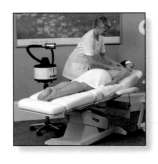 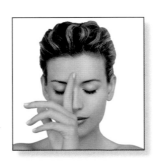 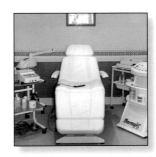

Professional basics

The **Professional basics** section draws together all of the common threads running through the practical units. The basic principles that will underpin all your knowledge and understanding are included here. As you learn each new skill area, you will need to refer back to this section. You will be directed to the relevant pages in **Professional basics**.

Understanding the basics is very important to your development within the role of a professional beauty therapist and will help you to achieve your NVQ qualification. It sets the highest of standards, which you should always aspire to. This is your transition from student to employee, and your employer will have a very high expectation of the new Level 3 recruit!

There are four main topics in this section:

- You – the therapist
- You and your client
- You and your working environment
- You, your client and the law.

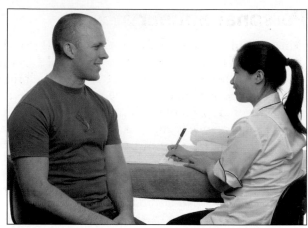

A thorough consultation before treatment is important to develop a good relationship with your client

You – the therapist

You will learn about	
• personal appearance • your salon's requirements • personal safety and security	• personal risk assessment • managing resources within the limits of your authority.

Before beginning any new training or learning new skills, you will need to go back to the fundamental basics of beauty therapy and start by looking at yourself – the beauty therapist. While not a novice at beauty therapy – you already have qualifications – it is very important that you assess yourself in a slightly different light and re-evaluate yourself in all aspects of professional life.

A mental 'spring clean' and re-think will eliminate any bad habits which you may have and encourage you to develop the good practices you have adopted. Sometimes senior students become complacent – you should be setting an example to students just starting, as they really do look up and aspire to be like you, and not fall into careless habits, which can be hard to break.

NVQ Level 3 work requires a thorough approach as the electrical equipment used, if handled incorrectly, could cause your clients harm and you will need to be fully aware of health and safety implications. At this level, clients will also have a greater expectation from their treatments.

Personal appearance

When you meet someone for the first time, what is the first thing you are likely to notice? Our first impressions of people usually involve judging their appearance. Aspects of appearance include clothing, body adornment (jewellery), hairstyles and physique, especially relevant when people seek to achieve a particular style such as a body builder or as a professional in the creative field of hairdressing or beauty therapy. Appearance is combined with spoken language, and with non-verbal communication, to convey a variety of messages – an important thing to remember when greeting and dealing with clients.

In particular, people's appearance helps to develop their identity and will reflect:

- their occupation – a uniform or business suit representing what they do
- their membership of a social group, such as punk rockers
- their status, e.g. a judge's gown and wig
- their self image – whether the person has high or low self-esteem
- their setting or image – think about dressing for a party.

Your professional appearance says so much about you, your business, and your abilities. All this is reflected in your personal appearance, body language and attitude, and the client will visually weigh up all this information within ten seconds of meeting you. So you have just ten seconds to make the right impression, and convince the client that you are the therapist for his or her needs, while giving a caring and competent reflection of your abilities!

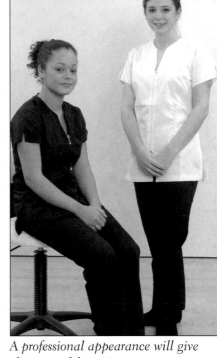

A *professional appearance will give clients confidence in you*

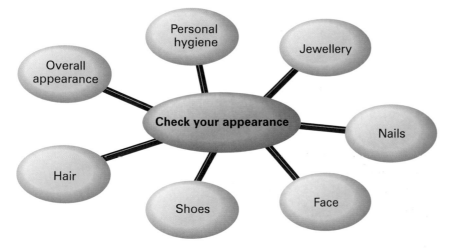

You have just ten seconds to make the right impression!

Appearance guidelines are laid down by both the awarding body of your qualification and your professional therapist association. Their codes of practice are quite specific regarding professional appearance and are of prime importance for competent assessment achievement.

Overalls

Be critical about your overalls. If you have had them since you first started training, they may not be as immaculate as they once were. Level 2 treatments can take their toll on overalls. Do you have tint splashes or wax stains on your overalls, which never seem to quite fade away, or has the whiteness of your overalls simply faded after so many hot washes?

Many training establishments encourage a different look for the more senior students, and it is possible to invest in some professional work wear, which is a little more reflective of your new status. Trousers and tunic tops are encouraged by lots of salons as uniforms, and are both comfortable and very practical – you may change tops more than trousers.

Hair style

Are you as particular about your hair at work as you were when you first trained, or have you developed the habit of holding it back with a band or clip, as it really needs washing but you did not have the time? Bad habits start to creep in, almost unnoticed! Is your hair in good condition, or in need of a trim and colour? Nothing makes the hair look dirtier than obvious re-growth, when the true hair colour is growing through the highlights, and even if freshly washed, the hair still looks in need of attention. Ask yourself this: would you wear your hair out to a party as you wear it to work? If the answer is 'No, of course not', then you need to re-think. Hair up in a professional style is both attractive and practical, so go back to the good habits of your initial training. Fresh, clean hair also enhances the overall hygiene of a person.

Footwear

Are your feet safe and comfortable? Are your shoes in need of a clean or repair, or do they look worn out? Feet need the protection of safe shoes – with toes covered and no high heels – for your own safety and to maintain a good posture. Work shoes should meet industry standards and your college regulations, but students often forget to change from outdoor shoes into appropriate salon footwear.

If your training centre has allowed senior students to change uniforms, what about new footwear? There are some very comfortable, closed-in shoes, which are also fashionable, available in most high streets.

Beware! Some work-wear companies advertise clothing with the models wearing an open toe, or flip-flop style shoe. This is not suitable salon wear, and will probably not be approved by either your awarding body, or the insurance company for your training centre.

Face

While you do not need to wear full make-up to look professional, you should remember that Level 3 treatments are all about skin improvement and that your face can be used to advertise your abilities. Start by taking a look in good daylight at your face, skin and eyebrows. Are they in need of some attention? The old proverb is often true – 'The cobbler is worse shod'; in other words, as a therapist, you may be too busy to have an eyebrow shape or a facial, but how does that reflect on your image to the client?

A therapist with congested skin is hardly in a position to advise a client which treatments to have, and the home care routine to follow, if she is not taking her own advice! The advice you give to clients also applies to you – enough sleep, a sensible diet, a little exercise, reduced coffee and alcohol intake and plenty of water, which will pay dividends with a clear skin, plenty of energy and a positive glow. You will help to inspire the client to look after her skin by setting the example, and looking good.

Check it out

Look in trade magazines for adverts for salon work wear. Phone or write for brochures. Compare three different styles and prices, and put forward a proposal to your salon manager/lecturer about the possibility of wearing a new style for client sessions.

Remember

Leather shoes allow the feet to breathe and are more hygienic as they prevent a build-up of bacteria, which may cause odour problems and lead to athlete's foot.

Oral hygiene

Regular dental care will protect against tooth decay and will prevent bad breath. Regular brushing, mouth sprays, sugar-free mints and breath fresheners are also advisable to prevent stale breath being passed over the client. Remember that bad breath can be a sign of illness, so it may be worth having a dental/medical check-up if your think you may have a problem.

It is only polite and courteous to your client to avoid strongly flavoured foods such as curry, garlic and onions. Cigarette smoke can also cling to the breath and clothing, so avoid smoking in working hours.

Nails

Nails reflect both your hygiene standards and your profession. Short, unvarnished nails are always best for giving an intuitive massage, without fear of stabbing the clients' skin, and for maintaining a clean appearance. Always wash your hands after a toilet visit, handling food or stock, and after handling money, the worst offender for spreading dirt and germs! If you accompany the client to the till and handle money, just check and see how dirty your hands have become.

Always wash your hands at the beginning and the end of a treatment – the client will expect to see you do this. You will also need to wash your hands during a treatment, for example if you have blown your nose or touched your face. Certain procedures such as extraction will also require a mid-treatment hand wash. If you train to become a nail technician, then your clients will expect to see beautifully manicured nails, but it would be impractical to take massage assessments with nail extensions on.

Jewellery

Jewellery is neither safe nor practical within Level 3 treatments. Rings can scratch the clients' skin, ruining the relaxation of the treatment. They are also dangerous to wear when carrying out electrical procedures, as metal is a good conductor of electricity. A minimal amount of jewellery is recommended by most awarding bodies – a wedding band, small earrings and nothing else. It is not safe to have necklaces and earrings dangling when working, and it may affect any insurance entitlement if negligence is claimed. There is also the risk of your best jewellery getting lost at work, or ruined by products and wear and tear.

Your salon's requirements

Salons vary in uniform codes and the expected dress for work, so you must always check exactly what is expected of you within your own training establishment. Different dress codes are acceptable, and you should try to be flexible as long they are safe, comfortable and easy to maintain. Some fabrics are totally unsuited for uniforms, such as silk which is not hard wearing and requires dry cleaning. Polyester and cotton mixtures wear and wash well, and many companies are incorporating linen blends in their fabrics, which look very professional.

Overalls for large groups of employees or students need to suit all figure types. The most important function of any uniform is to allow the wearer a free range of movement. When trying on a uniform, put it through its paces – stretch out your arms as you would if you were performing a massage to make sure the uniform allows plenty of give across the shoulders. It is often a good practice to buy a size larger than usual, just to be able to work comfortably – as long as the overall does not swamp you

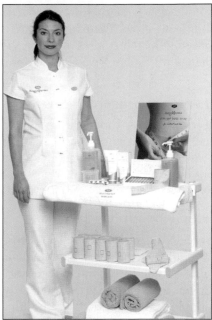

A smart, tidy uniform and trolley reflects good hygiene and high professional standards

and is safe. Looking trim in a fitted overall to look the part may be nice but is highly impractical! For this reason, trousers and tops make a flexible uniform, as you can mix and match colours and sizes. Try to shop around and get a uniform you are really happy with – but always check your salon requirements before purchasing.

Personal presentation

Presentation is about the whole package – not just the uniform or face, make-up and nails, but your entire image, facial expressions, body language and attitude. It is not only personal appearance that makes a professional beauty therapist, but his or her attitude too.

Preparing for the day ahead

It takes organisation, care and dedication to be ready to work effectively. You should aim to be calm, relaxed and to ignore any personal problems and focus your whole attention on the client. The beauty therapy industry is a service industry. The general public are your clients and they pay for your service and expertise. Therefore, they should also be entitled to your full attention and care.

It is not just the décor of a salon that creates atmosphere; it is the ambience created by the people within it. How the therapist mentally prepares for work goes a long way to producing the calm, relaxed atmosphere of a salon which allows the client to gain maximum benefit from the treatment.

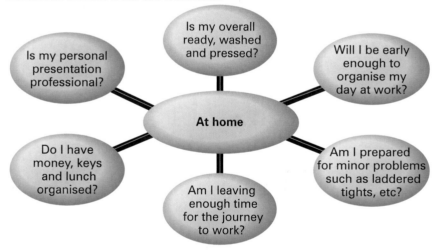

Preparing for work – at home

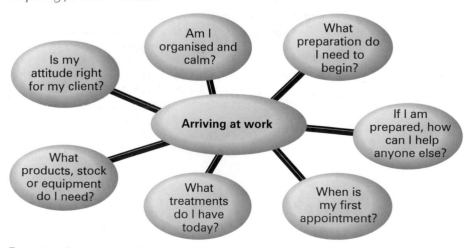

Preparing for work – at the salon

Keys to good practice

- Be totally attentive to the client and his or her needs.
- If you do not show interest in the client, then he or she may not return to the salon for other treatments.
- As you prepare your working area, clear your mind of all angry thoughts. The client does *not* want to hear about *your* problems.

In the salon

All through school and college, Hayley was known as a scatterbrain. She would forget lunch money and have to borrow from friends but then forget to pay it back. She missed exam deadlines and sometimes overslept on salon days. Her forgetfulness was not too serious and because she is a sweet-natured girl, her friends and lecturers at college would raise their eyebrows in despair, but she was nearly always forgiven.

Now Hayley is in the world of work, and she is employed in a smart salon, but on the other side of town from where she lives. Her trade test was fine as her treatments are good, but her disorganisation has not really improved since college.

So far, she has been late on several occasions, lost the keys to the stock cupboard, left the payment book at the bank and broken a couple of teacups. Twice, she has left her uniform on the bus coming to work. Her employer is beginning to get fed up loaning her money for lunch, or bus money, and having the extra cost of replacing keys, cups, etc. On the other hand, the clients like her, and although she has been late, she does not understand that she is in the wrong.

- As her employer what would you do?
- Do you recognise any of Hayley's traits in yourself?
- Are you able to accept the responsibility that employment brings?
- Should Hayley's employer sack her?
- Is there anyone in your group who has the same life pattern?

Personal security and safety

This is about you taking responsibility for yourself, your actions and for others. The Health and Safety at Work etc. Act 1974 (HASWA) states, 'Employees have responsibilities to take reasonable care of themselves and other people affected by their work and to co-operate with their employers in the discharge of their obligations' (see page 67). It is absolutely essential that you remember this when dealing with electrical equipment, the wet area and body treatments. You must *never* jeopardise the safety of your client (or yourself), as the consequences are serious.

Each piece of equipment used in the practical units has its own risk assessment and safety regulation, safe use and storage guidelines, and so on. The **Professional basics** section refers to you, and your attitude to working, to keep you and everyone around you safe.

Beauty therapists often work very long hours and may be on the go all day. They are usually in a busy salon environment, with other people present all the time – clients, other beauty therapists, sales representatives, managers, receptionists, cleaners, etc. If the therapist does not have a sense of personal safety and respect for the safety of others, accidents will occur.

Remember

It is not only the employer's responsibility to provide health and safety management. It is also the responsibility of each employee to follow the rules.

Informing others of your whereabouts

Ensure that someone in the salon knows where you are or what you are doing, regardless of how simple a task it may appear. If you stand on some steps to change the light bulb, then make sure that another member of staff is with you, to prevent you being knocked off, and to take the old bulb from you. Do not be tempted to stand on a chair, or an old delivery box, or anything else remotely unstable.

If you go to the local shop for lunch, pop to the bank or run an errand, tell someone when you will be back, and where you are going. You may wish to carry a personal alarm but make sure that you keep it handy, in a pocket of your coat for example (not at the bottom of your bag), ready to be activated in an emergency.

The salon should have a list of telephone numbers by the phone in case of emergency, such as the local police station or security guard room. This will save time when it really counts.

Do not be unprotected. For example, do not leave outside doors open when working in a treatment room, do not leave the till draw open, etc. Do not be naive enough to think that it could not happen to you! If unsure, seek professional advice from the local crime prevention officer or local police station, both for building security advice and also for personal safety hints for staff and clients.

As a professional therapist, always follow your professional guidelines:

- Do not treat a male client alone in the salon late at night.
- There should be a minimum of two people working in the salon on winter evenings when it gets dark early.
- Always lock up the premises together.
- If you drive a car to work, think about the best place to park it. Always choose an area that will be well lit after dark.
- Do not park in a multi-storey car park if you know that you will be going home late and in the dark.
- Do not travel home after work alone in the dark – phone a taxi, family member or friend.
- Do not put yourself at risk in any way.

Personal security for staff

The salon should provide lockable staff storage cabinets or similar so that personal belongings can be locked away. Handbags and purses are always vulnerable to the opportunist thief, who may slip in and out of the salon undetected. Staff should be discouraged from bringing large amounts of cash into work and should avoid wearing expensive jewellery, which has to be removed during treatments and is therefore vulnerable to loss or theft.

The salon's takings should be transferred to a bank or night deposit daily. Avoid taking the same route to the bank at the same time of day. Someone may be watching!

Be very aware of clients' jewellery. Let them see that this is placed in a bowl on the trolley, do not forget to return it when finishing the treatment and do not put yourself in danger of being called a thief by slipping it into your overall pocket!

Be aware of suspicious packages left unattended. Inform a supervisor and if necessary, call the emergency services.

Remember

There are many types of potential harm – verbal, mental or physical – and they can come from many sources, often unexpected ones.

Remember

If the therapist does not have a sense of personal safety and respect for the safety of others, accidents will occur.

Your posture

Good posture can protect you from aches and pains, as well as the development of more permanent back problems, repetitive strain injury (RSI) and time off work due to illness. Try to avoid stooping and slouching, and this will prevent back problems occurring.

Maintain a good posture and evenly distribute body weight by standing correctly with the feet slightly apart. This will prevent accidents and injury. A full body massage is a very demanding treatment to give, and you may treat several clients on the same day, so good posture is essential to avoid muscular problems in the shoulders and lower back. Poor posture may lead to discomfort and, in the worst cases, can cause permanent problems with vertebrae. It is common for therapists to suffer from RSI in both the wrists and the lower back, especially if the therapist specialises in massage, and does five or six treatments in a day. Prevention is so much better than cure – and often there is no cure for a bad back, just rest and avoidance of the activity.

For this reason, try to work with a couch or bed which is set at the correct height for you. It should be at a comfortable height so that you do not have to bend at the waist nor bend your arms at the elbow. When trying out a couch you will need to take into account the added height of the clients' body, so when purchasing, ask a colleague or friend to lie on the couch to allow you to judge the correct height.

Hydraulic adjustable couches are ideal for suiting all therapists, but are expensive to purchase. It may be possible to raise the couch by using wooden blocks under the legs, but these must be approved by your health and safety officer, put under the couch before the client is on it, and of a suitable size and material to support the weight of the client. If the block is not solid, or the couch leg is perched on the edge of the block, an accident might happen.

You will also need to ensure that your equipment is posture friendly. Do not position your trolley or machine so far away from you that you are continually leaning over to reach it. This would mean that you are over-extending, and you will not be in full control of the machine for safety and client comfort.

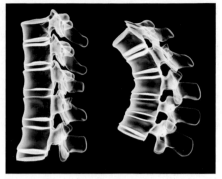

Poor posture can lead to spinal damage

Protection and personal cleanliness

- Always wear the correct protective clothing provided to shield a uniform.
- Always wear gloves when using chemicals or if there is a possibility of coming into contact with body fluids.
- Always follow the correct disposal regulations for gloves and waste materials.
- If an establishment provides a uniform as part of a corporate image, then wear it!
- Hair should be tidy. Clip back loose hair. Avoid long hair styles as these are considered unhygienic and may be unsafe (see the table on the next page).

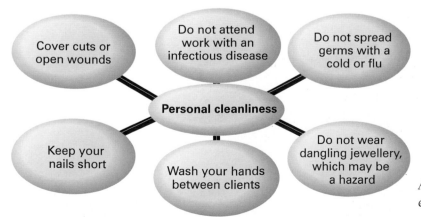

A high standard of cleanliness will ensure no cross-infection can occur

Personal risk assessment

Unit G1, Ensure your own actions reduce risks to health and safety, is all about being safe and responsible throughout your working day, and you will be referring back to that unit for all your practical treatment applications. You will also need to carry out a personal risk assessment which involves considering your dress code and presentation, how you handle electrical equipment and the way you deal with clients and carry out your duties.

Dress code and presentation

The table below looks at some of the reasons why it is essential to present yourself professionally and some of the possible consequences for the therapist if she fails to do so.

Definition of terms

A **hazard** is something that could cause harm, such as an electrical cable trailing across the floor.

A **risk** is the likelihood of the hazard actually causing harm, for example the therapist tripping over the cable and injuring herself.

Presentation	Hazard (What can go wrong?)	Who could be harmed?
Shoes	High heels may cause you to be unstable on your feet. They may cause you to trip over or fall sideways off the heel. If you trip while carrying equipment, you could injure yourself and damage the equipment. Open-toed shoes provide no protection if equipment or products should fall on your toes.	Yourself Other therapists Members of the public Other staff Visitors
Overalls	Baggy sleeves may catch on handles, products and equipment. Overalls too tight will restrict movement which will inhibit safe conduct. Trousers which are too long may cause you to trip.	Yourself Other therapists Members of the public Other staff Visitors
Hair style	Long hair dangling in the eyes may distract you or prevent you seeing clearly and may cause eye irritation. Hair is a conductor of electricity, and if you make contact with a client via your hair while he or she is having a galvanic facial, you may cause the current to short cut, causing sparking and pain for the client. Not regarded as hygienic.	Yourself Other therapists Members of the public Other staff Visitors
Nails	Long nails or jagged nail edges will inhibit massage movements and can cause skin damage to clients if you scratch or jab them. If not kept scrupulously clean, may harbour germs and pass infections.	Yourself Other therapists Members of the public Other staff Visitors

Risk assessment: hazards connected with appearance

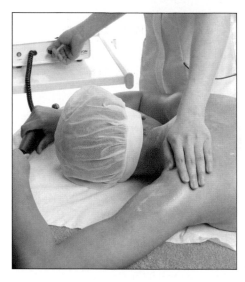

Always handle electrical equipment with care

Prevention (How can I prevent this?)	Monitoring (How can I check?)	Corrective action (What should I do if things are not right?)
Adhere to your salon dress code and the code of your professional body. Buy a safe, sensible pair of shoes with closed-in toes.	Try on the shoes before purchase and walk around in them. Are they comfortable and safe? Do you feel unstable or as if you are tottering around?	Keep sling-backs, high heels and open-toed shoes for evening wear and non-work occasions.
Adhere to your salon dress code and the code of your professional body.	Try on overalls before purchase and stretch and move as in treatments. Are they comfortable and safe?	Stop wearing a tightly fitting overall and purchase a larger size. If your overall is far too large, either alter it yourself or ask a professional seamstress to alter it for you.
Practise putting hair up at home into a style which suits you and feels comfortable. There are lots of hair accessories available to help.	Does your hairstyle feel comfortable? If it is scraped back and too tight, it will give you a headache and may make you feel irritable. Make sure that your choice of style does not cause you to constantly fiddle with your hair, which is distracting and unhygienic. Check your hair from all angles using a mirror.	Seek advice. Your manager will tell you what is acceptable and what isn't. Go to a hairdresser and ask for a lesson on putting hair up. Invest in a good haircut, which will provide you with a professional look.
Keep nails very clean by scrubbing with a suitable antibacterial cleanser. Keep nails at a workable length to prevent damage to clients' skin.	Look at your fingers with the palm towards you – if you can see the free edge of the nail plate, over the fingertip, then they are too long!	If you cannot work safely with longer nails, then file or cut them to a suitable length.

Handling electrical equipment

How you handle electrical equipment can have consequences for health and safety. The table below gives an overview of the risk analysis you should carry out before working with any item of electrical equipment. Individual equipment will have specific hazards, and these are explained within each practical unit.

Hazard (What can go wrong?)	Who could be harmed?	Prevention (How can I prevent this?)
Misuse of equipment can cause: • serious injury – electric shock, burns • damage to the equipment • fire • scarring as a result of negligence – the client may seek damages from the therapist, which could cost you your business, or your salon owner a hefty fine • loss of earnings • trailing leads – which may cause an accident if someone trips over them	Yourself Other therapists Members of the public Other staff Visitors	Never abuse the equipment Never operate equipment you have not been trained to use Follow manufacturers' guidelines Arrange regular maintenance checks – these should be carried out by a qualified electrician (refer to Electricity at Work Regulations 1989) Report faulty equipment Never use equipment which you think may be defective Attend regular updates for training and safety Follow salon safety guidelines – e.g. never use equipment with wet hands

Monitoring (How can I check?)

Always complete a full consultation and check for contra-indications
Always test the equipment on yourself before the client
Always explain the treatment to the client
Always follow manufacturers' instructions
Never overload the plug socket

Corrective action (What should I do if things are not right?)

Remove the defective equipment from use
Clearly label the equipment as unusable
Make sure all staff are aware of the problem
Have the equipment repaired by an authorised repairer
Return new equipment that is found to be faulty to the manufacturer

Risk assessment: hazards for the therapist working with electrical equipment

Your conduct in the salon

When you work in a salon you may have a manager who supervises what you do, or you may have junior staff for whom you are responsible throughout the working day.

When working under a manager:

• you will need to accept that he or she is in charge
• you should be able to take instructions and act upon them
• you will need to communicate effectively
• you will need to take responsibility for your job role and do it to the best of your ability.

Working together as a team:

- means supporting each other, not being in conflict with one another
- gives the salon a good atmosphere which the client senses
- provides a reliable service
- gives excellent results.

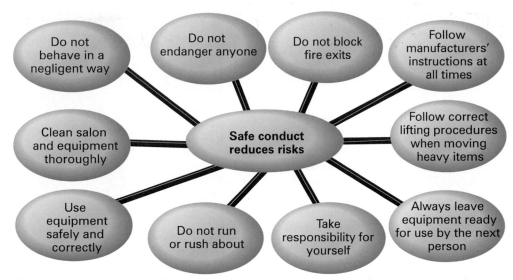

The importance of safe conduct in the salon

Unacceptable behaviour

Whatever your position within the salon, there is a certain etiquette which must be followed, and respect for colleagues is top of the list.

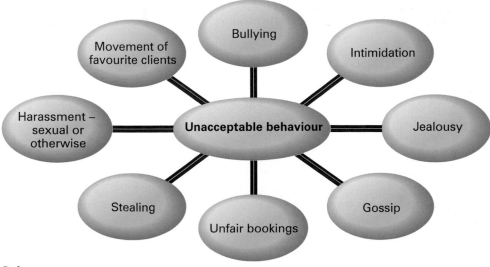

Salon etiquette

There may be a certain rivalry between staff if treatments and product sales are organised on a commission basis and the therapists are in competition with one another, but if the therapists are made to feel part of a team and the division of labour allows everyone to succeed, then serious rivalry can be avoided.

> **Remember**
>
> As an employee, you are expected to be responsible about your work, reliable, and dependable. You are accountable for all your actions and the possible consequences of irresponsible action.

A sense of pride should be instilled in all staff, with regular training and positive feedback. A strong management structure will ensure that minor problems never get out of hand, and that staff morale is good. This can be encouraged in the salon by showing the staff that they are valued and treated with respect, for example through shared tips, rewards of products or treatments and through social events such as Christmas lunches and charity events.

Dealing with conflict

If you find yourself in a situation, either in the salon, at college or at work, where you feel victimised or undermined in some way, then you should deal with it quickly. It is important to maintain a sense of proportion, and to be mature in your reaction.

Ask the person involved for a private talk, and avoid spreading rumours or innuendo among other members of staff. There is a danger that if the issue gets blown out of proportion, it will become a bigger conflict than it needs to be, so act quickly and sensibly to sort out the problem. Often, a one-to-one discussion will clear the air if it is handled correctly. If it is a conflict with another student, go to your tutor and ask for a meeting with your tutor present.

Avoid apportioning blame, and try not to be either aggressive or defensive – tears are not appropriate in this type of meeting and they make the atmosphere very emotional. It is better to begin with something like 'I don't know if you are aware of it, but I feel very undermined when you talk to me in front of clients', or whatever the problem is. This then allows the offender to say that he or she was not aware of this and to apologise, and gives you the opportunity to clear the air and move on. Your aim always is to build a better working relationship.

Before the meeting, practise what you are going to say, and be clear and as factual as you can. The problem may not be something that the other person has recognised, and if an apology is offered, then be gracious and accept it.

At the meeting, remember to keep calm and follow these guidelines.

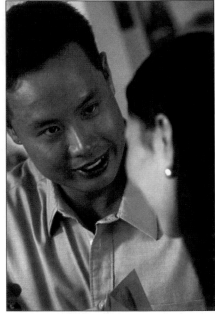

A private talk is a positive way of resolving conflict

- State your feelings clearly. The other person cannot dispute that you may feel undermined or devalued. Your feelings are personal to you; it is the other person's behaviour which is making you feel a certain way, and this needs to be looked at.
- Avoid blackmail, emotional or otherwise. Being negative and stating that you will have to seek employment elsewhere is a risky strategy. Your bluff may be called, and you may find yourself job hunting. Only use the threat of resignation as the very last resort, if this and subsequent meetings fail to resolve the problem.
- Be receptive. The person may understand your side of the problem and realise his or her behaviour is unacceptable to you, but he or she may also want you to understand that your own behaviour may have contributed to the situation. It could be that if you have not said anything before, it was assumed that you accept the situation. For example, if a manager regularly teases you, he or she will not know that you find it irritating unless you say so.
- Be clear in what you are asking for. State firmly that you wish the behaviour to stop. If you do not say this, then the meeting will be a waste of time.
- Be positive and upbeat. You all have to work together, so be encouraging. State clearly that you are pleased to be able to clear the air and move forward.
- Have closure. This American phrase sums up how to end the conflict. Do not drag it up at every available opportunity. Forgive and forget, and respect others as you wish to be respected.

Managing resources within the limits of your authority

When managing your resources there are two main areas to consider:

- what you are responsible for, and expected to do
- what you are not responsible for, and should not attempt to do.

Knowledge and good management are essential in working within your job limits and not exceeding your own authority. Knowing what you are not allowed to do is as important as knowing what is expected. (See also Unit G11, Contribute to the financial effectiveness of the business, for guidance on financial resource management.)

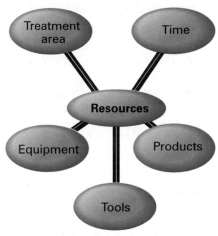

Resources in the salon

Tools

The tools of your trade are precious resources and should be kept in pristine condition – not only for hygiene reasons and reducing the possibility of cross-infection but also because they are expensive to replace. Your tools reflect your professionalism. Whose job is it to see that they are clean, sterile, and ready for use after each client? Yours. From mask brushes (for applying conductive gels) to tweezers to electrical equipment, even your hands for massage could be considered tools of your trade. Look after them, and they will serve you well for years. Abuse and mistreat them, and not only will you lose customers but you will also be replacing expensive tools more often than you would wish.

Replace small items such as sponges and mask brushes before they disintegrate on the client's skin! By having a number of sponges and mask brushes, you will be able to rotate their use and prolong their life. It will also allow you to have some in the autoclave, while using others.

In the salon

Saskia had only one mask brush – she could never find the time to visit the wholesalers to buy extra ones. In her hurry to sterilise the brush between clients, she soaked it in a very strong antibacterial solution from the hairdressing section of the salon. She did not realise that the solution had not been diluted and was dissolving the glue which bound the bristles into the handle. As she started to apply desincrustation gel to the client, the bristles started to come loose and fell on to the client's face. After explaining what had happened and carefully removing all she could, she applied her rollers with current flowing. The current gravitated towards the bristles (made of hair) and the client had several concentrations of current, which made her face tingle and became increasingly uncomfortable. The treatment had to be stopped.

- What should Saskia have done to prevent this happening?
- How would you react as the client?

Products

Products are the lifeblood of any therapy business – no therapist can work without them, and they are one of the most expensive ongoing outlays for the salon (along with the premises, insurance and staff wages).

Always treat products as if you personally had paid for them. Do not be wasteful. For example, when decanting a product into a small bowl prior to application, only use what you need – you must not re-use or pour back the product into the container because of the risk of contamination. On the other hand, do not use too little of the product – you should always use the correct amount or the product will not perform its function. With experience, you will find that you can judge exactly how much you need. However, you cannot, for example, always estimate how much oil a very dry back will soak up during massage. If you pour only a small amount into a bowl, you can always add more, but if you start off with too much, you cannot pour it back in.

It is inevitable that accidents will happen, and you may find that your salon runs a policy of breakage being paid for by the member of staff responsible for the accident.

Try to avoid having expensive products on show or on display near the reception area and doorway, where they are easy to steal. Displays and stock for sale should be kept under lock and key, and dummies used for open display areas.

Remember

Giving clients good aftercare advice and recommending the correct products to use at home will re-enforce the benefits of salon treatments and continue your good work! For example, if the client is not cleansing her face properly at home, or if she is using an incorrect product, then all improvements an electrical facial gives will be lost. If, however, you have recommended the correct skin care routine, she has purchased the products and you have instructed her on the correct usage, then her skin will improve enormously, and she will be delighted.

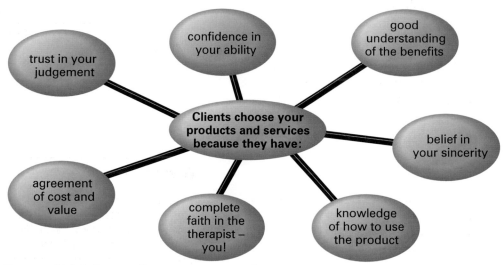

Factors which influence clients to use your products or services

Client understanding of product use

(See also the information on clients' rights in **You, your client and the law** beginning on page 67 below.)

To get the best from a product, clients should fully understand how to use it, or when to apply it, and its benefits and advantages. For example, a rich eye cream needs a delicate application using the ring fingers of both hands, with a tiny amount of product warmed between them, before patting on, starting from the outer eye and working inwards. Too much product and the eye area absorbs it, becoming puffy, and using heavy strokes to put it on will pull the fragile skin around the eyes, causing damage.

When talking application through with clients, or demonstrating, look for lots of eye contact and nodding, which you will see if clients have understood your instructions. If clients look confused, bored or distant, you have lost their interest, they are unlikely to use the product and may even return it.

Ask clients to repeat back to you what you have said. Check understanding by asking questions such as:

- When do you apply it?
- How is it put on?
- How regularly?
- How much do you need?

This will confirm that clients have fully understood how and when to use the product. Write any product purchases in clients' record cards and the next time you treat them remember to ask them how they got on and if they are pleased with the results. Be interested in clients' efforts and comment on the effects of their product use, as this will confirm your recommendations were correct.

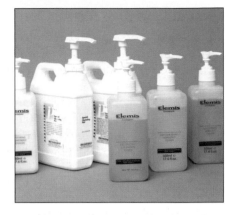

Product displays

Product displays are generally included in the job role of the receptionist. However, if you have a spare hour and wish to promote your own range of products, say for electrical treatments, then you may be asked to be 'hands on' with displaying and promotion of products.

Retail sales will always boost a salon's profits and are a key factor in enhancing the benefits of the clients' salon treatments by encouraging use of the correct products at home. Therefore, running out of a popular line of stock or having poor displays of products makes neither good business sense nor gives the reception area a professional look. Nothing looks more off-putting than empty shelves!

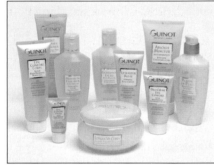

Product displays may be organised by product type

By taking regular stock checks, the salon can see exactly what is required, which products are the most popular and sell well and those which are slow moving and may require a promotion to boost sales. Keep product displays simple, clean and neat. No one is going to be tempted to buy a dusty pot of cream, or one which looks as if it is past its sell-by date.

Product displays may be organised in two ways:

- by product type
- by design.

If there are many products in the range, then use the display cabinets to double up as storage and display the products in a logical order, that is by size or by product type, for example all cleansers together, toners together, and so on. Display by height and size so that clients can easily compare the value of buying the larger economical size (always a good selling point – the larger the product, the better the saving).

Products can also be displayed to look attractive – usually using 'dummy' (empty) boxes, and organising them in an artistic display, with flowers or ribbons to complement the colouring of the display cabinet. The boxes are usually clustered to form a small display within a glass case, and stock is held in a cupboard below for easy access.

Remember

Whichever display type is used, the products need to be locked up to avoid pilfering of stock – security should be an important factor.

Check it out

Visit a local department store and investigate the way its beauty product displays are designed. Is security a factor? Can you touch the displays? Which one did you prefer and why?

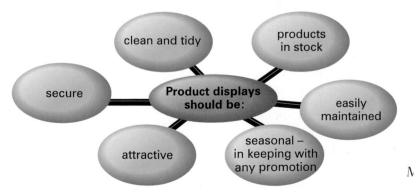

Maintaining product displays

Prompt delivery of goods

If, following your advice, clients wish to purchase either a product or treatments, you will need to ensure they understand the time constraints or delivery expectations. When you order stock the time taken to deliver it will vary between suppliers, depending on their resources and stock levels, and whether the supplier is based in your area. It may be a next-day delivery if the company is local, or it might mean a wait of several weeks if the suppliers are themselves awaiting a shipment. The client may be enthusiastic about the product, but if it needs to be ordered, make sure that you keep the client fully informed about delivery dates, to avoid misunderstandings. Be honest with your client and you will keep your integrity!

When ordering products ensure you know how to order the correct goods, or refer to the staff member who is responsible for the salon's purchasing. Take responsibility for your actions – if you make an effort to get it right, the client will appreciate this.

Refer clients to alternative sources

There are times when you cannot recommend or offer clients want they need. This could be because you are not yet trained in the particular treatment or it may be that your salon does not offer the recommended treatment. For example, should a client require a sunbed session and the salon does not have one, or the client would like a specialist epilation treatment (hair removal) and the salon does not offer it, then you may recommend a *reputable* therapist who can provide the treatment required.

There is the possibility that you will lose the client altogether, but he or she may approve of your professionalism and remain loyal to you for other treatments. At the same time, you could take the opportunity to recommend to the manager or owner that the salon should investigate the possibility of offering the required treatment to expand business opportunities, if there is sufficient demand and the salon is losing clientele by not offering it.

Try to do your own research on costing of equipment and training needs, profit margins and expected returns, and then make a short presentation to the staff – you will learn a lot and so will they, as well as being impressed by your initiative!

Time

Client time management

Time management is easy to grasp in theory but often very hard to put into practice! Your time as a therapist is expensive: you give one-to-one treatments and this should be reflected in the treatment price. For example, a full hour's body massage is labour intensive. You stay with clients throughout the treatment and they receive a full hour of your time. A one-off treatment is very easy to time manage, and if the client takes his or her time getting undressed, falls asleep on the couch, and takes time getting dressed, then that is fine. But you do not give one-off treatments. Your working column is full for the whole day, and you are probably going to give a variety of treatments, say three body massages, a galvanic facial and a couple of tanning treatments, along with epilation and a sauna and body treatment.

Good time management involves working out the amount of time each treatment needs. There are a number of things that you will need to take into account.

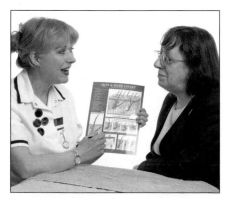

Good time management includes explaining treatments within acceptable times

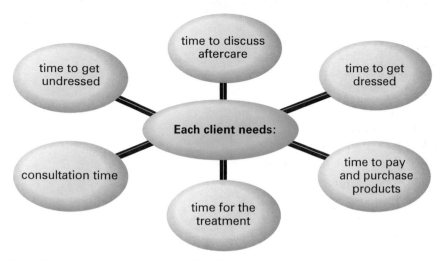

Calculating how much time is needed for individual treatments

Each client deserves the same professional attention, and may also like to chat and extend the treatment time because he or she has enjoyed it so much. So the problem is although you think you are responsible for your own time management, you really are not – the client structure dictates how long you have for the whole day. A good receptionist (or the person who books in the appointments) will understand this, and make allowances for the consultation and dressing and undressing, but you still cannot afford to go over time. If each booking runs over by just ten minutes, by the end of the day your last client is likely to be waiting for up to an hour for his or her appointment as the time lost has accumulated through the day!

Organising your time

As well as organising client time management, you will need to allow time to:

- prepare the working area
- clean tools
- dispose of waste products
- sterilise necessary equipment
- gather new equipment, if required
- leave the working area as you would wish to find it.

For the newly qualified therapist, this can be quite a daunting task. Experience will help with spreading the workload. Remember to ask for help if you need it – there may be a spare pair of hands willing to help, and you can return the favour. This is all part of good team work.

Poor time management leads to stress, the feeling that there are not enough hours in the day, and job dissatisfaction, as you feel you cannot cope well, and seem to do nothing right. Ask for help before you get to that stage, and at an appraisal with your line manager you should be able to put into place a routine that will save you time. Often, it takes someone else to observe your working routine to be able to spot time-saving remedies.

The key is to be organised and prepared. Work at least one client ahead:

- What will I need next?
- Where is the galvanic unit – who is using it?
- How long have I got?
- Could a junior member of staff help me prepare something?

Remember

When you are at work, time is money! The profit margins of the business will be eaten away if you do not remember this.

Good communication also helps. No client will be offended if you say politely 'I'd love to stay and chat, Mrs Brown, but my next client is due in soon, and I need to prepare for her. Why don't you go into the sun lounge and have a drink to help you relax after your treatment?' Be calm, but firm with the client who hovers and does not seem to want to go. The client may have time to spare, whereas you have several more clients to see.

Ensuring that you have enough resources will also help to improve your time management. For example, getting a fresh brush from the autoclave saves time, as do spare sponges, spare turbans and fresh towels. Having only one set of everything is really hard work and it is virtually impossible to keep up a safe level of hygiene.

Do not be tempted to cut corners in order to save time. You cannot afford to compromise either the safety or hygiene of the client and this could be a very expensive problem in the long run, should negligence be proven.

The other main problem with time management is the unforeseen event, which you cannot be prepared for, such as:

- a sick member of staff
- a piece of equipment becoming faulty and needing to be removed from service
- the client who turns up late and still expects to be treated
- the staff member who cuts herself badly and has to go to hospital for treatment
- the client who wants an extra treatment for which you have not allowed time.

One or any combination of these problems and your time management collapses as easily as a pack of cards! The solution is to have regular planning meetings and ensure that strategies, or contingency plans, are in place to cope with the unforeseen event. Staff will then know what to do in the case of cover being required and what is expected.

To make life easier all staff should implement salon policies and staff training on time management. Late arrivals and no-show clients should be made aware of the salon's policy. Some salons state that charges will be made if an appointment was not attended. Training should be given on covering staff absent due to illness – who is the flexible stand-in, or who has the necessary skills to cover, and who would be able to cancel clients if needed. A good manager will fully support all staff decisions because he or she has put procedures in place, and the therapist will be acting in the knowledge that her decisions are the views of the management.

If the problem is a faulty piece of equipment, and there is no other available, then honesty is the best policy, and perhaps an alternative could be suggested, or the appointment rescheduled.

Team work and good communication through the day, by the 'front of house' team who deal with appointments and bookings, will provide updates and progress reports for the therapists working in their therapy rooms. Good team players make all the difference to time management.

Equipment

Managing your own equipment is not so easy when you are sharing the bigger electrical machines with others – this equipment is not then solely for your use, and professional teamwork is needed here, too.

Remember

Where possible, avoid lending or borrowing small equipment. Try to be self-sufficient as this will make you independent and you will then not need to rely on others to provide for you. It will also prevent your precious (and expensive to replace) equipment getting lost!

Again, it is largely a matter of having enough of the right equipment to go around. Some smaller salons have, for example, three or four facial steaming units as this is a popular treatment, but they may have only one galvanic unit as this is an expensive piece of equipment to purchase.

Planning the day is essential, and a morning staff meeting, with the booking-in sheet for the day, should allow the team to stagger the use of equipment so that all client needs are accommodated. Very soon it will appear which equipment is most in demand and will therefore require further investment by the salon.

When sharing equipment remember the following:

- Leave the equipment as you would wish to find it – clean and ready for use.
- Set dials and settings to the '0' position – what is suitable for one client may not suit the next person.
- Unplug the equipment from the wall socket, so the therapist moving the equipment does not accidentally pull the lead out of the socket.
- Remove any heads or tubes which you have used but are as yet unable to clean or sterilise – the next client should not make contact with these.
- Ensure the equipment is placed safely on the trolley, and not balanced precariously.
- Do not clutter the equipment trolley with waste materials, used brushes or sponges – the next client does not need to see your rubbish!

The same principles of time management should be applied to your own personal small equipment: make sure you have enough small items to allow flexibility for sterilising and washing items. Turbans and small towels, brushes, tweezers and sponges should be plentiful to allow rotation, and avoid the need to waste time waiting for them.

> **Remember**
>
> You must manage your resources within the limits of your own authority – it may not be your decision to purchase new stock or equipment, change the staff rota or alter the running of the salon. Know your place, and stay there! There may be reasons unknown to you as to why certain things do or do not happen. Follow the management hierarchy within the salon and observe the correct protocol. If you have suggestions to make and recommendations which you think may help, then use the correct procedure for suggesting them – perhaps at a staff meeting. Try not to jump up the ranks, and go over people's heads – it is not professional and can be very undermining.

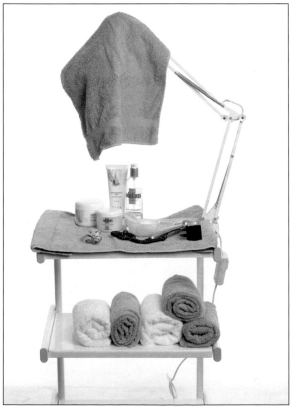

Leave equipment as you wish to find it, ensuring safety. For example, placing a towel over a hot infrared lamp safeguards the therapist from getting burnt

You and your client

You will learn about

- communication
- body language

- the consultation
- hygiene and avoiding cross-infection.

This part of **Professional basics** considers the client, the all-important consultation and how to get the best out of the consultation to match your client's needs. The specific consultation details for either face or body treatments are covered within the **Facial treatments** and **Body treatments** sections. This is a general introduction and is intended to refresh your consultation techniques.

Before you can assess individual clients for treatment, you will need to have a lot of information about them. Based on this knowledge, you will then be able to make an analysis.

Much has been written about the treatment of clients in a holistic manner. *Holistic* is a medical term and describes 'an approach to patient care in which the physical, mental and social factors in the patient's condition are taken into account, rather than just the diagnosed disease'. As you are not a medical practitioner and may not deal with pathological disease (it is a contra-indication to treatment), beauty therapists have adapted the term to cover the clients' differing conditions. Usually, in beauty therapy the holistic approach is applied to the clients' spiritual well-being as well, especially in reflexology, aromatherapy and massage – treatments which are very calming and replenishing. But you can also use the holistic approach to include small treatments to the client, for example if the client requires an eyelash tint, manicure or leg wax. Just remember to keep them separate from the Level 3 assessments – but do not refuse the business for your salon!

Communication

Communication can be:

- verbal
- non-verbal.

Verbal communication

Verbal communication is what we say and is full of different expressions, which can be used to convey many emotions to suit the occasion. The words can be made to sound different by altering the pitch, tone and volume and the emotion behind the words – the same words can be said with kindness, harshness or sarcasm. Even a simple phrase like 'Thank you' can sound like a criticism.

Aspects of speech include the following:

- **Intonation** is the tone of speech and it can significantly alter the meaning of words. 'Well done' can be made to sound sarcastic, or be genuine praise. The variation of tone enlivens speech, which would be very boring if it was all monotones, and the different speech patterns and accents add shades of meaning or emotion, and help retain the listeners' attention. Flat boring tones will not engage listeners and will not help them understand what is being said to them. Intonation also helps distinguish

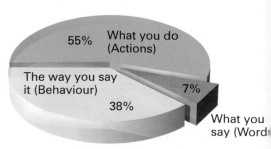

Speech is only 7 per cent of all communication; 38 per cent is the way you say something and 55 per cent is your actions, or what you do

people's home country, e.g. southern hemisphere accents from New Zealand and Australia tend to go up in tone towards the end of the sentence, almost like a question, and are easily recognisable.

- **Pitch** is most noticeable when it is either high or low, and easily reflects the emotional state of the person. A depressed person often talks quite slowly in a low, falling pitch, whereas a raised pitch conveys excitement, enthusiasm or anxiety. Voice coaches recommend to people in the public eye, who have to make lots of speeches to a wide audience, to lower the pitch slightly and slow down their normal rate and rhythm of speech.
- **Pace** is literally the speed of the words. A calm, slow, measured speech reflects reassurance and confidence – the speaker is pondering over getting the message right. In contrast, interest and enthusiasm are often reflected in a more rapid delivery. Panic, anxiety and lack of confidence can produce fast, muddled speech.
- **Pauses** can be either a comfortable silence, allowing reflection upon what has been said, or can be very awkward, even menacing. Judging a pause and knowing when to break it takes a little patience and skill. Hesitation in speech patterns may indicate uncertainty or stress, or just tiredness, where the brain function is slowing down.
- **Volume** can reflect attitudes and emotional states and varies from a polite request – 'Please get my coat' – to an angry demand. Volume can also denote the hierarchy within a structure or situation. People in authority are far more likely to raise their voices to a subordinate than the other way around. It can also be a sign of showing off, or feeling superior, or being a bore!
- **Stress** patterns in speech can draw attention to the point of the sentence for extra emphasis, and can change the meaning entirely. For example, HE gave the money to me, he GAVE the money to me, or he gave the money to ME.

All of these effects (called prosodic effects) in speech can influence the message the speech is to convey. So it is not just what you say, it is the way in which you say it, and emphasise it, which gets the right or wrong meaning across.

There is also some relationship to voice quality and personality types. Extroverts, for example, tend to speak more loudly and more rapidly than introverts, with fewer pauses and at a higher pitch. Confidence plays its part in making speech clear and if you wish to come across as competent in your job, then reflect that in your speech patterns.

Speech pointers

- Avoid jargon where possible. Jargon is verbal shorthand for the professional. It can seem as if you are showing off, and while it may be appropriate in the staff room to ask for the UV lamp for example, you will confuse the client if you talk about a galvanic facial. If you explain the treatment as a deep cleaning and rehydration of the skin, the client will be far more receptive to having the treatment.
- Avoid slang, bad language and lazy speech. Slang is acceptable in your own social circle, where everyone knows what is meant, but if you were to refer to money as 'bread', the client may not understand you! Bad language (swearing and blasphemy) is inappropriate in the salon. It is easy to fall into the habit of bad language, but remember that some clients may be offended. Lazy speech includes dropping Hs and missing Ts in the middle of words, which makes it hard to understand.
- Always be respectful to clients. Use titles and surnames where appropriate, e.g. Mrs Smith, Dr Patel, and so on. Do not view this as using language to give the client power; view it more as a recognition of their importance to you and the salon.

Check it out

Listen carefully to people on television and judge their speech patterns. For example, do younger presenters talk more quickly than older presenters? How does the news delivery change with each topic? Who would you consider to be a very good public speaker, and why?

- Be aware of people's sensitivity and never be offensive. Sexist, racist and ageist terms are not acceptable – your salon could find itself the subject of a lawsuit and a hefty fine if you use such terms. If you avoid all ethnic, age, gender and sexual orientation terms, then you cannot offend anyone!

Politeness in your job role

To build up a rapport with clients and establish a relationship, you will need to have respect for them, and this is shown in politeness, a broad term for the sensitivity that we should all show one another in conversation.

Examples of politeness include:

- using the appropriate forms of address
- speaking to others in a way that is fitting to the social relationship you have with them
- speaking with a degree of formality if required, especially for new clients
- showing an understanding of the conventions of speech – knowing when a conversation is beginning or ending
- listening carefully to what clients are saying – or not saying, which is often just as important.

Conversation support

It takes two to hold a conversation! To make sure that your conversation with a client is a two-way street, you will need to use supportive conversation techniques, otherwise the conversation may become stilted and stop altogether. To support conversation, try some of the following techniques.

- Ask more questions – show interest in what the client thinks, and encourage him or her to participate.
- Give lots of supportive feedback when listening, e.g. through 'back channel' noises such as 'mm' and through expressions of agreement and understanding like 'Yes, I know'.
- Pay compliments where appropriate.
- Initiate more topics of conversation.
- Make an effort to bring others into the conversation – general family topics are usually safe, and pets and social activities are interesting to talk about (the client's – not yours!).
- Use 'you' and 'we' more often as it involves the client in the treatment and what is being said.

Try not to:

- interrupt
- express strong disagreement or criticise the client for expressing an opinion, e.g. 'You can't really like so-and-so's singing'
- ignore the client's utterances
- show reluctance to pursue the topic the client is initiating.

Questioning techniques

Asking questions is a skilled task if you really want to find out what your client thinks and needs from you. How you ask, what you ask and the type of question will dictate the reply you get, so it is important that you give some thought to your questioning technique.

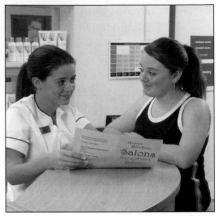

A supportive conversation involves good eye contact

The information you obtain should be included on the client's record card, which you will be filling out as you discuss details during the consultation. Use the record card as your guide. Verbal questioning will determine all the personal details – refresh your memory by going back to the record card.

There are two types of questions – open and closed.

Open questions help to make the conversation flow, as they require a fuller response than a simple yes or no reply. For example, 'How did your skin feel after your facial last week?'. Open questions are good to break the ice.

Closed questions usually need only one-word answers. For example, 'Have you ever had high blood pressure?' These questions are intended to confirm or eliminate information. Sometimes you have to use a closed question if you just require facts, but try to keep their use to a minimum.

Non-verbal communication

Non-verbal communication (NVC) is a broad term, and refers to the way we all interact with one another, excluding the actual words. It includes not only body language (gestures, facial expressions and physical contact) but also appearance and non-verbal aspects of speech itself.

The functions of NVC include the following.

- Accompanying speech – to reinforce what you are saying, using gestures as you go along.
- Replacing speech – as in a sign, such as a thumbs up for OK, or a wave, or a horizontal shake of the hand to denote something uncertain.
- Betraying attitudes or feelings – unfortunately, when you tell a lie, your speech is saying one thing, but your unconscious body language is saying another! Expressions and closed gestures such as crossing the arms may give away your true thoughts, as will avoiding eye contact and touching the nose or ear when lying.
- Self-presentation – NVC contributes to the way you choose to present yourself, e.g. wearing a smart suit to an interview or the professional uniforms worn in the salon.
- Social rituals – people formally shaking hands upon meeting, or the less formal European greeting among friends of kissing both cheeks.

Body language

Body language may be broken down into the following categories:

- proximity
- orientation
- facial expressions
- eye contact

- gestures
- posture
- head movements
- touching.

Proximity

This refers to the physical distance between people.

- The smallest is the intimate zone of about 50 centimetres, used only by close family members and partners.
- The personal zone is 0.5 – 1.5 metres, used when chatting at a party or with people whom you feel very comfortable with.
- The social zone 1.5 – 4 metres is used in a business setting, dealing with shop assistants, and trades people.
- The public zone 4+ metres is used when delivering a speech or public address.

Remember

In beauty therapy you are breaking into a person's most intimate space to deliver treatments, so the relationship between therapist and client has to be built upon trust, confidence and total rapport, otherwise the relaxation and benefit of the treatment is wasted.

Orientation

This refers to the way you position yourself in relation to others.

- If you turn away from a person while in conversation, this shows either a lack of interest or that you wish to be separated or disassociated from that person.
- People who face towards each other, and even mirror each others' actions or position, signal interest and friendliness.
- Sitting on opposite sides of a desk, or couch, facing each other, may be interpreted as competitive or a sign of confrontation, whereas sitting side by side in a personal zone is much more harmonious and suggests empathy and cooperation. This is most useful to know when carrying out a consultation: you may think that being on the other side of the couch is fine – your client may perceive your signal differently!

Facial expressions

The face is a true reflection of what you are thinking and can convey all emotions, but remember to concentrate, as a look of boredom or tedium is very difficult to hide! In western cultures facial expressions tend to mean the same, and expressions are used to give feedback and show interest, with eye contact and smiling to offer encouragement. (However, conventions can differ around the world. In China, for example, sticking out the tongue shows surprise and delight at something.)

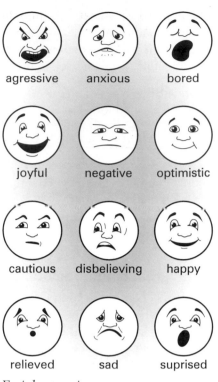

Facial expressions

Eye contact

Eye contact is very important, not only at the beginning and end of a conversation, but to judge someone's level of self-esteem, and to show confidence and interest. Lack of eye contact may just be shyness, but if it happens continually, it usually indicates the person is intimidated, frightened or lacks self-assurance.

Gestures

These can be used for clarification, to demonstrate or point to something or to emphasise a point. Jabbing an index finger at a person, invading their intimate space, during an argument would be a sign of aggression. Pointing can be a pre-signal to attack with a fist, and politicians are taught not to use such a bullying gesture during speeches. By contrast, shaking hands with someone originates from showing you have no concealed weapon in the palm of your hand and is a friendly gesture. Any gesture showing the palm is very good and can be used to show a client around, but flicking a thumb to show where the toilet is would be considered ill mannered.

Posture

Posture can reflect the emotional state of a person. Sitting on the edge of a seat shows tension and anxiety. A person with head hung low, drooping shoulders and a shuffle as he or she walks would be easy to read as being in a depressed state. A confident extrovert would have head held high, making eye contact easily, with a positive stride and shoulders back.

Head movements

The slightest inclination of the head can mean many things. Nodding forward and back shows both agreement and understanding, and side-to-side shaking can mean disbelief or disagreement. Tossing the head and shaking the hair usually accompany a

Remember	

There is a saying 'Fake it 'til you make it' and that is so true of posture. If you look confident and in control, people will believe your body language, even if you are quaking like a jelly inside! Soon your bluff of confidence will become real, especially when you get good feedback from others.

bout of laughter, or can be part of the subtle mating ritual, showing interest, if aimed at an attractive partner! Tossing the head over the shoulder, if used to indicate where something is, can show lack of interest.

Touching

Touching is vital for us all to bond, especially as babies, but as we grow up our personal space becomes more pronounced and we become more inhibited. This is, of course, a generalisation – some families are great huggers and kissers, both male and female, and the Continental Europeans are less inhibited than the British. Who we touch, how, and in what way, will depend upon the situation. Women tend to kiss more; men shake hands. We are more likely to touch in relationships familiar to us – you would not kiss your clients in the salon as it would not be appropriate, but if a family member came to visit you at work, you would be far more likely to.

Touching is, of course, the very basis of beauty therapy treatments, especially in all forms of massage, so it has to be appropriate, carried out professionally and in the correct context. Massage has been recognised as being very beneficial in the healing process, and is soothing and comforting for all ages.

> ### Remember
>
> Only massage or treat a client who is undergoing medical treatment with the approval of his or her doctor. While beauty treatments can be very therapeutic, therapists are not medically trained and may be creating more problems for the client.

The consultation

A successful and profitable business will earn its reputation by providing an excellent personal service. It starts with a good consultation. The very first impression that you give to the client, the care and attention he or she gets, and the feeling of being comfortable and secure will last indefinitely, creating repeat business and expansion of clientele, as your excellent reputation will be spread through recommendation.

The consultation should be carried out in complete privacy, be complimentary (free of charge), and carried out when both parties have the time to be thorough and establish a good rapport with one another. Your manner should be polite, sensitive and supportive, encouraging clients to feel able to ask questions, especially if they are unsure of anything.

Often a consultation is used by a potential client to vet the staff and premises, before deciding to go ahead with a treatment or course of treatments, and therefore business can be lost or gained in an instant. The key words of professionalism, integrity and honesty sum up all the traits required during a consultation – any insincerity, talking about treatments of which you have no real knowledge, or general lack of interest will be detected and you will lose the client.

Position of the client

One of the key functions of the consultation is to determine if the client is suitable for treatment, as well as deciding upon the client's needs. Therefore, it makes sense to conduct the consultation with the client before he or she is prepared for the treatment, undressed and on the couch.

The client is normally taken into the working cubicle, which is quiet and private, and the record card and pen should already be prepared in anticipation. Make the client feel comfortable, ask him or her to remove outer clothing and to be seated. Some salons have a private room, which is separate from the working cubicles, off the main reception for consultation, in which case you must ensure the clients are given a conducted tour of all of the facilities, to familiarise themselves.

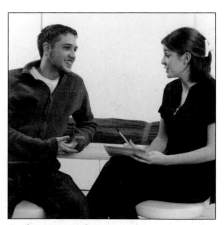

A client consultation

Some training establishments have the client on one side of the couch, and the therapist on the other. This may be to save space in a large training room, if the beds are quite close together. Ideally, there should be no barriers between you and the client. Seating side by side is ideal, and it allows you to touch the client should the need arise. Clients can feel very vulnerable in the initial consultation, and become emotional – it is nice to be able to reach out and hold the client's hand, to offer reassurance, if appropriate.

Not only is the 'how' of the consultation important, all the other skills required will make the process successful.

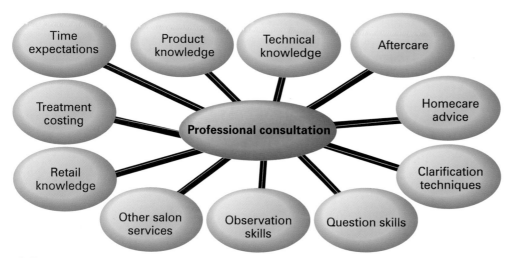

Skills required during a consultation

A good therapist will use a combination of all the skills to gain the information required for the consultation. However, it may take several visits before all the information is given freely; after all, a lot of the detail required is very personal, and the client may hold some things back until a rapport has been built up.

The consultation is the time for you and the client to agree on:

- the treatments
- the time span involved
- the total treatment costs
- the expected outcomes
- the client's contribution in the programme.

This treatment plan should be written, rather like a contract between you and the client, on the consultation form. If a treatment plan is not suitable for the client, for example because of time constraints and financial limitations, you will lose the client to a salon which can give a more realistic treatment plan.

Knowledge

In all parts of the consultation, it is very important that the therapist understands what she is talking about. If in doubt, ask a more senior therapist who has more experience, or who has the training in the treatment, to talk to the client. Do not make up benefits of a treatment, deliberately mislead the client in any way or give false information about the time or cost involved. Legally, the salon is not permitted to make untrue claims about treatments, and your salon would be liable to prosecution under the Trade Descriptions Act and the Supply of Goods and Services Act, if you did so (see **You, your client and the law**, page 77).

Statements like 'miracle anti-wrinkle cream removes all signs of the aging process' or 'G5 treatment promises instant slimming results' or ' Lose ten pounds in the sauna' are just not true, and cannot be proven – which could result in a hefty fine from your local Trading Standards office.

Be careful when using technical terms, or jargon, as your client may not understand them, and you could be perceived as showing off, or be thought patronising. Keep information straightforward and easy, and talk about benefits, rather than just how the equipment works.

Be honest with your product knowledge, too. Selling an unsuitable product, just because it happens to be the only one in stock, is very poor practice, and that all-important trust you have built up will be lost.

When giving advice, keep to the specific problem, rather than being too general, or giving too much advice. You are the professional, but only in beauty therapy; your client may have previous or professional knowledge equal to or greater than your own, so never patronise.

The first few questions on a record card will be the personal details of name, address and so on. This is an ideal ice breaker, to build up a rapport with the client, leading into conversations about how easy it was to get to the salon and so on. It is also important to record details of the client's GP.

Literature

HEALTH & BEAUTY PACKAGES

Luckam Park Top to Toe Day £195.00

Full Body Massage

Clarins Personal Blend Facial

Jessica Manicure

Jessica Pedicure

Clarins Professional Make-up

2 course lunch and a glass of wine in the Spa

Full use of the Spa facilities

Pregnancy Package £155.00

Over 3 months

Clarins Blissful Beginnings Face & Body Treament

Jessica Luxury Manicure with Le Remidi Hand Treatment

Jessica Luxury Pedicure

2 course lunch and a glass of freshly squeezed fruit juice in the Spa.

Full use of the Spa Facilities

Thalgo Top to Toe Day £195.00

Detoxifying Exfoliation

Marine Algae Body Wrap

A Thalgo Marine Facial to suit your skin type

Full Body Massage

2 course lunch and a glass of freshly squeezed fruit juice in the Spa. Full use of Spa facilities

Holistic De - Stressing Package £175.00

Clarins Personal Blend Facial

Body Exfoliating Treatment

Aromatherapertics Aromatherapy Massage

Reflexology

2 course lunch and a glass of wine in the Spa

Full use of the Spa facilities

Price list

It is a very good idea to give the client your full brochure, or price list. Treatment explanations and approximate timings should be included – clients do not retain all the verbal information you give them in the consultation, so it is useful to have something to take away to read at leisure. Again, be careful that the treatment explanation is correct and gives an accurate picture, with no hidden costs.

Working with the client

During the consultation, it is a good idea to emphasise the client's active participation in the chosen programme of treatments – the salon treatments are only half of the story. To see real benefits for either facial skin improvement or body toning treatments, or a slimming programme, the homecare and long-term commitment should be stressed to the client.

If the client uses the wrong products, fails to remove her make-up or eats an unbalanced diet, then expecting the therapist to work miracles in the salon is unrealistic, and the client would be wasting money. This is where the holistic approach is needed. The consultation should view the wider picture of the client's lifestyle and nutrition, which play a large part in the body functioning efficiently and healing and repairing itself.

Contra-indications and GP referral

The contra-indication checklist will tell you whether the client is suitable for the treatment. Although you may be knowledgeable and able to recognise certain symptoms, the qualification you hold is not a medical one. As a beauty therapist, you are not permitted, nor should you attempt, to give an opinion about any symptoms the client divulges during the consultation.

A general contra-indication checklist is found on most record cards. Manufacturers often produce a specific contra-indications list to be used with individual items of equipment. A completed contra-indication checklist is shown on the next page.

If a contra-indication is present, then the treatment must not go ahead, both for health and safety reasons and because the treatment might aggravate the client's condition. Without causing any undue alarm or concern, the client should be referred to his or her GP and, often with a permission letter, the treatment can take place at a later date.

If the contra-indication is a small one, such as a cut or broken skin in a small area, then the treatment can be performed if the area is covered with a plaster, or avoided altogether. If the problem is on a part of the body which is not being treated, but there is current flowing through the body, then use some petroleum jelly to protect the damaged area.

If any clients are particularly nervous, you could ask them to read the contra-indications checklist, and tick any problems that relate to them, and then discuss these. This provides the client with something to focus on and he or she is actively participating. However, clients are notoriously forgetful – they may tick 'No' in all of the boxes to say there is nothing wrong with them, but then reach the 'Medication taken' section and you will find that they are on medication for all sorts of things! The card will then need to be amended.

Remember	

- For assessment purposes, it is best to talk through all of the contra-indications with your client, as your assessor will want to hear that as evidence!

- If you do your consultation with the client undressed and on the couch awaiting the treatment, and *then* discover a contra-indication which prevents treatment from taking place, your client will have to get dressed. You will have wasted time, and the client will be very disappointed to get so close to having a treatment, only to learn that it cannot take place.

Record Card

Condition – please ✓ if present and use comments box

Condition		
Skin conditions/disorders, e.g. eczema, psoriasis	✓	
Muscular or skeletal problems	☐	
Varicose veins or thrombosis	☐	
Metal plates or pin inserts	☐	
Oedema (swellings/kidney problems)	☐	
Circulatory disorders; e.g. high or low blood pressure	☐	
Systemic disorders or infections, e.g. hepatitis	☐	
Heart conditions: angina, pacemakers	☐	
Diabetes	☐	
Epilepsy	☐	
High or low blood pressure	☐	
Sprains, strains or undiagnosed lumps or bumps	☐	
Respiratory problems, e.g. asthma	☐	
Digestive or abdominal complaints, e.g. irritable bowel syndrome	✓	
Hormonal or menstrual difficulties	☐	
Are you currently menstruating?	☐	
Serious medical conditions, e.g. cancer	☐	
Nervousness, stress or anxiety	☐	
Thrush or urinary problems	☐	
Hereditary conditions or genetic defects	☐	
Recent surgery	☐	
Alcohol intake within 24/48 hours	☐	
Known allergies/medication taken for allergic reactions	☐	
Localised skin damage, i.e. cuts or bruising	✓	
Medication taken and state reason	✓	

Contra-indications

Slight eczema in the elbows and behind the knees. Skin not broken, no infection present

IBS present, especially during the week prior to the beginning of a period or in times of stress at work

Bruise on the ankle, caused by open dishwasher door – no break in the skin and healing well
Anti-spasmodic drugs for tummy cramps when IBS flares up

A general contra-indication checklist found on most record cards

Thermal and sensitivity testing

As well as going through the contra-indication checklist, it is important to check that the skin is receptive to electrical treatments, and that no nerve damage is present, causing a lack of sensitivity. This can cause injury, as the client can feel no depth of current, or sensation.

It is very important that tests are carried out in the area to be worked upon, not just a general test on an arm or leg. So, if a facial is being given, the tests must be carried out on a clean, grease-free face; if it is to be a cellulite treatment on the thighs, then the tests must be carried out on the legs.

- The **thermal test** for the differentiation between hot and cold involves placing test tubes containing hot and cold water alternately on the skin, so that the client can tell you which is which. Ideally, the client should have his or her eyes closed, but if the test tubes are identical, it will not be possible to distinguish temperature just by looking.
- The **sensation test** will enable you to tell whether the client can feel the difference between sharp and soft objects. The client will need to close his or her eyes for the test. Use a cotton wool pad stroked over different areas of the skin, and the end of an orange stick provides a sharp enough sensation for the client to tell the difference. Just put slight pressure on the skin; do not stab the client to cause pain (or draw blood!).

These tests are very important, as they inform the therapist that the nerve endings in the skin for temperature and sensation are working properly. Should the client be unable to distinguish hot/cold and soft/sharp, do not commence the treatment but refer the client to his or her GP.

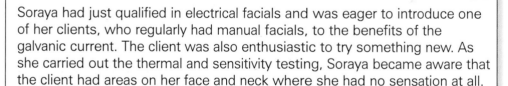

In the salon

Soraya had just qualified in electrical facials and was eager to introduce one of her clients, who regularly had manual facials, to the benefits of the galvanic current. The client was also enthusiastic to try something new. As she carried out the thermal and sensitivity testing, Soraya became aware that the client had areas on her face and neck where she had no sensation at all.

Twice she went over the areas and the client could feel nothing. Soraya explained to her client why the treatment could not go ahead, but that as she had no medical training she was unable to comment on why this was occurring. She suggested her client visit her GP.

About a month later, the client came into the salon with a bunch of flowers to thank Soraya for her time and trouble. The client's GP had referred her to a neurologist who diagnosed a disease of the nervous system. Although serious, early diagnosis had allowed prompt treatment to take place.

Analyse the client for treatment

Regardless of whether you are carrying out a consultation for a facial or body treatment, some of the consultation will have a common theme; other parts will not. For example, your questions will be similar, but your observations will differ – it is unlikely you will be looking for a varicose vein in the face, or comedones on the legs!

Your consultation techniques will include:

* questioning
* observing
* manual examination.

Questioning

Follow the questions within your record card as a guide to what you need to ask. Be polite, and clarify any points which you feel need further investigation. Be prepared to answer the questions clients have – they may (quite rightly) want to know why you need the information. You will need to reassure clients that the reasons are for their safety and health, not just because you are being nosy! You should also understand the effect the treatment may have on particular conditions and why the treatment cannot go ahead. For example, if the client has epilepsy, then an electrical current may stimulate the brain into triggering a seizure, so cannot be offered as a treatment option. It is possible to offer non-electrical facials and body treatments, so alternatives are available. As long as the explanation offered is full, then clients should understand and be open to other options.

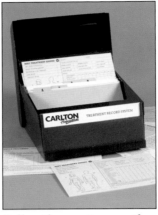

Follow the questions on the client's record card to help you remember what to ask

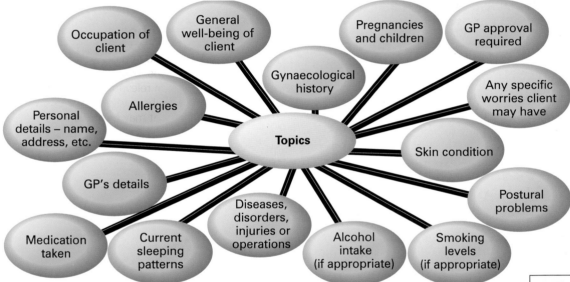

Topics to be discussed at a consultation

Client modesty

The client's modesty must be preserved, and behind a closed cubicle ask the client to remove all outdoor and heavy clothing for the initial verbal consultation. Protecting the client's privacy is not only about personal modesty but is also about safeguarding personal information and maintaining client confidentiality. The topics you discuss with your client, and their possible medical nature, are private to them, and should not be discussed outside of the cubicle, unless it is in a consulting, professional manner (should you need to seek clarification on something you are unsure of). Even then, ask the client's permission to consult with a more senior colleague or your lecturer.

Once the initial consultation has been completed, and you are happy that no contra-indications are present, you are ready to begin a facial or body analysis, which means you can prepare the client for treatment and instruct him or her to lie on the couch or bed. (For in-depth analysis, client positioning and client modesty for facial or body treatments, refer to pages 33-4.)

Keys to good practice

What *you* decide for individual clients may not necessarily be their goal – it is therefore their decision which treatments and home care they opt for. Being too dictatorial and not working with clients may mean that they decide not to have any treatments with you. For example, putting the client on a very low carbohydrate diet to lose three stone in as many months may not be what the client wants, and this will affect motivation, results and ultimately will cost you the client's business. Talk to clients about what *they* want to achieve in their time with you – and allow that to happen, rather than being forceful and dogmatic in your treatment approach.

Hygiene and avoiding cross-infection

Hygiene and avoiding cross-infection are of the utmost importance within beauty therapy, as the therapist has personal bodily contact with clients, and many of the benefits of the treatments would be ruined if protective clothing and gloves were to be worn. For example, imagine giving a full body massage with gloves on!

The professional bodies' codes of practice state clearly that all members are expected to abide by a standard of good practice in relation to hygiene. Special care must be taken to ensure that cross-infection does not occur and official guidelines are respected.

Hygiene is not just about passing your assessments but should be regarded as a protection against disease and illness. As a professional therapist, good hygiene practices will:

- maintain your own health
- maintain your clients' health
- maintain your colleagues' health
- protect your business reputation, and ultimately your business.

Good hygiene practices are also a legal requirement.

Expert advice on hygiene can be confusing, and sometimes there are conflicting reports in the media. The most valuable information can be gained from the professional body's code of ethics or practice (refer to your own awarding body for more details). These guidelines have been drawn up after a great deal of research on behalf of the beauty industry and are most likely to be current.

It is important also to understand the responsibilities you have under the Health and Safety at Work etc. Act 1974 and the Control of Substances Hazardous to Health (COSHH) Regulations 2003 (see **You, your client and the law**, pages 67 and 72.).

In order to maintain the highest hygiene standards, you will need to understand how infection can occur. An infectious disease is one which can be passed from one person to another. A therapy room creates an ideal breeding ground, supplying warmth and moisture, especially if there is a wet area, showers and heat from infrared lamps and sunbeds, and so on.

Disease can be spread by:

- direct contact, as in touching
- infection from droplets
- indirectly, by contact with an infected object (towels, shower mats, etc.).

Infection is caused by three different groups of micro-organisms. A micro-organism is any organism that is too small to be seen by the naked eye. They are ever-present in the environment and include:

- bacteria
- viruses
- fungi.

Bacteria

Bacteria are classified according to their shape, as shown in the table on the next page.

Shape	Description	What they look like	Diseases they cause
Round – cocci	They can protect themselves by forming tough outer coats, and in this condition they are known as spores		This is the dormant stage of the life cycle in cases of adverse conditions. Not suitable for multiplication – but tetanus is caused by spores in soil, and enters the body through cuts. May be present in pot plant soil.
Round in couples – diplococci	They bond together in pairs		Parasitic bacteria including pneumococcus causing pneumonia
Round in bunches – staphylococci	When cocci bunch together they form clumps		Acne, boils, barbers rash
Round in chains – streptococci	Cocci link together at the ends to form chains		Impetigo, sore throats
Rod-shaped – bacilli	Separate rod shapes		Scarlet fever
Spiral shaped – spirochaetes	Single threads form in a spiral, lack a rigid cell wall and move by muscular flexions of the cell		Diphtheria and typhoid, tuberculosis, whooping cough
Comma shaped – vibrios	They have thicker bodies and a tail-like structure		Venereal disease such as syphilis
Cholera

Classification of bacteria

The beauty therapist may avoid the bacterial infection tetanus through an injection of antitoxin. Tetanus causes violent muscle spasms and, in extreme cases, may be fatal. The tetanus jab needs boosting every ten years, and should be given after a suspect injury such as a cut from a rusty blade. Cutting your hand while gardening and then getting the spores in the cut may lead to tetanus.

Bacteria need a number of conditions to survive and thrive, as shown below.

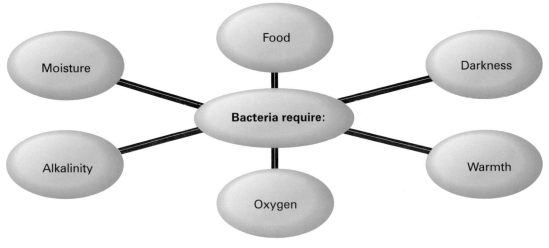

Conditions for growth of bacteria

Viruses and bacterial infections

A virus consists of a protein shell, which has in it particles of genetic material, either DNA or RNA. The virus infects a cell and uses the host's genetic material to reproduce itself. Viruses can then leave the host cell and invade other cells.

Most viruses enter the body through the mouth or skin and then spread to cells throughout the body, via the blood stream. Because the cells can multiply only in living cells, they cannot survive in the horney layer of the epidermis – they need to be deeper within the epidermis to find a living host cell.

Viruses cause:

- the common cold
- flu
- cold sores (herpes simplex)
- warts
- measles
- rubella (German measles)
- mumps
- chickenpox
- hepatitis A, B and C
- HIV.

Boils

This bacterial infection forms at the base of the hair follicle. Bacteria can spread through an open scratch in the skin. The area is raised, red and painful. Pus may be present.

Impetigo

Highly infectious, this bacterial infection starts as small red spots, which then break open and form blisters. Most common around the corner of the mouth and if picked, will spread. It can be spread through use of unsanitised equipment.

Cold sores

The cold sore virus appears on the lips, cheeks and nose. Blisters form, the skin is broken and painful. The blisters are likely to spread when open and weepy and then crusts form.

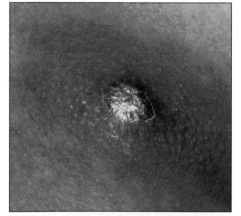

A boil

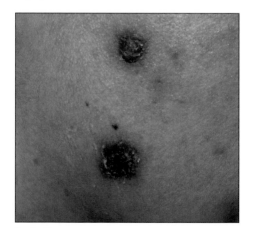

Impetigo

Cold sores

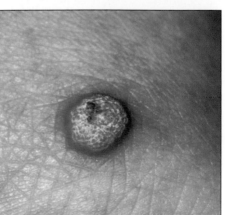

A wart

Warts

Warts are caused by a virus. They are small, compact raised growths of skin. They can be light or brown in colour.

Measles

Measles is an accute, highly contagious viral disease causing fever and a blotchy rash. It can cause more serious complications.

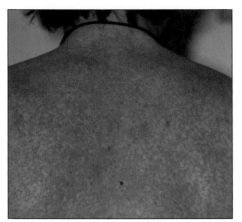

Measles

Chickenpox

Chickenpox is a mild, specific contagious disease of childhood, caused by a virus. It causes crops of spots which scab and are itchy, and may cause scaring.

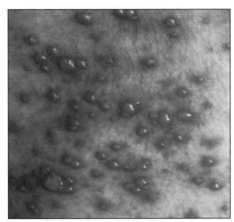

Chickenpox

Oral thrush

This can be seen as white spots in the mouth, which often form ulcers. It can be brought on by poor nutrition, a weak immune system, or the long-term use of antibiotics.

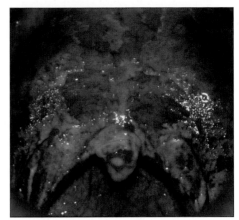

Oral thrush

The common cold

The common cold is caused by a virus and is easily spread. Streaming eyes and nose, coughing and sneezing are its symptoms.

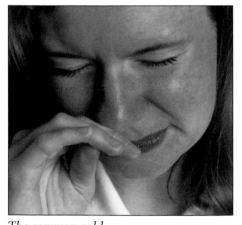

The common cold

Conjunctivitis

This is a nasty eye condition. The eyelids are red and sore, with itching. It is mainly caused by bacteria present, but can be irritated by a virus or an allergy.

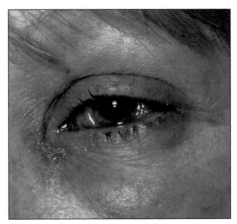

Conjunctivitis

Stye

This is a small boil at the base of the eyelash follicle, which is caused by a bacterial infection. It is raised, sore and red, and there may be considerable swelling in the area.

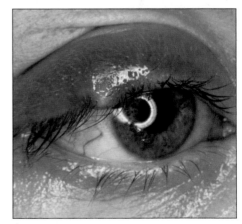

A stye

Fungi

Fungi/yeast infections cause:

- ringworm of the foot, body, head and nail
- thrush
- infection to the heart and lungs, which may prove fatal.

Protozoa (large group of microscopic single-cell animals) cause:

- diarrhoea
- malaria
- amoebic dysentery.

Micro-organisms enter the body through any route they can:

- through damaged, broken skin
- through the ears, nose, mouth and genitals
- into hair follicles
- into the blood stream via a bite from blood-sucking insects.

Ringworm

Ringworm is a highly contagious fungal infection. Red pimples appear and then form a circle, with clear skin in the middle. Scales and pustules follow. It can be spread on to the face from any other area of the body, and can be passed to humans by contact with animals.

Blepharitis

This is a fungal infection of the eyelid causing inflammation. The eye looks sore and red. Depending on the severity of the condition, it may be better to avoid eye make-up.

Remember

The symptoms and severity of an infection or disease will depend on the type of invasion, the ability of the person's immune system to defend the body and his or her general health. If a person is run down, then the micro-organisms have more chance of multiplying rapidly. They also thrive in poor hygiene. The best method of avoiding infection is prevention, through good hygiene practices.

While some of these diseases may be life threatening, many are not and can simply be prevented by good hygiene. For example, protozoa can be transmitted from contaminated food and water into the bowel where they multiply and cause diarrhoea.

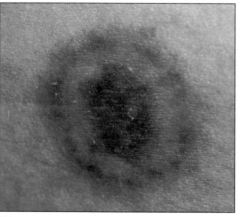

Ringworm

Blepharitis

Vaccination can offer protection against a number of diseases, for example hepatitis B and tetanus, and is recommended for beauty therapists. Most school children are immunised against measles, mumps and rubella, unless there are medical complications preventing the injections. Whooping cough has been dramatically reduced by the same method of immunisation.

Remember

Hygiene practices should be continuously carried out in the salon to ensure no cross-infection takes place. This will give the client total confidence in the salon, and ensure the best results are gained from every treatment.

Maintaining good hygiene practices in the salon

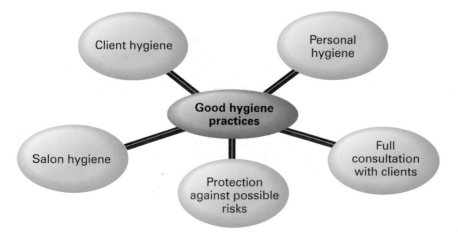

Hygiene practices in the salon

Risk assessment for hygiene

Refer to Unit G1, Ensure your own actions reduce risks to health and safety, to support your risk assessment knowledge.

The best way to prevent infection occurring in the salon is to look at the systems and procedures in place regarding personal hygiene, client safety and sterilisation methods. Prevention is always better than cure, and sterilisation is the only sure way to destroy organisms, so it is worth investing in some modern and efficient equipment.

Keys to good practice

- If you intend to set up your own business, either as a mobile therapist or a salon, purchase the best sterilising equipment you can afford, and which is practicable.

- When going for an interview in a salon, check its hygiene standards by asking lots of questions and looking for the right equipment. If a salon has poor hygiene, is it really the type of place where you would want to work?

The table below and on the following pages considers the effects of poor hygiene practices on you – the therapist, the client and the salon environment.

Poor hygiene practice	Hazard (What can go wrong?)	Who could be harmed?
You – the therapist	Infections spread through open wounds, harboured in jewellery, long nails or on clothing Bringing infection into the salon	Yourself Other therapists Members of the public Other staff Visitors

Prevention (How can I prevent this?)

Wash hands before and after every treatment – use bactericidal gel if possible
Wear disposable gloves for treatments if there is a possibility of an exchange of body fluids, e.g. waxing
Wear personal protective equipment (PPE)
Cover cuts or broken skin with a waterproof plaster
Keep nails short and scrub under them with a nail brush
Do not come to work if you know you have an infection or disease likely to put anyone else at risk, e.g. impetigo
Wash hands thoroughly after every visit to the toilet
Follow guidelines on personal presentation and clean overalls, etc. (see page 9–11)
Attend training programmes for hygiene and use of sterilising equipment
Do not use equipment that is cracked or broken as germs will be present (includes chipped cups, plates or glasses)

Monitoring (How can I check?)	Corrective action (What should I do if things are not right?)
Constantly check your own hygiene – are my nails clean and short? Get into good habits Report lack of cleansing facilities, e.g. running out of soap Carry out spot checks on each other in the staff room Keep up to date with vaccinations Report any incidents of infection	Take preventative measures – seek expert advice Report unhygienic practices Hold regular staff meetings to ensure all staff have the same procedures for hygiene and prevention of infection Contact your local federation for advice and guidance on the latest information on hygiene and the latest legislation

Poor hygiene practice	Hazard (What can go wrong?)	Who could be harmed?
The client	Bringing infection into the salon Having a treatment knowing a contra-indication is present Not washing hands after using the toilet Not using protective steps put in place by the salon, e.g. not treading upon the couch roll when getting out of the shower	Yourself Other therapists Members of the public Other staff Visitors

Prevention (How can I prevent this?)

Display a notice in the reception area asking clients to check that they are not knowingly suffering any contagious diseases

Always carry out a full consultation to discover any contra-indications

Always perform a physical check of the area to be treated. Do not treat if any unrecognised problems are present

Ask the client to sign the declaration on the record card stating that all medical and other information is correct to date to avoid possible repercussions later

Always wipe the area to be treated prior to commencement with appropriate lotion, e.g. surgical spirit, Hibitane or the recommended choice of your training establishment

Provide all possible protection for clients and insist they use the provided procedure, e.g. treading on the couch roll if feet are bare to avoid touching the floor surface

Discourage clients from having a treatment if they have the beginnings of an illness – explain that you would not wish to infect other clients

Monitoring (How can I check?)	Corrective action (What should I do if things are not right?)
Constantly look and ask clients Carry out spot checks on clients' record cards Keep up-to-date record cards Insist clients follow your directives for maintaining hygiene standards Seek GP approval for clients with any contra-indications or who may present a slight risk	Stop the treatment immediately and refer clients to their GP Disinfect the area where the client has been Sterilise the equipment which was being used

Poor hygiene practice	Hazard (What can go wrong?)	Who could be harmed?
The salon environment	Infection from equipment, towels or products may cause multiple infections with many clients becoming infected	Yourself Other therapists Members of the public Other staff Visitors

Prevention (How can I prevent this?)

Sanitise equipment used as fully as possible. This means following manufacturer's instructions for individual equipment, e.g. using the recommended cleaner

Invest time and correct training in the use of sterilisation equipment such as an autoclave or sanitising unit

Clean the treatment area/room daily and wipe generally after each treatment has taken place

Clean all work surfaces regularly with hot water and detergent

(continued on the next page)

Use couch roll and towels as a barrier between blankets and the clients – these can then be disposed of and fresh ones put on for each client

Tuck tissues into the headband or turban – these can be disposed of after use and keep the turban looking fresh

Wash towels after use – so your training salon needs to invest in towels to ensure you do not run out!

Wash towelling robes for clients

Decant creams and oils, using a spatula, into a smaller bowl and throw away any excess

Never pour back into the original container any product that has been in contact with the hands and the client. To be cost effective, be careful not pour out too much, which may be wasted

Use disposable spatulas for massage creams, that is, one use from pot to client, to avoid contamination

Do not accept products from the manufacturer which have been opened or the seal broken

Never use products past their shelf life

Monitoring (How can I check?)	Corrective action (What should I do if things are not right?)
Regular cleaning sessions	Stop all treatments immediately
A duty rota signed when the tasks have been completed	Close the salon for a whole cleaning day
Spot checks carried out	Enrol professional help – employ professional cleaners to steam clean areas, if necessary
Return faulty products to manufacturer and seek their assurances for fresh products – or change suppliers	Buy new sterilising equipment – a new autoclave will be an excellent investment

Risk assessment: infections

Sterilisation

The three main methods of sterilisation are:

- heat
- chemical
- radiation.

The advantages and disadvantages of each method are shown in the table on the next page.

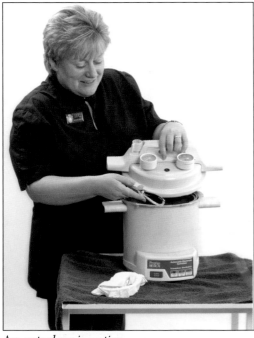

An autoclave in action

Method	Suitability	How it works
Dry Heat		
Oven	Not very practical in the salon, and only some items can go in an oven – plastic bowls, for example, would melt. The oven would need to be in constant use and be very large	An object needs to be the oven for one hour at 160°C – this will destroy even spores
Naked flame	Not practical – risk of fire, especially with so many inflammable chemicals in the salon Can only be used on metallic equipment Blunts the instrument, so cuticle nippers would be rendered unusable in a short time	Flame needs to be red hot to destroy all the germs – a small metallic object such as a needle will then be sterile
Burning	Not practical to burn salon's paper refuse in a bonfire – risk of fire getting out of control, pollution (environmentally unfriendly) May be illegal in some areas	
Glass bead steriliser	Small electrically heated box with a cylinder full of small glass beads. Because of its size the steriliser can only hold small items – not practical. Items to be sterilised should be inserted deep into the glass beads and removed with a clean pair of forceps	Temperatures vary from 190–300°C. It takes from one to ten minutes to sterilise, but the steriliser takes up to one hour to reach the correct temperature (the unit cannot be used for at least 30 minutes after being switched on), so this method may have time constraints
Moist heat		
Boiling	Washing machine hot wash cycle will destroy germs in towels, robes, turbans, etc. Not suitable for items which rust or melt in hot water	Most germs destroyed at 100°C (boiling point of water) within 15 minutes; spores are more resistant and take longer
Autoclave	Similar to a pressure cooker; used to sterilise equipment. Most suitable for small metal equipment, e.g. eyebrow tweezers, manicure tools Refer to individual manufacturer's instructions for use Remove instruments with a clean pair of forceps and place in a kidney bowl with tissue soaked in isopropyl alcohol or similar	By heating water under pressure to a higher temperature than 100°C, creates an environment where germs cannot survive
Chemical vapour	Most useful for sterilising non-metallic tools as metal tools may develop pitting in the surface, and can also cause bluntness Unpleasant fumes Equipment must be washed with soap and water prior to sterilisation	A foam strip is soaked in 5 per cent formalin liquid, which is heated, releasing fumes, becoming formaldehyde. The fumes circulate in the sterilising box, which has open shelves for storage. The formaldehyde destroys the germs
Radiation	Only suitable for sterilising equipment without body fluids on it, so tweezers need to be put into the autoclave As the ultraviolet waves travel in straight lines, the tools need to be turned over to allow both sides to be sterilised Equipment must be washed with soap and water prior to sterilisation Useful to store small items, but not very powerful	A mercury vapour lamp emits ultraviolet (UV) radiation inside a cabinet which has perforated wire shelves on which to lay the equipment. The process works by irradiating the equipment with UV light at a wavelength of 254 nanometres (1 nanometre = one-millionth of a millimetre). When a suitable dose has been delivered, bacteria are made inactive. (Refer to individual manufacturers' instructions, and see tanning unit for electro-magnetic spectrum in Unit BT30 on website page 3) The cabinet must be kept very clean as grease is a barrier to UV radiation The lamp must be changed after 2000 hours' use, the equivalent of one year's use at eight hours per day, five days per week

Advantages and disadvantages of methods of sterilisation

A guide to controlling micro-organisms

There are a great many commercial products on the market for cleaning and sterilisation, under a variety of trade names. Below is a general guide. Please check the manufacturer's instructions for each individual piece of equipment. Most companies have their own particular favourites that they recommend. Also investigate the recommendations from beauty wholesalers and suppliers.

Ammonium Commonly used as a base for trade liquids used to kill bacteria, e.g. Barbicide is used to soak suitable instruments in salons.

Antibiotics A chemical substance that destroys or inhibits the growth of micro-organisms. Usually used to treat infections that respond to them, e.g. fungal or bacterial. Prescribed to humans and some animals for treatment.

Antiseptic A chemical agent which destroys or inhibits growth of micro-organisms on living tissues, thus helping to fight infection when placed on open cuts and wounds.

Bactericide A chemical that will kill bacteria but not necessarily the spores, so reproduction may still take place. Can be called either biocide, fungicide, virucide or sporicide. Biocides destroy bacteria, fungus, viruses and spores.

Chlorhexidine Trade names for chlorhexidine include Savlon and Hibitane. Widely used for skin and surface cleaning and for cleaning some sunbed canopies. Check individual manufacturers' instructions for cleaning.

Disinfectant A chemical that kills micro-organisms but not spores – most commonly used to wash surfaces and used in drains.

Detergent A synthetic cleaning agent that removes all impurities from a surface by reacting with grease and suspended articles, including bacteria and other micro-organisms. Needs to be used with water but is ideal for cleansing large surface areas.

Phenol compounds Ideal for large areas that need cleaning, but it does have a chlorine base and should not be used on the skin. Used in industrial cleaning preparations and the old carbolic soap!

Sanitation Used to describe conditions favourable to good health and preventing the spread of disease.

Sterilisation The complete destruction of all living micro-organisms and their spores.

Surgical spirit Can be used for skin cleansing and the removal of grease on the skin. Widely used, and available from pharmacists. Comes in varying strengths of dilution. A 70 per cent alcohol base concentration is acceptable for cleansing.

You and your working environment

This part of **Professional basics** looks at where you work – a cubicle, a room or a large salon space – and how you manage it. This includes health and safety within the area, managing your resources, and using your surroundings to create the right setting for a pampering and relaxing treatment.

Hygiene in the treatment area

When preparing and managing your treatment area, you will need to ensure that your working environment meets the legal, hygiene and treatment requirements, as set by both your awarding body and government guidelines.

Hygiene is important for:

- the **permanent fixtures** in the salon, that is:
  - walls
  - flooring
  - doors
  - windows

- the **portable equipment** you use, including:
  - the couch
  - machines
  - small equipment
  - products.

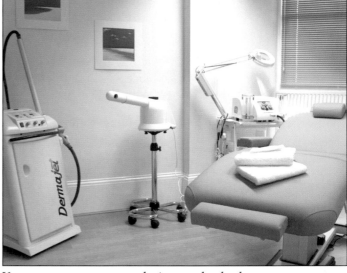
Your treatment area must be immaculately clean

You will need to refer to the Health and Safety at Work etc. Act 1974 for full guidance (see **You, your client and the law**, page 67) and also to work to the specifications of the Workplace (Health, Safety and Welfare) Regulations 1992, which require all premises used as work places to have effective means of:

- lighting
- ventilation
- temperature control
- providing adequate work space
- maintaining cleanliness
- arranging safe salon layout (see **You, your client and the law**, page 70).

(See **You, your client and the law** for a full list of treatment and working regulations, and below for environmental conditions for creating the right atmosphere.)

Hygiene for permanent fixtures

The salon should be regularly cleaned to prevent the spread of infection, and to make it welcoming for the client. A dirty salon will be judged on its appearance rather than on the treatments carried out.

Most colleges and training establishments employ a cleaning firm, usually on a fixed contract, which provides staff to do the daily chores for hygiene maintenance: floor cleaning, emptying of general waste bins, sweeping the stairs, and so on. More staff may be employed to carry out longer-term spring cleaning of windows, paintwork and re-sealing of the floors.

Small salons do not normally subcontract their cleaning duties – it tends to be done on a rota system, with junior staff doing most of the jobs. Any idle pair of hands will be asked to get on with some cleaning duties, and all staff can expect to share the workload – it is almost part of the job description. It would be unrealistic to expect otherwise.

Salon décor needs to be attractive yet practical, with suitable surfaces. There is a fine line between the clinical décor of a hospital and a welcoming salon which is easy to keep clean.

Check it out

Who does your company/training establishment employ to do the cleaning, if anyone? How much does the service cost? Who is responsible for checking the job is well done? What happens if it isn't?

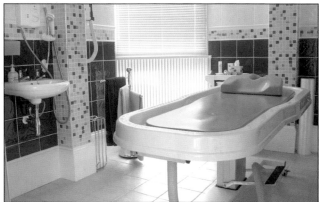

Ensure your salon's surfaces are attractive and easy to clean

- **Flooring** should be made of non-slip material, such as vinyl tiles or a softwood finish, which is easy to sweep or vacuum everyday. Carpet or carpet tiles may look good to start with, but can be high maintenance when getting old, and are not practical for spillage or keeping in pristine condition. A good disinfectant and mop will lift most dirt and grease from a floor, which should be cleaned nightly.
- **Walls and doors** should be painted for two reasons: they are easier to wipe with a disinfectant or abrasive cleaner such as sugar soap, and it is easy to maintain a high standard of décor, as redecorating is a quick coat of paint! Any household preparation or spray cleaner will clean off finger marks or dirt from paintwork, using a damp cloth. Sugar soap (granules which dissolve in hot water) will cut through long-term grease and make a good preparation of the surface for the new coat of paint.
- **Light switches and dado rails** tend to collect finger marks and general dirt, so they also need a spray with a household cleanser – but spray the cloth, rather than the light switch, and wipe over, to avoid getting the electric cable behind the switch wet.
- **Ceilings** can get very grubby – especially the old swirl-effect artex ceilings, where dirt can accumulate in the grooves, and if the room has been used as a smoking room, the ceiling can become very dirty. Washing ceilings should only be done when the salon is empty, and by using the correct ladder, or wide steps, for health and safety reasons. If the salon has subcontracted its cleaning, the contractor would normally have carried out the correct risk assessments and training for this task. Ceilings are actually quite a focus for clients as they often lie in the supine position (facing upwards) and a dirty ceiling will certainly catch the eye, and be very off putting! Always remember to look up when vacuuming the carpet, so that you can vacuum up those long cobweb formations which accumulate in corners, with the nozzle of the vacuum cleaner.
- **Windows** are as hazardous as ceilings to clean, and should be left to an outside contractor, especially the high, external ones. When cleaning the insides of windows the old-fashioned recipe of vinegar diluted in hot water and rubbed with newspaper is highly effective! Never open a big window which is high up to try and clean the outside, or lean out to clean – that is an accident waiting to happen! Vinegar works equally well on mirrors, and modern window cleaning sprays have vinegar additives in them, as it cuts through greasy smears, leaving windows and mirrors streak free.
- **Shelving and worktops** can collect dust very easily and need regularly stripping and wiping with disinfectant – a flick with a feather duster will remove the dust particles but should the dust mix with grease or moisture, dirt forms and cannot

be just waved away. If you use a scouring powder on some surfaces, then tiny scratches will be engrained onto the surface and bacteria will soon breed in them. Some salons have worktops over their units, which is very practical as these are hardwearing and easy to clean.

- **Basins, sinks and toilets** need to be kept extra clean, as they are a place where germs and bacteria may breed and flourish. The ideal conditions of heat and moisture make sinks and toilets very appealing to bacteria. Any household bleach containing chlorine is ideal for work surfaces, toilets and sinks. Be careful not to mix bleach with other toilet cleansers as a reaction will occur and poisonous fumes can be given off. Having bins for paper towels, and providing covered waste bins for sanitary items is essential. Pump-action soap dispensers in the showers and hand basins stop contamination from multiple users, as do disposable paper towels rather than a shared towel on a roll.

Remember

Many people judge the cleanliness of a toilet as a good indicator of the standard of hygiene in an establishment, whether it is a restaurant, hotel or a salon. Unsatisfied customers will leave and take their business elsewhere, rather than be somewhere they consider to be unclean. Always make sure that your toilet/washroom facilities pass the hygiene test.

Hygiene for portable equipment

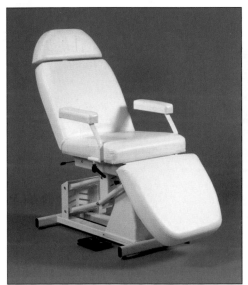

Adjustable facial chair

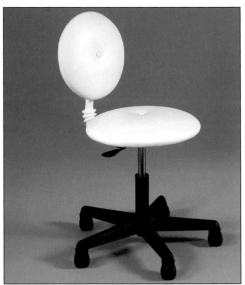

Therapist stool with gas-lift pump

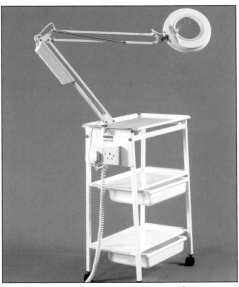

Multi-purpose trolley with magnification lamp

- **Couches** need to be cleaned at the beginning and end of the working day. Remove the fitted couch cover or towelling material and wash the vinyl covering with a disinfectant solution. When dry, the couch cover should be placed over the top, and the couch set up for the next treatment. The cover can stay on all day, as it tends to be covered by bath-sized towels and couch roll, and does not attract a lot of dirt because of this. However, if there is a spillage, the couch will need to be stripped, cleaned and a fresh cover fitted. Most salons buy fitted couch covers to match the towels and general décor, which gives a calming and soft effect.
- Ideally, **chairs** should be covered with a washable vinyl, which can be wiped. Cloth covers look lovely until they get dirty and then they will need to be cleaned with a special upholstery cleaner. Clients' outdoor clothing may bring in dirt and grease from outside (they might have brushed against a dirty car), with the likelihood that the dirt may transfer on to the salon chairs. Tell the client, as he or she will probably not be aware of it, and remove the offending mark as soon as possible. If the therapist's chair is an adjustable one, be careful of the accumulation of grease around the two pistons underneath, used for height adjustment – that can get on clothing, too.

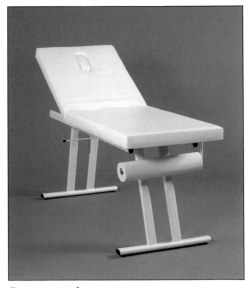

Beauty couch

- **Trolleys** should be made of metal or strong moulded plastic and have removable trays for easy access and cleaning. Avoid purchasing glass-topped trolleys as these are unsafe – if the glass gets hot from equipment on it, it may shatter. Covering trolley tops with towels and couch roll prevents them getting too dirty, and you can change the couch roll after every client, which looks smart and hygienic. Like couches, trolleys only need a cleaning morning and night if they are covered all day – except in the case of spillage. Trolleys seem to gather dust in their corners every day, from the cotton wool fibres and tissues used, so they do need emptying and thoroughly cleaning at the end of every day.

- **Towels, turbans and couch covers** can be washed in a hot wash cycle in the washing machine, and tumble-dried. The salon should have a plentiful supply of these, so there is no shortage while dirty ones are being washed and dried. Always check washing instructions to avoid shrinkage and avoid mixing dark and light colours together to prevent colour runs. Ideally, whites should be washed separately – one dark item in a white wash can turn the whole load 'grey'. When changing the décor in the salon, some salons will invest in a clothes dye, which can be used in a washing machine, and then all towels, turbans and gowns can be dyed the same shade – it can be very effective, and may give tired towels a new lease of life.

- **Machinery** should always be cleaned following manufacturers' instructions, to prevent damage and avoid accidents. Never immerse a machine in water to clean it, nor scrub the surface as you could rub off the dial markings which show heat intensity or strength of current. If that happens, you cannot be in control of the machine and it should be removed from service. Rubber will perish if cleaned with strong products, such as alcohol-based cleaner, and glass will develop scratches and not work well if an abrasive cleaner is used. If in doubt, ask, and if necessary, contact the manufacturer for advice.

- **Equipment** needs to be sterilised according to manufacturers' instructions as not all small equipment is suitable for immersion, or the autoclave. (See 'Hygiene and avoiding cross-infection', pages 47–8, for more details on sterilisation methods.)

Remember

The same rules you learned in your Level 2 assessments apply also to Level 3 assessments. Good working practices will ensure that your treatment area is fit for every client, every time!

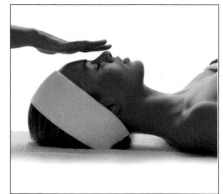

All equipment should be kept clean – including headbands

Keys to good practice

Here are some golden rules to managing your treatment area:

- Be hygienic by wiping down all surfaces and equipment with your chosen anti-bacterial cleaner, and then use couch roll on trolley tops, and on the floor to keep the area clean.
- Inspect the area both before and after treatment – would you like to have a treatment there?
- Be tidy! Tidy as you go, use a bin for waste products, tissues, and so on – never accumulate them in a heap on your trolley.
- Wash up as you go. If the working area has a sink and you can wash out your applicator brush, for example while the client has a facemask on, then do so. But do not leave the client unattended, and if the client is disturbed by the noise, then wash up later.
- Be organised! Have one trolley for products and small equipment, which is separate from the equipment trolley, and return them to place where they came from.
- Keep it simple! If all the product labels are facing you, then there can be no mistake in product application and you are safeguarding the client.
- Be methodical! Replace lids immediately after you have decanted the product to prevent spillage. Be economical with products – only put out what you will need. This also stops products and gels drying out in the hot salon atmosphere.
- Leave the room or area as you would wish to find it. Another therapist may be using the treatment area after you, and the client would be most put off by your mess not being cleared up!

Setting up required resources

When setting up your treatment area for the day, you may have an indication from the booking-in page about the treatments you will be carrying out, but you do not yet know if the client is suitable for them. You may have new clients, without known treatment requirements/expectations, and you may have the unexpected client who appears without an appointment. So preparation is the key, both for assessment criteria and so that you do not leave the client unattended, or waste time setting up because you were not organised.

Below is a suggested bed and trolley lay out which will allow you to complete a facial electrical treatment, body massage or a body electrical treatment. However, it is up to you to manage your resources well because some of the equipment, such as the body testing equipment, is likely to be shared between several therapists. In the case of assessments taking place in the salon, inform your salon manager of your need for the equipment and, with good communication and teamwork, all students should have access to suit their needs. (Refer back to 'Managing resources within the limits of your authority', page 21, to refresh your knowledge on sharing equipment and working with others as a team.)

> **Remember**
>
> If you have to leave the client unattended while you go off to seek a turban which you lent to a colleague, it may cost you your assessment, because you were not fully prepared in the first place.

Suggested
treatment area equipment

~ Couch or massage plinth/stool
~ Stool or chair
~ Trolleys (x 2)
~ Magnifying lamp
~ Towels, large and small
~ Towelling robe/gown and disposable footwear
~ Headband/turban
~ Cotton wool rounds or squares
~ Sponges
~ Tissues
~ Couch roll
~ Containers for client's jewellery and spatulas
~ Spatulas
~ Mask brushes
~ Waste bin with liner
~ Record card and pen
~ Test tubes (for thermal testing)

~ Sharp and smooth objects (for sensitive testing)
~ Gloves
~ Talcum powder
~ Petroleum jelly
~ Products – depending upon treatment

~ Eye goggles and shower products if giving a tanning treatment
~ Tape measure, fat callipers, peak flow and blood pressure machine (sphygmomanometer)

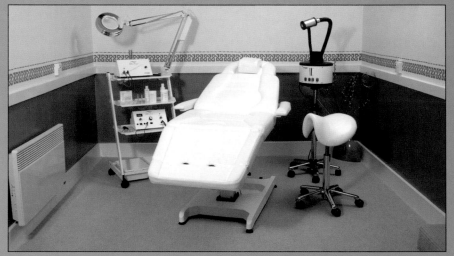

A treatment room layout

(Refer to Unit G1, Ensure your own actions reduce risks to health and safety, for potential risk assessments for equipment and your working area.)

Environmental conditions

Most treatment objectives are primarily for relaxation and a sense of well-being for the client, regardless of whether the treatment is on the face or body. For clients to relax and enjoy the treatment, they need to feel safe, confident in your capabilities and to be in an environment conducive to relaxation.

Many factors influence the relaxation dynamics in the salon, including:

- lighting
- heating
- ventilation
- general comfort
- suitable music and sound
- atmosphere.

Lighting

Lighting is one of the most instant mood enhancers – get it right and the client is encouraged to relax tense muscles, the eyes are soothed and the stress begins to melt away. Get it wrong and the facial muscles contract – harsh, strong lighting makes the client wince and the atmosphere is spoilt.

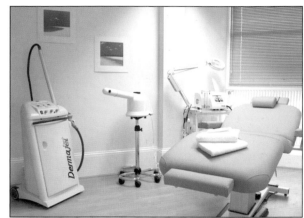

It is important to get the salon lighting just right, so the client can relax and you can see to work

Natural daylight is very good for mood enhancement, as everyone loves sunshine streaming through the window, but on winter days there is not enough natural light to illuminate the salon all through the working day. Big windows, such as a shop front, will allow natural light in, but are impractical for treatment areas as they would allow the client little privacy. There needs to be enough light to work by, but at the same time ensure that the client is not distracted by too much light. It is important to be able to see what you are doing, and inadequate lighting over a period of time can cause eyestrain, so you certainly need enough light to write out the consultation card comfortably.

For health and safety reasons, sufficient lighting is essential in some areas, for example the stairwell, and when using electrical equipment, mixing chemicals or during epilation. In the treatment area, avoid direct lighting where possible. A ceiling light or strip fluorescent lighting is quite harsh, and shines into the eyes when the client is in supine position (face up) on the couch. Soft wall lights spread the light and are soft and relaxing. Up-lighter shades, which allow the light to be arched towards the ceiling, are ideal, and are relevantly inexpensive to purchase. Corner lighting from tall standard lamps, or modern wrought-iron stands, has the same effect – although there is always the danger of knocking them over. Ideally, a corner position means that they are not in the way of traffic flow through the room.

For a general body treatment involving electrical equipment, good lighting is essential so that you are able to see and be in control of the machine, but for massage, where the aim of the treatment is relaxation, softer lighting is appropriate. Many salons have dimmer switches on the wall lights enabling the lighting strength to be adjusted to suit the individual treatment.

If you are unsure of the comfort of the lighting in your treatment area, try lying on the couch. Can you close your eyes comfortably? Do you have harsh lighting in your eyes? If necessary, make some adjustments where you can – a darker lampshade perhaps, or turn off the strip lighting for the duration of the treatment.

There is a medical condition called SAD (seasonal affective disorder) where a person suffers from a type of depression to which lack of sunlight contributes, due to a drop in the chemical reaction in the brain related to sunshine. Although a therapist cannot offer an opinion on SAD as it is a diagnosis for the doctor, it is probable that clients will be prescribed a course of treatment on the sunbed to help the condition and may come into the salon with a doctor's referral.

Heating

Correct levels of heating are essential in the salon, as temperature has a direct effect on the body, and the effectiveness of the treatment depends on the correct, comfortable temperature.

If the treatment room is too cold:

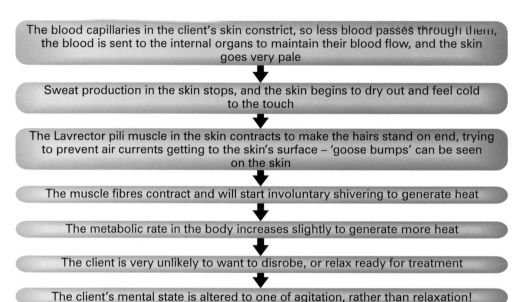

The blood capillaries in the client's skin constrict, so less blood passes through them, the blood is sent to the internal organs to maintain their blood flow, and the skin goes very pale

Sweat production in the skin stops, and the skin begins to dry out and feel cold to the touch

The Lavrector pili muscle in the skin contracts to make the hairs stand on end, trying to prevent air currents getting to the skin's surface – 'goose bumps' can be seen on the skin

The muscle fibres contract and will start involuntary shivering to generate heat

The metabolic rate in the body increases slightly to generate more heat

The client is very unlikely to want to disrobe, or relax ready for treatment

The client's mental state is altered to one of agitation, rather than relaxation!

If the treatment room is too hot:

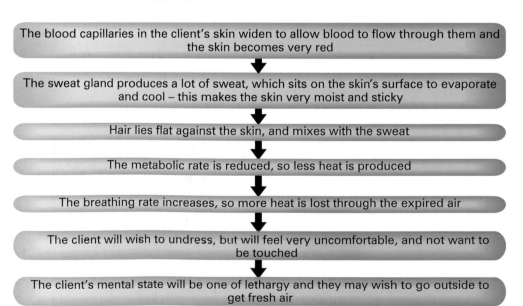

The blood capillaries in the client's skin widen to allow blood to flow through them and the skin becomes very red

The sweat gland produces a lot of sweat, which sits on the skin's surface to evaporate and cool – this makes the skin very moist and sticky

Hair lies flat against the skin, and mixes with the sweat

The metabolic rate is reduced, so less heat is produced

The breathing rate increases, so more heat is lost through the expired air

The client will wish to undress, but will feel very uncomfortable, and not want to be touched

The client's mental state will be one of lethargy and they may wish to go outside to get fresh air

Neither of these scenarios is conducive to a pampering treatment, and the client will want to leave as soon as possible!

> ### Remember
>
> Under the Workplace (Health, Safety and Welfare) Regulations 1992, the minimum temperature in the workplace should be 16°C one hour prior to work commencing (see **You, your client and the law**, page 70).

The core body temperature should be maintained at 37°C, which allows the body to function and the enzymes involved in metabolism to work efficiently. Should the temperature drop to 27°C, then the enzymes work half as fast, which is insufficient to keep the body alive. If the temperature rises to 41°C, the enzymes die in the heat and are unable to work, stopping bodily functions.

It is reasonable to expect that if the salon is offering body treatments, has a wet area, with showers, spa bath, and sauna or steam cabinets, the client will be warm in a swimming costume or with very little clothing. No one wants to get undressed in the cold, the body is not receptive to treatment and does not respond well, and the client's frame of mind is not ready for maximum relaxation.

Most modern buildings have gas-fired central heating, with a central boiler and radiators placed in every room, much like a domestic heating system, only on a larger scale. The boiler needs to be well maintained. The hot water supply will also come from the boiler, and the salon would cease to function without either heating or hot water.

Temperature control is governed either by:

- a wall-mounted control panel for all the radiators, with a temperature dial, or
- individual thermostatic controls on each radiator, which can be adjusted to suit the room and its needs, e.g. it can be turned up for clients coming in from the wet area, or having massage.

There are other methods of heating, including storage heaters, gas fires, electric under-floor heating and electric plug-in radiators, but gas central heating is the most economical and most preferred method in the modern salon. It is also the safest method for fire prevention.

Heat may be lost through:

- poor insulation
- walls and ceilings
- single-glazed windows.
- open doors and windows.

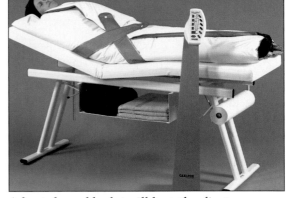

A heated over-blanket will keep the client comfortable and warm

As it is expensive to heat the salon, make sure that you do not waste money by leaving doors or windows open on a cold day – you may also create a draught on the client.

Keeping the client warm is essential, and you should have adequate bedding – blankets and large, warm bath towels – to wrap the client in. Muscle fibres relax in heat and constrict in cold, so you will be undoing all the benefits of heat treatment if the client is allowed to become cold. Once the client is on the couch, there are a number of electronically heated under- or over-blankets which offer safe, professional individual heating, designed to suit the client. These are similar to an electric blanket on a bed at home, and offer a cosy and gentle sedation prior to massage and body treatments. The client is literally cocooned in a warm envelope of blanket, heated to his or her own optimum level.

Ventilation

Air movement is essential to comfort, and ties in with the heating of the salon. Too little air movement in the salon or one room can create a stuffy atmosphere, while too much can make a room seem draughty. All humans exhale carbon dioxide and if this builds up in a busy salon, combined with heat and odours, clients and the therapists will feel very lethargic and may develop a headache.

> **Remember**
>
> In hot, humid countries therapists work in air-conditioned rooms, which are quite cold, and clients prefer pre-cooled or iced towels on the body. It is only salons in colder conditions which require heating.

Good ventilation also prevents a build-up of chemical fumes (if your salon has a nail extension bar) and stops unpleasant odours accumulating, especially if there is a staff room or relaxation area where clients are permitted to smoke. (Most salons would discourage smoking, on health grounds.)

Ventilation can be:

- natural
- mechanical or artificial.

Natural ventilation

This takes place when windows and doors are opened and also occurs with the movement of air through cracks or gaps in windows and doors. The obvious disadvantages to natural ventilation are possible cold draughts, noise and odours from external sources coming in and ruining the atmosphere, and draughts blowing papers about.

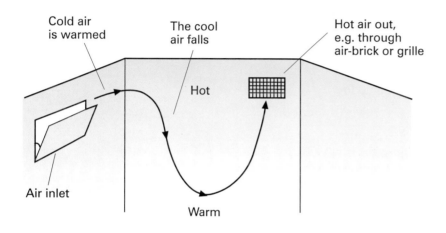

Natural ventilation by convection

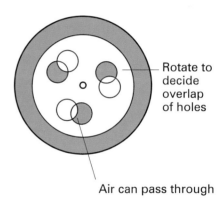

A coopers disk allows natural ventilation

Natural convection can be used for ventilation. This is where a small window, high up on a wall, is open, which allows cold air into the room. As it is high up, the cold air is warmed by the hot air it meets (heat rises) and the warmed air then drops into the room. As this air heats up, it rises and a ventilator grille, or airbrick, on an opposite wall draws it out. This keeps the air circulating without creating draughts.

Older windows sometimes have a double disc cut into them with two sets of holes (called a coopers disc). When the holes line up, the airflow is allowed to enter into the room.

Louvre windows were a feature of many buildings of the 1970s. The slates of glass can be opened as widely as is required and are easy to clean. However, they are also easy to remove, making them a security risk.

Mechanical or artificial ventilation

Mechanical or artificial ventilation using electric extractor fans is more desirable as it is a controllable system, more efficient and cost-effective to run, with no draughts on the clients. Most modern extractor fans can take air in from outside, as well as extracting the stale air in a room. Ideally, they should be fixed to an outside window or wall, but not near open windows or doors, as otherwise they will simply extract the fresh air coming in.

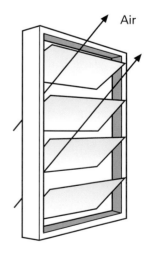

A louvre window can be used to direct airflow into the room

Free-standing fans can be used to refresh a room or salon on a hot day, but these are not very safe as they are not stable and may be knocked over easily if in the main traffic flow of a room.

Air conditioning, which passes air over filters and coolers, is a very effective method of ventilation but is the most expensive.

General comfort

If the salon has appropriate heating, lighting and ventilation, the environment is well on the way to being suitable for a pampering, relaxing treatment. The general comfort of the client should also be considered, and often makes all the difference to a treatment.

- Towels, bedding and gowns can be warmed on a radiator, just before the client arrives, for that extra luxurious feeling of warmth.
- Ensure that the salon has a pleasant aroma, neither too chemical nor antiseptic based. Plug-in air fresheners are very acceptable, and you do not need to be qualified in aromatherapy as you would if you use an oil burner. Flower-based fresheners such as rose or lavender are associated with relaxing, so can be used throughout the salon.
- The salon décor should be soothing on the eye, with colour coordination and matching bedding, towels, and so on. Warm colours such as pink, peach and lavender are harmonious, and create a calm and enticing look to the treatment rooms. Harsh, loud colours are not conducive to relaxation. If you are aiming to attract a male clientele, avoid an image that is too feminine in your colour scheme and accessories, as male clients may be put off by such a setting.
- Be ruthless with things past their best, such as chipped cups, old towels and threadbare gowns! Not only are they unhygienic, they create a poor impression. Throw away odd cups and invest in matching china. Keep cutlery and china in mint condition – no one wants to drink from a dirty cup and saucer. When offering the client water after the treatment, use a glass, rather than an old beaker, and regularly wash glasses so they shine like crystal!
- A selection of up-to-date magazines in reception will make a good first impression.
- Replace failed light bulbs as soon as they go, both for safety reasons and to maintain the professional image of the salon.
- To enhance the look of the salon, invest in some good quality houseplants, but remember to tend them well – poorly kept, or dying, house plants, look depressing. If you are not green-fingered, then invest in some nil-maintenance, artificial plants.
- Clients appreciate good quality toilet paper and soap dispensers.

It is the attention to detail which makes the difference to clients. They need to feel cosseted and cosy, and valued.

Suitable music and sound

Music and listening to relaxing sounds, such as whale calls, can create a relaxing atmosphere, but always ask individual clients for their preferences. Musical choice is personal, and while one client may like the sound of a cascading waterfall to fall asleep by, another client may find it irritating.

Some large training salons have piped music put through to all salons via a central sound system, from a CD player, usually in reception. The disadvantage to this is that you have to listen to the receptionist's choice of music, rather than the client's choice.

Remember

In a busy salon the air change should be three or four times per hour, depending upon the size of the room. Ventilation is especially important in the wet area, where clients will be wet – they should not be allowed to get cold through draughts and poor heating facilities.

A small sound unit in the treatment room is better, allowing volume and choice to be personalised, and some clients just prefer to have complete quiet, so they can really drift away.

There are several things to remember when choosing music:

- Use of music in the treatment room, reception or in exercise groups is classed as a public performance. Phonographic Performance Ltd (PPL) collects licence payments on behalf of artistes and record companies from people wishing to play recorded music in public. Legally, all salons and exercise/aerobic instructors must purchase music that has a built-in licence (see **You, your client and the law**, page 79, for information on the Copyright, Designs and Patents Act 1988). While more expensive to purchase (a CD can cost about £30), it will prevent liability to a heavy fine. Most good specialist music shops have a section of licensed music – ask the shop assistant if in doubt.
- Compilation CDs can be very repetitive when played over and over, as the brain starts to anticipate the next track. This can be very irritating to the client. It is far better to vary the music and invest in several different CDs.
- Look at the length of time the music runs for. Nothing is more disruptive than the music ending just as the client is floating away and you are halfway through the treatment. You may have oily hands and should not break contact with the client, so you will have to end the treatment in silence. If you are doing a full body massage, check you have at least a one-hour CD playing before you start the treatment.
- Remember that your choice is not always the same as the client's. Always ask.
- Radio stations are not very suitable for easy listening as there is too much variation in the sound: the DJ may talk, adverts come on, weather, news and traffic are regular slots, and the client may be listening to roadworks information, instead of mentally relaxing.

Atmosphere

A salon can have perfect facilities, be pretty and chic, with all essential ingredients in place, and yet if there is a poor atmosphere between staff, with tension and bad feeling, the client will pick up on it immediately. Often, the client will say, 'I don't know, it just didn't feel right' if the overall ambience of the working environment is poor.

The atmosphere in the salon needs to feel friendly. The staff should be approachable, work together as a team and make the client feel wanted and a most important person. No clients equals no business, so you will need to work hard to create a good working atmosphere, which encourages clients to enter, stay and recommend you to others. (For more information on working together, solving difficulties and being mature in your working outlook, see **You – the therapist** page 20.)

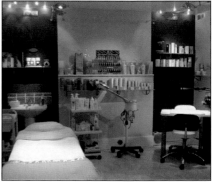

A soothing colour combination is vital in creating an appropriate atmosphere

Fire precautions and evacuation procedures

Using electrical equipment means there is a higher risk of a fire starting, so all Level 3 therapists should know the legislation involved, and the actions to take should a fire occur. (See Unit G1, Ensure your own actions reduce risks to health and safety, for the risk assessment for hazards involving electrical equipment.)

Fire Precautions Act 1971

This Act is concerned with fire prevention and the provision of escape routes should an evacuation be required. The employer is responsible for fire safety in the workplace and he or she must ensure the workplace complies with the fire regulations.

The employer should have a fire certificate if:

- there will be more than 20 people working on the premises at any one time
- there will be more than 10 people working anywhere other than the ground floor.

Fire Precautions (Workplace) Regulations 1997 (amended 1999)

The regulations require all premises to undertake a fire risk assessment. If five or more people work together as employees, the risk assessment must be in writing. Employers must also take into account *all other persons* on the premises, not just employees.

There must also be a fire and evacuation procedure. In every period of one year there must be at least one fire drill, which involves everyone. All staff must be fully informed, instructed and trained in what is expected from them and some people will have special duties to perform. Employees, trainees, temporary workers and others who work in any undertaking must, by law, agree to cooperate with the employer so far as is necessary to enable them to fulfil the duties placed upon them by law. This means cooperating fully in training courses and fire drills, even when everyone knows they are only a practice!

Most large training establishments will have their own policy on fire evacuation procedures and may carry out a fire drill once a term, that is three times per year. This is especially important with large groups of people or students, and any disabled persons who will need special consideration. Many fire-training exercises are organised with a fire safety officer from the local fire station. Often the fire engines will take part in the exercise to test their own attendance time from the station to the premises. Everyone should be made aware of his or her own particular rules for evacuation.

When joining any business/establishment the new employee should be briefed regarding all health and safety issues, and especially fire evacuation procedures. It is standard practice to include the information in a handbook containing all the establishment's policies.

On the next page is an example of an evacuation procedure.

Emergency procedures

Fire drill relevant to the working area

- Switch off all electrical equipment.
- Close windows.
- Clients should be led by the therapist to a safe area. If necessary, wrap clients up warmly using blankets and towels – this is especially important where a client has been having a body treatment.
- If possible, clients should take their valuable possessions with them, such as handbag and jewellery, but not if these are safely locked away, or if it puts the client or therapist in any danger. (Usually clients' belongings are kept under the trolley and therefore are within easy reach.)
- Be aware of the treatment being performed during the evacuation – if the client has chemicals on the skin, it may be easier to remove immediately. (This would need to be at the judgement of the lecturer in charge of the workshop – certainly a client having an eyelash tint will need to have it removed before being able to proceed to the assembly point.)

Building evacuation procedures in the event of fire or bomb alert

The following procedure has been agreed and must be followed. Any staff member who does not comply is committing an infringement of the college disciplinary code. Whenever a fire occurs, the main consideration is to get everybody out of the building safely. Protection of personal or college property is incidental.

Raising the alarm

Anyone discovering a fire must immediately raise the alarm by operating the nearest fire alarm and report to the controller the fire location.

On hearing the alarm the receptionist will immediately contact the emergency services and then evacuate the building.

In the event of a fire being discovered when the reception is unmanned – the premises officer on duty will contact the emergency services and assume control.

On hearing the alarm

All those in senior positions proceed to the control point, normally at a main entrance to the building – where one person must take control of the proceedings.

All other staff: close windows; switch off machinery and lights, and close doors on leaving the room.

Assist less able colleagues, leave the building by the nearest marked route and proceed quickly to the appropriate assembly point. Staff must supervise their class.

Staff evacuating the building must check their locality is clear.

Assembly points

Everyone must remain at assembly points well away from buildings and clear of access roads.

Report to control in person or via two-way radios where allocated.

Everyone must remain at assembly points until further instructions.

DO NOT re-enter the building until you are told it is safe to do so.

An evacuation procedure

- Take appropriate remover and damp cotton wool or tissues to remove products on the skin such as facemasks. While not dangerous to the skin if left on, the client will probably be more comfortable, and the skin less dry if it can be removed.
- Be aware of the client's footwear, and if possible encourage the wearing of shoes to prevent an accident during the evacuation.

Bomb alert

Act quickly if an abandoned parcel or bag arouses concern. Follow the procedures for a fire drill. Do not look inside a suspicious package.

Gas leak

- Open all windows.
- Evacuate the building following the fire drill procedure.
- **Do not turn off or switch on any electrical equipment (including light switches) – this may cause a spark which could ignite the gas.**

Sensible fire precautions

Be informed – know what to do and where to go when the evacuation begins.

- Be sensible and do not panic – this will only make the client feel panicky, too.
- Make sure that you know the location of the fire bell, fire extinguishers and fire exit.
- Never ignore smoke or the smell of burning – it is far better to have a false alarm. Better safe than sorry!
- Do not misuse or mistreat electrical appliances that are a potential hazard – a healthy respect is needed.
- Do not ignore manufacturers' instructions for the storage and use of highly flammable products, which are very common within the salon.
- Do be sensible with naked flames and matches or disposal of cigarette ends – a smouldering tip can burst into flames that would destroy the salon in minutes.
- Check that all clients have been evacuated – the appointment book can be taken outside, as a check on which clients should be present. A college lecturer or trainer should do the same with the class register to check that the right number of students are present.
- Do not use a lift for the evacuation – it may be that the fire affects the electric mechanism and that then becomes another emergency.

If you are not at the correct location for the fire evacuation, report to your allocated assembly point. Otherwise you may not be accounted for. This may mean a fire fighter risking his or her life to go into a burning building to check – when all the time you were around the corner!

Fire fighting equipment

Fire extinguishers

Not every fire extinguisher is suitable to fight every fire, and using the wrong one can make the situation worse.

Only a person specially trained in the use of a fire extinguisher should attempt to use one. Never put yourself at risk; personal safety is more important than saving material items that can be replaced – a human life cannot be replaced.

Extinguisher	Type	Colour	Uses	NOT to be used
Electrical fires	Dry powder	Blue marking	For burning liquid, electrical fires and flammable liquids	On flammable metal fires
	Carbon dioxide	Black marking	Safe on all voltages, used on burning liquid and electrical fires and flammable liquids	On flammable metal fires
	Vaporising liquid	Green marking	Safe on all voltages, used on burning liquid and electrical fires and flammable liquids	On flammable metal fires
Non-electrical fires	Water	Red marking	For wood, paper, textiles, fabric and similar materials	On burning liquid, electrical or flammable metal fires
	Foam	Cream / yellow markings	On burning liquid fires	On electrical or flammable metal fires

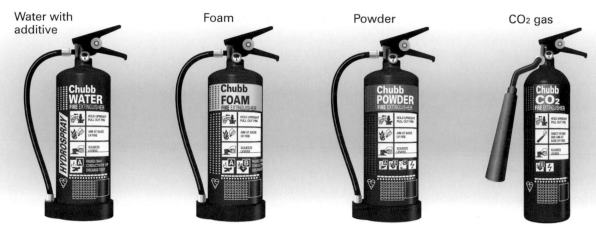

| Water with additive | Foam | Powder | CO₂ gas |

Fire extinguishers

Fire blankets

Fire blankets are made of fire-resistant material. They are particularly useful for wrapping around a person whose clothing is on fire. A fire blanket must be used calmly and with a firm grip. If the blanket is flapped about, it may fan the fire and cause it to flare up, rather than put it out. The hands should be protected by the edge of the cloth and the blanket should be placed, rather than thrown, into the desired position.

Fire blankets conforming to British Standard BS6575 are suitable for use on small fires. These will be marked to show whether they should be thrown away after use or used again after cleaning in accordance with manufacturer instructions. Fire blankets are best kept in a central location for easy access.

Sand

A bucket of sand can be used to soak up liquids which are the source of a fire. If the fire is too large for you to contain, or you are in any doubt, **never risk injury, get out and phone the fire and rescue service**.

Even small fires spread very quickly, producing smoke and fumes, which can kill in seconds. If there is any doubt, do not tackle the fire, no matter how small.

First aid

The Health and Safety (First Aid) Regulations 1981 set out the essential aspects of first aid that employers must address, because people at work can suffer injuries or fall ill. It does not matter whether the injury or illness is caused by the work they do. It is important that they receive immediate attention and that an ambulance is called in serious cases.

First aid can save lives and prevent minor injuries becoming major ones. First aid in the workplace is the initial management of any injury or illness suffered at work. It does not include giving tablets or medicines to treat illness.

Remember
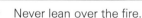

- Never lean over the fire.
- If you cannot control the fire, leave the room, close the door and phone the fire and rescue service.

Remember
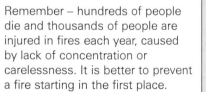

Remember – hundreds of people die and thousands of people are injured in fires each year, caused by lack of concentration or carelessness. It is better to prevent a fire starting in the first place.

This means that sufficient first aid personnel and facilities should be available to:

- give immediate assistance to casualties with both common injuries and illnesses and those likely to arise from specific hazards at work
- summon an ambulance or other professional help.

This will depend upon the size of the workforce, the type of workplace hazards and risks, and the history of accidents in the workplace.

Two aspects of first aid need further consideration: trainees and the public.

- **Trainees** – students undertaking work experience on certain training schemes are given the same status as employees and therefore are the responsibility of the employer.
- **The public** – when dealing with the public these regulations do not oblige employers to provide first aid for anyone other than their own employees. This means the compulsory element of public liability insurance *does not cover* litigation resulting from first aid to non-employees. Employers should make extra provision for this themselves. Education establishments must also include the general public in their assessment of first aid requirements.

First aid kits

The minimum level of first aid equipment is a suitably stocked and properly identified first aid container.

First aid containers should be easily accessible and placed, where possible, near to handwashing facilities. The number of containers will depend upon the size of the establishment, and the total number of employees in that area. The container should protect the items inside from dust and damp and must only be stocked with useful items. Tablets and medications should not be kept in there.

There is no compulsory list of what a first aid kit should contain but the following would be useful:

- a leaflet giving general guidance on first aid (such as the HSE leaflet *Basic advice on first aid at work*)
- 20 individually wrapped sterile adhesive dressings (assorted sizes) appropriate to the type of work
- two sterile eye pads
- four individually wrapped triangular bandages (preferably sterile)
- six safety pins
- six medium-sized individually wrapped wound dressings
- two large sterile individually wrapped unmedicated wound dressings
- one pair of disposable gloves
- antiseptic cream or liquid
- eye bath
- gauze
- medical wipes
- a pair of tweezers
- cotton wool.

Do not forget that if in doubt, do not treat – phone for an ambulance immediately.

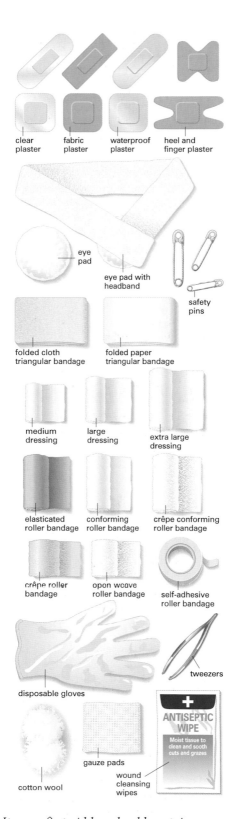

Items a first aid box should contain

First aid training

First aid certificates are only valid for a certain period of time, which is currently three years. Employers need to arrange refresher training with re-testing of competence before certificates expire. If a certificate expires, the individual will have to undertake a full course of training to be re-established as a first-aider. Specialist training can also be undertaken if necessary.

Records

It is good practice for employers to provide first aiders with a book in which to record incidents which require their attendance. If there are several first aiders in one establishment then a central book will be used.

The information should include:

- date, time and place of incident
- name and job of the injured or ill person
- details of the injury or illness and what first aid was given
- what action was taken immediately afterward (e.g. did the person go home, go to hospital, get sent in an ambulance)
- name and signature of the first aider or person dealing with the incident.

Accident reporting procedures

Accidents happen, even to the most careful of people. The key is to react in the correct manner, stay calm and follow the establishment's accident procedures. You should be aware of every possible risk in all aspects of salon life, as shown in the diagram below.

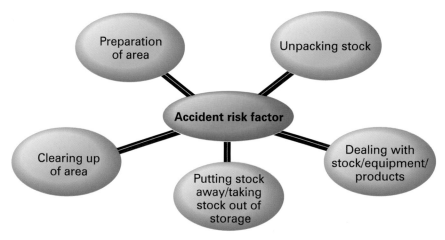

Risks in the salon

Remember

- All activities should be continuously reviewed for accident potential.
- If equipment is continually being broken because of lack of storage space or because a trolley is too close to a windowsill, then a review should take place. If the same accident repeatedly occurs, then it is important to ask why.

Check it out

Find out your establishment's set procedure to follow in the event of an accident.

You, your client and the law

You will learn about

- legislation
- insurance
- industry codes of practice or ethics
- salon guidelines.

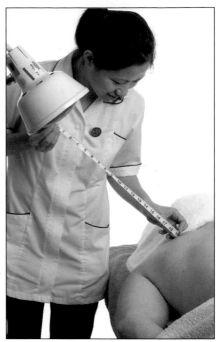

Health and safety legislations are created to protect you and your client

This part of **Professional basics**, together with Unit G1, Ensure your own actions reduce risks to health and safety, is essential to your duty as a professional therapist. It will enable you to protect everyone in the salon, including yourself, colleagues, clients, visitors to the salon and even passers-by.

Legislation

It is vital that you are aware of current health and safety legislation and how it relates to you, and your responsibilities within the salon. Your working life is controlled by two sets of external laws – Acts and regulations.

An Act is laid down by Parliament as law. It usually contains general objectives that employers, employees and others must achieve. A regulation is a statutory instrument – in other words, a detailed means of meeting the general objectives of an Act.

Health and Safety at Work etc. Act 1974

Most health and safety law is derived from the Health and Safety at Work etc. Act (HASWA)1974.

This Act requires employers to:

- provide and maintain a safe working environment
- provide adequate welfare facilities
- provide safe systems of work
- provide information, training and supervision
- ensure the safe handling, storage and transportation of goods and materials
- provide and maintain safe equipment.

These requirements are also included in other regulations, some of which will be discussed later in this section.

The enforcement of health and safety regulations is carried out by inspectors who are employed by the Health and Safety Executive, a government-appointed body. Inspectors may enter and inspect a workplace at any reasonable time, following an accident or complaint, and can do so without warning. For example, they may:

- offer informal advice
- offer informal advice supported by a formal letter
- issue an improvement notice
- issue a prohibition notice
- recommend prosecution.

An improvement notice will recommend actions to be completed by the employer within a certain period of time, whereas a prohibition notice will require immediate action and may well involve the removal of a process or item of equipment until these actions have been completed. Failure to comply with either of these notices will result in a criminal prosecution in either a magistrates court or crown court, depending on the gravity of the offence. Courts have the power to fine or even imprison for such offences.

As an employee, you also have duties under this Act. You must:

- not endanger yourself or others by your acts or omissions
- cooperate with your employer in order for the employer's duties to be fulfilled
- not misuse anything provided in the interests of health and safety
- report all accidents, incidents and unsafe conditions or practices.

As you progress through this section, you will see that many of your workplace activities relate to HASWA.

Employers' and employees' responsibilities

Employers' responsibilities include:

- planning safety and security
- providing information about safety and security
- updating systems and procedures where there are five or more employees.

Employees' responsibilities include:

- using systems and procedures correctly
- reporting flaws or gaps within the system or procedure when in use.

Employers and employees also have shared responsibilities which include:

- the safety of individuals being cared for
- safety of the working environment.

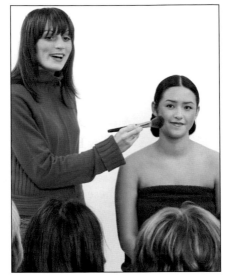

It is your employer's duty to hold regular training sessions on health and safety issues, such as posture while working

Employees have a duty to take reasonable care of themselves, colleagues, other people affected by their work and the general public and to cooperate with their employers in fulfilling their health and safety obligations.

The employer's duty is to provide:

- a safe place to work
- systems and equipment
- safe storage and transport of substances and material
- access to workplace exits
- good practices in the workplace.

The employer also has a duty to other persons not in employment but affected by his or her actions, to reduce their exposure to health and safety risks.

HASWA provides powers for the Health and Safety Commission and the Health and Safety Executive. It covers self-employed persons as well as persons who work alone away from the employer's premises. The Act allows for various regulations which control the workplace.

European Union directives

In 1992, European Union directives updated legislation on health and safety management and widened the existing Health and Safety at Work Act. These directives came into force in 1993. They cover six main areas:

- provision and use of work equipment
- manual handling operations
- workplace health, safety and welfare
- personal protective equipment at work
- health and safety (display screen equipment)
- management of health and safety at work.

The latest provisions include:

- the protection of non-smokers from tobacco smoke
- the provision of rest facilities for pregnant and nursing mothers
- safe cleaning of windows.

Manual Handling Operations Regulations 1992

The Health and Safety Executive (HSE) has drawn attention to skeletal and muscular disorders caused by manual handling and lifting, repetitive strain disorders and unsuitable posture causing lower-back pain. The regulations require certain measures be taken to avoid these types of injuries occurring.

In the salon, the regulations would apply to:

- stock unpacking and storage, e.g. lifting heavy objects
- couch height – needs to be adjustable for individual therapists
- chairs or stools used in the treatment rooms
- trolley height
- reception desk and chair
- rotation of job roles so that the therapist is not in the same position for every treatment
- height and size of nail art desk.

It is important to consider all of the above when purchasing equipment, as you will have to work with the consequences! For example, working at a couch at the wrong height may cause considerable discomfort and damage your back in long term (see **You – the therapist**, page 15, for information on posture and choosing equipment).

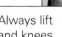

Remember

Follow the golden rule. Always lift with your back straight and knees bent. If in doubt – don't lift at all!

1 Think about the lift. Where is the load to be placed? Do you need help? Are handling aids available?

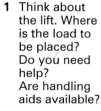 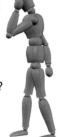

2 Get ready to lift. Stand with your feet apart.

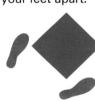

3 Bend the knees. Keep the back straight. Tuck in your chin. Lean slightly forward over the load to get a good grip.

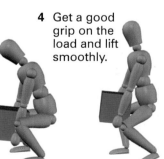 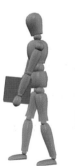

4 Get a good grip on the load and lift smoothly.

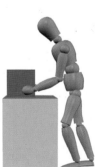

Safe lifting procedures must be observed

Management of Health and Safety at Work Regulations 1999

These regulations are considered to be the most important legislation relating to health and safety since the Health and Safety at Work Act. This is because they legally require all employers to effectively manage health and safety within their business.

Your employer is obliged to:

- carry out risk assessments to determine what health and safety measures are needed to protect you, the employee and others who may enter the business premises
- plan, implement and control whatever measures are thought necessary
- review these measures regularly
- provide health and safety training to all employees.

Provision and Use of Work Equipment Regulations 1998

Under these regulations, your employer is required to prevent or control the risks to your health and safety from any equipment you use at work. This applies to both new and second-hand equipment. The regulations state that equipment used at work must be:

- suitable for use and used for the purpose for which it is intended
- maintained in a safe condition for use
- inspected on a regular basis, by a competent person, and records kept
- used only by people who have been trained and instructed in its correct usage.

Written instructions must be provided if and when necessary.

Workplace (Health, Safety and Welfare) Regulations 1992

Your employer should ensure the workplace complies with the requirements of these regulations by:

- maintaining the workplace and all equipment and systems used there
- ensuring adequate ventilation
- keeping the workplace at a reasonable temperature (minimum 16°C)
- making sure you have sufficient light to work comfortably
- keeping the workplace clean and tidy
- ensuring you have enough room to work comfortably
- keeping floor and 'traffic routes' in a reasonable condition (no holes, slopes or uneven surfaces)
- ensuring workstations and seating are suitable
- providing suitable washing and toilet facilities (with soap and a means of hand drying)
- providing storage space for clothing (worn at work) and changing facilities
- providing facilities for resting and eating (if meals are to be eaten on the premises)
- providing clean drinking water and cups
- regularly removing waste material
- keeping you safe from falling objects
- making sure all doors and gates are suitably constructed and fitted with any necessary safety devices
- making sure windows are protected against breakage and display signs (or similar) where there is a danger of someone walking into them
- making sure escalators and moving walkways have safety devices fitted so they can be stopped in an emergency.

Heat stress

The most comfortable working temperature in beauty therapy is between 15.5°C and 20°C. Humidity – the amount of moisture in the air – should be within the 30–70 per cent range, although this will vary if your salon has a sauna and steam area, which should be in a well-ventilated area away from the main workrooms, while still being accessible to clients.

There should also be sufficient air exchange and air movement, which must be increased in special circumstances such as chemical usage. Treatment rooms used for nail art, aromatherapy, bleaching or eyelash perming will need specialist ventilation methods. (For more information on methods of ventilation, see **You and your working environment**, pages 57–9.)

A build-up of fumes, or strong smells, even from manicure preparations, may cause both physical and psychological problems which affect not only clients but staff too.

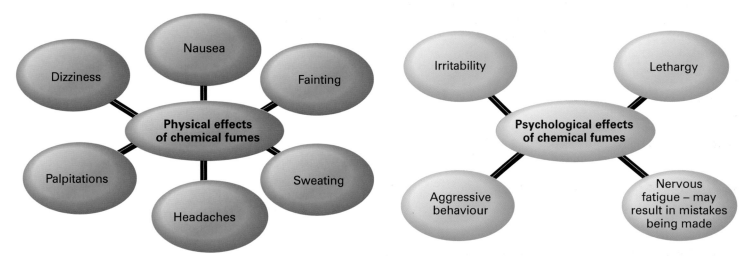

The effects of chemical fumes

Personal Protective Equipment at Work Regulations 1992

Employers and self-employed people must ensure that suitable personal protective equipment (PPE) is provided for themselves and employees where they may be exposed to a risk to their health or safety while at work. This is particularly relevant to epilation and milia extraction, where there is a risk of contamination by bodily fluids (see also Environmental Protection Act, Controlled Waste Regulations and Special Waste Regulations below).

These regulations cover both equipment and protective clothing provisions to ensure the safety of everyone in the workplace. They also provide that workplace personnel must have appropriate training in the use of equipment. Protective clothing, white overalls or work wear ensure cleanliness, freshness and professionalism.

For certain treatments it may be advisable to wear extra disposable coverings.

It is the employer's responsibility to:

- assess the need for the use of PPE
- supply protective clothing or equipment free of charge
- train staff in the use of personal protective clothing
- ensure it is fit for the purpose.

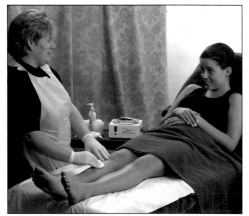

It is important to use the appropriate personal protective equipment

Check it out

What are your responsibilities under the Personal Protective Equipment at Work Regulations?

Control of Substances Hazardous to Health (COSHH) Regulations 2003

In the salon you will use many substances that may put your health at risk. The COSHH Regulations require employers to assess the health risks that arise from the use of hazardous substances within the workplace and to provide the controls that will be most effective in protecting employees and members of the public. The regulations apply to substances that have been classified as corrosive, explosive, harmful, highly flammable, irritant, oxidising or toxic. The COSHH classification symbols are shown on the right.

Your employer is required to:

- assess the risk to your health from the use of hazardous substances at work and what precautions are needed
- design and introduce appropriate measures to prevent or control your exposure to hazardous substances
- ensure that you follow the control measures and safety procedures, and use protective equipment when appropriate
- monitor your exposure to hazardous substances and carry out appropriate forms of surveillance to ensure you maintain good health
- inform and instruct you about the risks and precautions you need to take and train you to work in a safe way when dealing with hazardous chemicals.

Storage of hazardous chemicals

Products that are identified as hazardous must be stored in a cool, dark place, with good ventilation and away from direct sunlight. Always read the manufacturers' instructions when storing hazardous substances.

Handling and using hazardous substances

When using hazardous products you should wear disposable gloves and an apron (PPE). Some cleaning materials are classed as hazardous products, so gloves and an apron may be necessary. Look out for the COSHH classification symbols on the bottle or packaging and always read the labels to ensure your own safety.

Aerosols should be used away from any source of heat, especially a naked flame. Many styling and finishing products are classed as flammable substances and should not be used near any heat source.

- **Highly flammable** substances such as solvents, nail varnish remover or alcohol sterilisers are hazardous because their fumes will ignite if exposed to a naked flame.
- **Explosive** materials such as hairspray, air freshener or other pressurised cans are also highly flammable and will explode with force if placed in heat such as an open fire or even on top of a hot radiator.

 (a) Corrosive

 (b) Explosive

 (c) Harmful

 (d) Highly flammable

 (e) Irritant

 (f) Oxidising

 (g) Toxic

COSHH symbols

- **Chemicals** can cause severe reactions and skin damage. Vomiting, respiratory problems and burning could be the result if chemicals are misused.

COSHH precautions

Employers must, by law, identify, list and assess in writing any substance in the workplace. Not only does this apply to products in use in the salon but also to cleaning products, for example bleach or polish.

Keys to good practice

Read all the COSHH sheets used in the salon, and be safe: abide by what they say, never abuse manufacturers' instructions and attend regular staff training for product use – you never know when you might need it!

Remember

All substances must be given a hazard rating, or risk assessment, even if it is zero. Manufacturers have to supply COSHH data sheets for all their products. You should receive one for each product you purchase.

Sometimes a reaction may occur if the client is using products at home that may not mix well with salon preparations, for example home hair colourants.

Environmental Protection Act 1990; Controlled Waste Regulations 1992 (amended); Special Waste Regulations 1996 (amended)

These require all clinical waste to be kept apart from the general waste and to be disposed of to a licensed incinerator or landfill site, by a licensed company.

Clinical waste includes:

- waste which consists wholly or partly of animal or human tissue
- blood or other body fluids
- swabs or dressings
- syringes or needles.

Check it out

Obtain leaflets and the latest information regarding COSHH from your local HSE office.

Check it out

- Where is the notice of your salon's fire precautions and evacuation procedures displayed? Is it easy to follow and in a prominent place?
- When you next visit a hotel, check out the fire evacuation route and the information given on how to get out in case of fire.

Fire Precautions (Workplace) Regulations 1997 (amended)

New regulations require the small business owner to adequately assess the fire risks associated with work activities and to decide what needs to be done to control these. The steps to be taken for a fire risk assessment are similar to those taken for general risk assessments, though the business also has a general duty to the public (see Unit G1, Ensure your own actions reduce risks to health and safety).

Staff need to be aware of the procedures involved in the event of a fire (preferably through a displayed notice), and it is recommended that the salon should have some form of fire-fighting equipment – even it is just a fire blanket. Contact your local fire service for advice.

Remember

Gas fumes cannot be seen, are silent and very, very deadly.

Gas Safety (Installation and Use) Regulations 1994

These regulations relate to the use and maintenance of gas appliances. You may well think that this does not apply to you as a therapist, but read on! The Gas Safety (Rights of Entry) Regulations 1996 give gas and HSE inspectors the right to enter premises and order the disconnection of any dangerous appliances. The inspectors themselves are not normally trained gas fitters, so they will instruct you to contact your local service engineer.

Electricity at Work Regulations 1989

These regulations are concerned with the safe use of electricity. In the salon this applies particularly to the use and maintenance of electrical equipment.

Regulation 4 states:

- All electrical equipment must be regularly checked for electrical safety. In a busy salon this may be every **six months**.
- The check must be carried out by a 'competent person', preferably a qualified electrician. All checks must be recorded in a book kept for this purpose only.

A competent person need not be a qualified electrician but must be capable of attending to basic safety checks. Manufacturers may supply their own technical staff to attend to safety checks, as they will be trained in their own areas of expertise.

If electrical apparatus is found to be faulty, the equipment must be withdrawn from service and repaired.

A safety repair book should record the nature of the repair, the date the equipment was repaired and by whom. It should also contain a list of tests carried out on the equipment under inspection, the results of those tests and be signed by the competent person who carried them out. This is essential for insurance purposes for public liability and in case of legal action being taken for negligence.

Reporting of Injuries, Diseases and Dangerous Occurrences Regulations (RIDDOR) 1995

These regulations cover the recording and reporting of any serious accidents and conditions to the local environmental health officer responsible for dealing with beauty therapy and hairdressing salons. This will allow the officer to investigate the accident and to try to prevent it happening again. The officer can also assess the risk factors in each instance which should enable the salon to address these.

Types of incidents to report

- An accident or death at work – must be reported within ten days.
- An accident that does not require a hospital visit, but causes absence from work for more than three days.
- A work-related disease, e.g. occupational dermatitis, asthma caused through work, hepatitis.
- Accidents as a result of violence or an attack by another person.
- A car accident on company business.
- A dangerous occurrence even if no one was injured, e.g. the salon's ceiling collapses overnight.

Pressure Systems and Transportable Gas Containers Regulations 1989

Steam sterilising autoclaves come under these regulations. The salon is required to have a written scheme of examination carried out or certified by a competent person.

Employers' Liability (Compulsory Insurance) Act 1969

Employers and self-employed persons must by law hold employers' liability insurance. This will reimburse them against any legal liability to pay compensation to employees for:

- bodily injury
- illness
- disease

caused during the course of their employment.

Remember

If you are a mobile therapist working in someone's home and you have an accident or injure the client, you must report it.

Remember

Clients may be more susceptible to reactions if they are taking long torm medication, such as hormone replacement therapy (HRT) or the contraceptive pill. This information *must* be included on the client record card.

Employers must insure for at least £2 million per claim (check with your own insurance company). You should also follow the recommendations of your professional association.

A legal claim made against your salon could result in very large financial losses and possibly the sale of the owner's business or home. Damage to the salon could be so great that the business may never recover.

Some cases take up to ten years to come to court and with inflation, the claim against you could be very much more than your original cover if you only go for the minimum requirements.

Disability Discrimination Act 1995

Under this Act, you must not discriminate against any person with a disability. In October 1997, the government made public its commitment to developing comprehensive and enforceable civil rights for disabled people. From this, the Disability Rights Commission (DRC) was formed in April 2000. It statutory duties are:

- to work to eliminate discrimination against disabled people
- to promote equal opportunities for disabled people
- to encourage good practice in the treatment of disabled people
- to advise the government on the working of disability legislation (the Disability Discrimination Act 1995 and the Disability Rights Commission Act 1999).

The main function of the DRC is to assist disabled people to secure their rights. However, the commission will also provide information to employers and service providers, for example salon owners, about their rights and duties under the Disability Discrimination Act. It can advise on good practice and help to ensure that the obligations of the Act are met within the salon.

You have a duty within the salon to promote equal opportunities for disabled people. Your salon should be promoting good practice by widening its service provision depending upon the needs of the individual.

Under the Disability Discrimination Act, service providers such as salon owners must abide by the duties imposed upon them. From October 2004, service providers may have to make 'reasonable adjustments' to their premises so that there are no physical barriers making it unreasonably difficult for anyone with a disability to use their services.

If your salon is being refurbished, this would be a good opportunity to implement changes to the physical features of the salon. Otherwise the salon owner will need to consider a continuous access improvement programme. The salon owner has a responsibility to start preparing now, for changes in the law.

Consumer Protection Act 1987

This Act follows European law to safeguard the consumer in three main areas:

- product liability
- general safety requirements
- misleading prices.

Before 1987, an injured person had to prove a manufacturer negligent before suing for damages. This Act removes the need to prove negligence.

Check it out

Have a good look at your salon. Does it discriminate against disabled people in any way? Is there wheelchair access? Does anyone employed in the salon know sign language? Do you have a price list in Braille?

How could your salon better accommodate the disabled client? The Disability Rights Commission is there to give advice on these important aspects of law and good customer service.

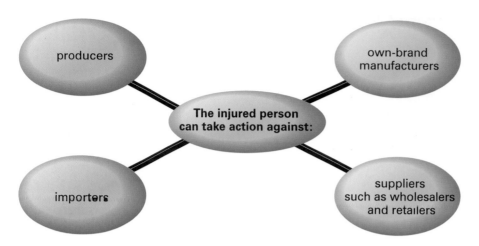

How the injured person may take action

In the salon this means that only reputable products should be used and sold.

Care should be taken in handling, maintaining and storing products so that they remain in top condition.

It is important that all staff are aware of the Consumer Protection Act when selling products and when using products in a treatment.

Consumer Protection (Distance Selling) Regulations 2000

These regulations were introduced to increase consumer confidence. They will apply to you if the salon where you work sells goods or services via the Internet, by phone, by fax, or mail order. The key points of the regulations are as follows:

- The consumer must be given clear information about the goods or services on offer. This information includes the price, delivery, costs, arrangements for payment, and so on.
- The consumer must be sent confirmation after making a purchase.
- The consumer must have a seven-day cooling-off period (this is meant to equate to the time the consumer would spend in the salon deciding whether to purchase).

It is unlikely that these regulations will apply to your salon if you do not usually supply clients in this way, but agree to do so as a one-off request. However, if the business regularly handles such requests, it is likely the salon should comply with these regulations. If this is the case, the salon should also ensure it has registered with and is fulfilling the requirements of the Data Protection Act 1998 (see page 79).

Cosmetic Products (Safety) Regulations 2004

These regulations are part of consumer protection. The EU has introduced strict regulations about the composition of products, labelling of ingredients, how the product is described and how it is marketed. American cosmetic companies have had to list all ingredients on their labels for years, and Europe is now following suit. This is useful for clients who may be allergic to certain ingredients such as lanolin.

Ingredients: alcohol denat. · aromatics perfume (parfum) · water (aqua purificata) purified · silica · mica · titanium dioxide (ci 77891) · iron oxides (ci 77491, ci 77492, ci 77499) [iln23089]

Ingredients in beauty products must be clearly labelled

Medicines Act 1968

This Act deals with the supply and use of topical anaesthetics and is enforced by the police and the Medicines Control Agency. Product licence conditions apply to medical application only and not to cosmetic use. Therefore, their use by a beauty therapist can be deemed unlawful.

Trade Descriptions Act 1968

This Act is concerned with the false description of goods. It is important to realise the relevance of this Act because it is considered illegal to mislead the general public. It also applies to verbal descriptions given by a third party and repeated. So, if you were to repeat a manufacturer's false description to a client, you could be liable to prosecution.

The law states that the retailer must not:

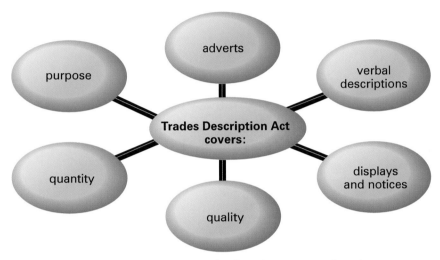

The Trade Descriptions Act covers misleading descriptions of goods

- supply information that is in any way misleading
- falsely describe or make false statements about either a product or a service on offer.

The retailer may not:

- make false contrast between present and previous prices
- claim to offer products at reduced price unless they have been offered at the former price for at least 28 days prior to the sale.

The retailer should also avoid making statements such as saying a product is offered at 'our price' and is worth 'double the amount'. Comparing prices can be misleading and may even be illegal – if making comparisons, make sure that the products are identical in every way.

It is also important to check that products are labelled with the country of origin.

Sale of Goods Act 1979 (amended); Sale and Supply of Goods Act 1994

The Sale of Goods Act has several others under its umbrella of protection, including:

- the Supply of Goods and Services Act 1982
- the Unfair Contract Terms Act 1977
- the Supply of Goods (Implied Terms) Act 1973.

The Act recognises the contract of a sale between the retailer and the consumer when purchasing a product. This applies when the salon sells a product to a client. It states that the retailer:

- has a responsibility to sell goods of the very best quality which are not defective in any way
- must refund the money for the purchase if the product is found to be defective (some retailers will offer only an exchange of goods if there is no receipt)
- must then make a complaint to the supplier.

Supply of Goods and Services Act 1982

This Act also deals with rights for the consumer and the trader's obligations towards the consumer.

The 'Goods' part of the Act allows the consumer to claim back some or all of the money paid for goods. When a consumer buys something in good faith, he or she expects it to be:

- of merchantable quality
- fit for the purpose for which it was sold
- as described in the advertising.

This applies to *all* goods, regardless of whether they are on hire, in part exchange, or as part of a service.

The 'Services' part of the Act requires the supplier of a service (such as a beauty therapist) to:

- charge a reasonable price
- give the service within a reasonable time
- give the service with reasonable care and skill.

If a client believes that he or she has a case against you, he or she can complain and may contact the local Trading Standards office.

Supply of Goods (Implied Terms) Act 1973

This Act deals with attempts to exclude or restrict statutory terms related to title, description and fitness of the goods.

Both of the above Acts covered consumer rights before the Sale of Goods Act 1979, when definitions became tighter and the law was well defined regarding consumer rights.

Local Government (Miscellaneous Provisions) Act 1982

Section 8 of this Act is concerned with local authority registration of any practitioners whose work involves piercing the skin, which applies to:

- acupuncture
- ear and body piercing
- tattooing
- epilation.

The Act applies to both salons and mobile therapists.

The concern of most local authorities is that through registration they will be able to keep some control of both hygiene regulations and try to ensure that practitioners have recognised qualifications. The enforcement of these regulations depends upon the individual authority, as does the amount of inspection that takes place, and the scale of fees for registration.

Other local authority bylaws

Other areas of beauty therapy are governed by local bylaws – laws decided by the local authority. Bylaws vary from region to region. For example, the Birmingham and London authorities have a register of salons offering body massage as a treatment. This is to maintain a professional qualified salon base, and to eliminate the 'massage parlour' image.

London Local Authorities Act 2004

This Act requires all premises in London that carry out treatments to be licensed by their local authorities. Out of the 32 authorities, 27 have adopted this Act, so you will need to contact your local authority to check whether you require a licence and what registration demands need to be fulfilled when setting up your own salon.

Copyrights Design and Patents Act 1988

Use of music in the treatment room, reception area or in exercise groups is classed as a public performance. This Act is designed to protect those who write and perform music but who do not get the royalty payments they should when the music is played. Phonographic Performance Ltd (PPL) collects licence payments on behalf of artistes and record companies from people wishing to play recorded music in public.

Under the Copyright, Design and Patents Act 1988, the PPL may take legal action against persons who do not pay a licence fee to use music. It can mean a considerable fine. So all salons and exercise/aerobic instructors must purchase music that has a built-in licence (for more information, see **You and your working environment**, page 60).

Data Protection Act 1998

This Act is there to protect the personal information that the business holds on individuals. You are required to ensure appropriate security measures are in place to prevent any unlawful or unauthorised access to data.

If your salon is holding personal data, it must be registered with the Information Commissioner. It is worth checking to find out if you should be registered, as failure to do so may result in prosecution.

The business must ensure that the information it holds is accurate and relevant to its needs and that the information is kept secure. The business must also comply with individuals' requests for information that it is holding on them. Failure to do so will contravene the Act.

Working Time Directive

Until the Working Time Directive was implemented in 1998, employers were free to set working times and holiday entitlements. Although many employers and employees negotiated terms and conditions, some employees were treated poorly. Since the introduction of the directive, an employer must take reasonable steps that are in keeping with the need to protect the health and safety of employees.

The main provision of the Working Time Directive relating to beauty salons includes:

- a limit on the average working week
- minimum daily and weekly rest breaks
- rest breaks at work
- paid holiday entitlement.

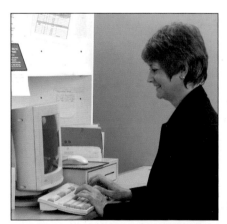

The Data Protection Act refers to all personal information held, like that on a database

The law applies to full-time, part-time and casual workers, which is anyone with a contract of employment (whether written or not). The directive does not cover self-employed people.

Key points of the Working Time Directive

- You should not be asked to work more than 48 hours a week, averaged over a 17-week period.
- You are entitled to a rest period of 11 consecutive hours between each working day.
- You are also entitled to a minimum of one day off per week.
- You are entitled to an uninterrupted break of 20 minutes if you work more than six hours per day. It should be a break in working time, not taken at the start or end of the working day.
- You are allowed at least four weeks' paid holiday per year. This is calculated on your right to take a twelfth of your holiday entitlement for each month worked (rounded up to the nearest half day). One week's holiday is equivalent to the time you would normally work per week, so if, for example, you work three days per week, your annual holiday entitlement would be 12 days. If your contract of employment is terminated before you have taken your leave entitlement, you have the right to payment in lieu.
- For staff aged 16 or 17, the law is slightly different. The rest period entitlement is increased to 12 consecutive hours' rest in every 24 hours, and they are entitled to an uninterrupted break of 30 minutes if they have worked for more than four-and-a-half hours.

Insurance

Professional indemnity insurance

All beauty therapists should have this insurance protection, regardless of how little or how many treatments they carry out.

The best deal for all insurance policies is usually found via your professional body. It is able to offer the best rates as it negotiates on behalf of members and is able to obtain a considerable discount.

As an employee, you will need to ask your employer whether you are covered under the business insurance, or whether you should organise your own cover. A salon owner/employer should include this liability in the public liability insurance policy (see below), so that all employees are protected against claims made by clients.

Professional indemnity insurance covers claims arising from:

- injury caused by treatment
- personal injury
- damage caused by treatment.

Having this insurance policy could save you a lot of money.

Public liability insurance

This is not compulsory, but it is certainly advisable. Public liability insurance will protect the employer should a member of the public be injured on the premises. It could be something as simple as a roof tile hitting the client on the way into the salon. If this results in the client being unable to work for a long period of time, the salon owner could be sued for compensation.

Industry codes of practice or ethics

There are several professional therapists' associations, each having their own code of practice, which offers a guide to correct procedures and etiquette. The professional body that you join is your own choice, and may depend upon the one favoured by your training establishment.

The cost involved in joining depends on your level of entry – a student membership is normally available. You will receive a joining pack which will contain a code of practice, or ethics. The code is a book of rules that the therapist agrees to abide by as part of the contract of membership. If these rules are broken or ignored, membership can be withdrawn.

There are benefits to being a member of a professional body, including:

- a good insurance deal negotiated on members' behalf
- support and advice upon leaving college
- regular legal updates, as they appear
- free legal help lines for all aspects of your business
- discount cards for suppliers.

Some professional associations publish a monthly magazine containing a recruitment section and adverts for equipment; some offer a business guide to help you set up on your own.

Salon guidelines

All the legislation mentioned above should be considered within your normal working life as a beauty therapist. Working safely and following the correct legal procedure are very important.

You will also need to follow the salon guidelines for the particular establishment you are working in, whether a training establishment, salon, health farm, ocean liner or renting a room in a health suite.

It is essential that you are aware of the policies on health and safety, safety training and what *exactly* is expected within your job role. Normally, salon rules are very similar, regardless of where the salon is located, but the safety procedures to follow if your salon happens to be floating in the Caribbean will be very different!

Salon expectations and the required behaviour should be set out at the beginning of your employment. This might be at your induction training, or even at the initial interview.

Regular review of policies and regular training for updates are essential, as is your attendance! If a member of staff continually ignores safety requirements, either through negligence or because of ignorance through failing to attend training, it could form the basis for dismissal. Even worse, should an accident happen through negligence, injury may occur, and the person responsible may be found liable.

Health and safety rules

These will encompass all aspects of the Health and Safety at Work etc. Act, COSHH and the Electricity at Work Act.

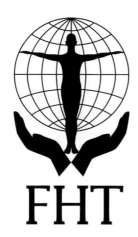

The FHT is a professional therapists' association

Remember

When you are in a training establishment there are many people who can give you help and advice – but when you are out in the working world you are on your own. It can be reassuring to have the support of a professional association behind you.

As a professional therapist, you should be in no doubt about:

- your responsibility
- the salon's procedures
- treatment safety
- equipment safety
- protection against cross-infection
- client safety, including:
  - positioning of client
  - appropriate couch height for getting on and off
  - correct use of equipment/products
  - correct diagnosis of treatments needed
  - correct evacuation procedures
- storage policies, including:
  - electrical equipment
  - chemicals
  - valuables
  - stock
  - money
- stock regulations, including:
  - COSHH
  - first aid procedures
  - stock rotation
  - spillage management
  - correct storage/containers.

Your employer or head of your training establishment should have all these standard procedures in place. If you are not instructed within the first few weeks, then ask!

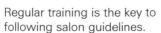

Remember

Regular training is the key to following salon guidelines.

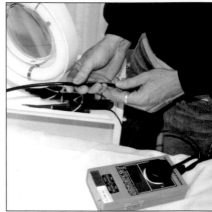

Ensure all electrical equipment is checked regularly

Knowledge check

1 Describe your responsibilities as a student under:
  a the Health and Safety at Work etc. Act
  b the Consumer Protection Act
  c the Electricity at Work Act
  d COSHH.

2 Why is it important for beauty therapists to be insured?

3 When would you need to wear protective clothing, and why?

4 Why is it important to follow manufacturers' instructions?

5 What are your salon guidelines on client safety?

6 Why should a salon have rules and regulations?

7 If a cream states on its label that it can guarantee weight loss, under which Act would the manufacturer be liable to prosecution?

8 Who provides a code of practice, or ethics?

9 Who makes bylaws?

10 Which Act states the correct lifting procedure?

11 If a treatment takes twice as long as it should, under which Act would you be liable to give the client a refund?

the workplace
ENVIRONMENT

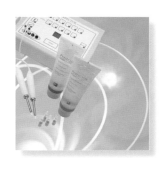
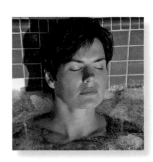
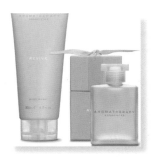

Ensure your own actions reduce risks to health and safety

Unit G1

This unit will help you to identify the hazards in your workplace, evaluate the risks and look at ways to reduce these risks.

The unit is for everyone at work, regardless of whether they are a paid worker, a volunteer, part-time or full-time employee, or a self-employed therapist in a mobile business. Everyone within the workplace has an obligation by law to secure their own and others' health, safety and welfare, and this unit is about identifying the factors that contribute to you becoming a responsible employee.

The Health and Safety at Work etc. Act 1974 covers the legal requirements of an employer and the Health and Safety Commission will give advice to those considering going into business and employing others.

But what about you? What are you responsible for? As a professional therapist, you are as liable as your employer, perhaps more so, as you have greater direct contact with the customer, and are therefore just as accountable should a client be able to prove any form of negligence on your part.

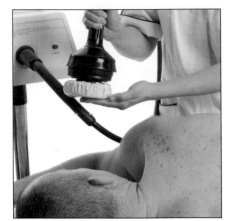

Testing equipment on yourself first helps reduce risk

Within this unit you will cover the following outcomes:

G1.1 Identify the hazards and evaluate the risks in your workplace
G1.2 Reduce the risks to health and safety in your workplace.

As a Level 3 student, you will be dealing with electrical equipment, which has a higher risk factor attached to it than manual treatments. The wet area, spa, sauna and steam cabinets also have risk implications, so this unit is very important to protect the safety of the client, yourself and others in the salon.

This unit is not a full guide to completing a full risk assessment – that should be done by a trained professional who specialises in that field. The purpose here is to give you an appreciation of the significant risks in the beauty salon, how to identify them and deal with them appropriately.

Each practical unit will have its own particular hazards which should be identified within the specific unit. General hazards in the salon and your actions are covered within this unit.

Remember

In Unit G1, the Health and Safety at Work Act etc. 1974 is the only piece of legislation specifically referred to as it is the main piece of legislation under which nearly all of the other regulations fall. You will need to study other legislation such as the Electricity at Work Regulations 1989 and the Environmental Protection Act 1990 to ensure health and safety in the workplace. For information on relevant legislation, see **You, your client and the law** on page 67.

Identify the hazards and evaluate the risks in your workplace

G1.1

In this outcome you will learn about

- hazards and risks
- promoting a safe working environment
- responsibilities – who does what?
- workplace policies
- identifying harmful aspects of the workplace
- reporting hazards
- dealing with hazards.

Hazards and risks

It has been said that all actions have a consequence, and that is very true when looking at possible problems that may compromise health and safety.

The two key areas to consider are:

- hazards in the salon
- the risk that the hazard will cause harm.

A hazard may be defined as anything that can cause harm, or which has the potential to cause harm.

A risk is the chance, however great or small, that the hazard will actually cause harm to someone.

For example, a galvanic unit has the potential to be hazardous – there is a danger of electric shock, chemical, electrical or heat burns to the body, and allergic or sensitivity rashes. However, the risk of damage would be greatly minimised in the hands of a fully qualified therapist, who is following the manufacturer's instructions, using equipment which is regularly maintained, following all safety rules, and has given a full consultation. For someone untrained, who has no qualification in beauty therapy, and has never used the machine before, the risk is much greater. This is the fundamental difference between a hazard and a risk.

The skill is not only to recognise the potential of the hazard to cause injury or harm, but to know how to act in the most sensible manner to neutralise or significantly reduce the risk.

Refer to **Professional basics** for:

- the legislation to support this unit – see **You, your client and the law**
- posture and manual handling – see **You – the therapist**
- sterilisation methods for equipment and the salon – see **You and your working environment.**

Carrying out and acting upon risk assessment does not have to be complicated, but it does need to be thought through thoroughly. Be logical and do not look too hard – the obvious route is often the right one to take. Imagine making a cup of tea. What is the most hazardous part? Boiling the water and pouring it into the teapot is the most obvious answer, as boiling water has the potential to seriously burn the skin. Other risks include: a stomach upset if the milk has gone off, the handle on the teacup breaking, the teapot spout leaking – but these are secondary possibilities. Go for the main hazard, even if you think it is probably too obvious, and you cannot go far wrong.

Check it out

Simple precautions can often be the most effective – and plenty of common sense should always help to prevent accidents. Ignorance is not an acceptable excuse, nor is it accepted as a defence against a misconduct or damage claim within a court of law. There is no justification for you not being fully aware of your responsibilities and your duty to yourself, clients and colleagues.

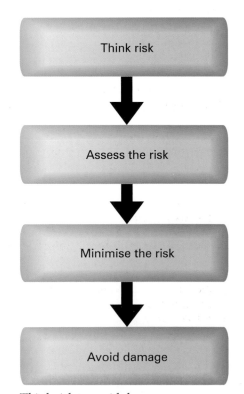

Think risk to avoid damage

Promoting a safe working environment

A question to ask when attending a job interview for any salon position is what staff training is available, not just for advancement of skill areas but also for health and safety training. Regular guidance for all levels of staff will help to identify and minimise the hazards.

A salon's workplace policy should include:

- workplace/environmental factors
- safe working methods and equipment use
- the safe use of all hazardous substances (not just for your particular job role)
- general policies for eating, smoking, drinking and drugs
- expected personal presentation
- what to do in the event of an accident, breakage or spillage
- all emergency procedures
- behaviour policies for all personnel
- corrective action where required.

If you are told at interview not to worry about any of the above, and that they really do not matter, then ask yourself, 'Do I really want to work in a place that has so little regard for the safety of its staff and clients, as well as breaking health and safety laws?'.

Responsibilities – who does what?

The Health and Safety at Work etc. Act 1974 is largely about employers' responsibilities and duties, but if you are planning to run your own business one day, then you will need to know about the Act.

The general duties of employers to their employees are set down in Section 2(1) of the Act:

> 'It shall be the duty of every employer to ensure, so far as is reasonably practicable, the health, safety and welfare at work of all his employees.'

In addition to responsibilities to employees, an employer also has a duty to protect other persons, for example members of the public. These are stated in Section 3(1) of the Act:

> 'It shall be the duty of every employer to conduct his undertaking in such a way as to ensure, so far as is reasonably practicable, that persons not in his employment who may be affected thereby are not thereby exposed to risks to their health or safety.'

Self-employed people also have responsibilities under the Act which are dealt with in Section 3(2):

> 'It shall be the duty of every self-employed person to conduct his undertaking in such a way as to ensure, so far as is reasonably practicable, that he and other persons (not being his employees) who may be affected thereby are not thereby exposed to risks to their health or safety.'

Even if you are not planning to set up your own business, as an employee you will still have responsibilities under HASWA (see **You, your client and the law**, page 68, for your own and shared responsibilities).

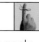

Remember

Health and safety regulations apply to all businesses, and they should not be something merely brushed up on where there has been an accident or near accident at work – it should be a full-time concern.

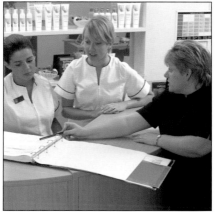

Divide health and safety responsibilties equally among the team

Check it out

Find out who covers which areas of responsibility in your salon. Compile a list so that in the event of an incident you will know who to report any health and safety issues to.

It is important for you to know who you should report any health and safety issues to in the salon. Salons will have different staff members covering various areas of responsibility, for example one or two staff will be trained in first aid, one person will assume responsibility for filling out the accident and report book and keeping health and safety records up to date, another will be responsible for building maintenance and replacement of light bulbs, and so on.

Workplace policies

All professional salons should have a set of rules and procedures for everyone to follow. This should be common knowledge within the salon for the safety and protection of all.

By law, the salon has to display:

- health and safety rules and regulations on the wall in a prominent position
- fire evacuation procedures.

Professionally, the salon will also have:

- codes of practice to follow from its professional body with regard to set procedures
- a set of standards to maintain for insurance cover to be valid – usually linked to the codes of practice.

Legally, the employer is responsible for putting into place the rules covering the health and safety of all employees and clients and ensuring that safe practice is followed by all staff. The employee is obliged to carry out these practices by law. This will involve:

- regular training, with staff meetings to update on safety issues
- clear outlines given at the initial interview as to what is expected
- maintaining records of injuries or first aid treatment given
- monitoring and evaluating health and safety arrangements regularly
- obtaining a written health and safety booklet
- consulting the experts and being knowledgeable – ignorance is not an excuse.

Workplace policies relevant to your working practice

A salon has a legal requirement to have written risk assessments and documentation if it employs five or more people, but the sensible salon owner will have these in place regardless of how many staff are employed. Many insurance companies insist on written risk policies before they will agree to insure the business.

The other health and safety requirements for a small business are:

- to inform the Health and Safety Executive's area office or the local authority's environmental health department of the business's name and address
- to inform the HSE's area office or the local authority's environmental health department of any new employees
- to display the health and safety law poster (available from the government's Stationery Office) or hand out leaflets containing the equivalent information
- to make an assessment of the risks in the workplace – which must be acted upon, and kept as a written record if there are five or more employees (this includes fire risks)

Check it out

- What does your beauty therapy professional body state regarding the use of gloves and aprons?
- What advice does it give on health and safety issues?
- How do you become a member?

Remember

Although the Health and Safety Executive (HSE) is primarily concerned with the salon owner, remember that the salon owner is your employer, and therefore health and safety regulations will have a direct effect on your working environment. It is advisable to be aware of the owner's commitment to protecting you – it might nfluence whether you want to work in the salon, or not.

- to bring to the attention of employees a written statement of the business's health and safety policy, and keep it up to date
- to register with the local health authority, if appropriate – this will apply in particular to therapists who carry out skin piercing such as epilation.

When you inform the HSE that you are setting up a business, it will probably wish to check out your business premises. This will depend on the authority within your own area, and the HSE's requirements would affect you whether you work from home or in a salon.

Workplace policies relevant to your job role

Take a closer look at your specific job role within the salon – could any part of your job harm yourself or others? This is not just about the treatments you carry out. For example, you could be in charge of changing light bulbs. When a bulb fails in a well-lit salon, it is not a problem, but if the only light bulb illuminating a dark stock room blows, then there is a greater risk of harm to everyone. Everyone has a responsibility to take their job role seriously – from the junior in charge of washing cups who may spread infection if her duties are not performed correctly, to the person in charge of maintaining the electrical equipment, with the potential to cause burns to a client.

Identifying harmful aspects of the workplace

How many hazards are there in a beauty salon? Here are just a few:

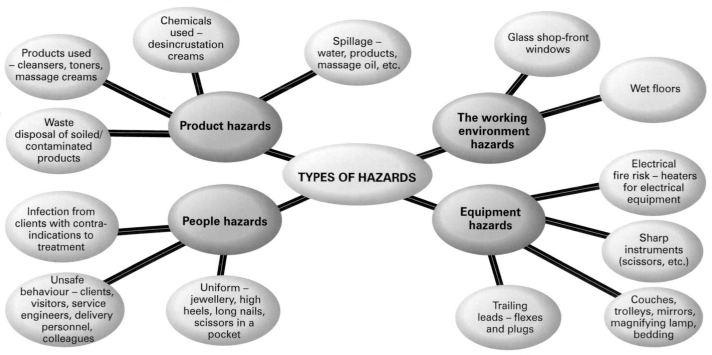

Identifying hazards in the salon

Although these are all identified as possible hazards, not all of them will occur, and certainly not all at the same time! Some may be low risk, others may be high risk. For example, an experienced therapist may never have experienced a fire caused by faulty equipment overheating and bursting into flames. The important point is that the therapist will have recognised the possibility of faulty equipment becoming a hazard and have her equipment checked regularly by a competent person, keep a safety log book with all equipment checks dated and signed (see Electricity at Work Regulations 1989 in **You, your client and the law**, pages 73–4). The risk will have been minimised, and should a fire start, the logbook will show that responsibility has been taken, and the therapist/salon owner has not been neglecting her duty.

The following table gives some examples of general hazards.

Hazard	High, medium or low risk	Checks
The working environment (the building)	High	Is the building safe and stable? Is there any asbestos present in the roof or walls? Is the outside of the building in good repair, with no likelihood of anything falling on the client or passers-by? Is the sign for the salon secure? Are there stickers on the large salon window to avoid anyone walking into the glass? Has safety glass been used to minimise damage should an accident happen?
Floors	High	Are they clean and dry? Is there any spillage? Are they over-polished to become slippery? Are there any loose carpet edges or rugs to trip on? Are they hygienic and easy to clean?
Doorways and hallways	High	Are they clear of obstructions? Is a fire exit being blocked? Are the doors too heavy to open safely?
Windows and curtains	Medium	Is any electrical equipment near to a curtain which could catch fire? Are the windows safe and lockable, both for security and for sufficient ventilation and airflow?
General décor and facilities	Low	Is the paint on the walls lead-free? Are the light fittings secure? Has the wiring for lighting and plug sockets been recently checked for safety? Is the boiler regularly maintained and serviced? Are there modern gas mains and water pipes, and are they working properly?

Identifying general hazards in the workplace

General hazards in the workplace are often out of the control of the therapist, and should be the responsibility of the salon owner, but if the sign to the salon was hanging off, ready to drop on to an unsuspecting passer-by or client, you would be neglectful if you did not report it and prevent an accident. Structural damage does happen to older buildings, and having a salon in an old building may mean that the amenities will not be modern. Older buildings can be very expensive to maintain and may present many more hazards.

The tables on the following pages give examples of hazards connected with equipment and products, and those connected with people.

Hazard	High, medium or low risk	Checks
Couch	High	Are the brakes on? Is it at the right height for the therapist to work comfortably, and not too high for the client to get on? Is the bedding a danger by being too long and trailing on the floor ready to trip someone up? Is the bedding easily cleaned, protected during the treatment and hygienic?
Chairs	High	Are they secured and at a suitable height? If hydraulic, are they regularly maintained? Are they stable? Are they on castors? Are they hygienic and easy to keep clean?
Trolleys	Low	Are they glass-topped and liable to shatter? Are they secure on their castors? Are they regularly cared for? Are they hygienic and easy to keep clean? Are they up to the job given to them – is the equipment too heavy?
Electrical appliances (refer to individual pieces of equipment within the facial or body treatments sections for specific dangers)	High	Are they regularly maintained by a competent person? Are they placed on a stable surface, rather than balanced on a windowsill? Are they used by qualified personnel only? Are they stored safely? Are they used with the correct products only? Were they bought from a reputable manufacturer, to ensure safety? Are they used at the correct socket with the right plugs and fuses? Are any leads trailing?
Disposal of waste products	High	Are the correct bins available for different waste products? Is contaminated waste separated from the rest (e.g. body fluids, blood, etc., from milia extraction)? Who is responsible for disposing of the waste products and how regularly? Is infection control in place to minimise risk?
Products	Very high	Are they clearly labelled? Are they stored safely and correctly (including toxic products)? Has a COSHH (Control of Substances Hazardous to Health) sheet been completed for each product? Do therapists know how to use them, and are they being used correctly? Are they stored in the proper containers, not in other bottles? Is the shelf life taken into account? Are lids secured properly? Is a designated first aider available in case of accidents? Do staff know what to do in case of personal injury caused by poor product use? Are correct patch tests being carried out to prevent allergic reactions? Is regular product training being offered?

Identifying equipment and product hazards

Hazard	Checks
You – the therapist	Do you lead others by showing good examples of safe working?
	Does your behaviour endanger others?
	Are you fully trained to use the equipment/products?
	Are you as hygienic as possible to avoid cross-infection?
	Do you follow the correct procedures for the workplace?
	Do you actively take part in regular training sessions for health and safety?
	Do you report possible hazards to the correct person?
	Is your uniform a health or safety hazard? Do you have safe shoes on? Are you wearing lots of jewellery?
	Do you walk around with sharp scissors in your pocket?
	Do you look out for the safety of others?
	Do you keep up-to-date client record cards?
	Do you use the correct lifting position when carrying heavy items?
Other people and visitors to the salon	Should they be there?
	Are they going to create a hazard? e.g. a service engineer carrying out a repair, with tools lying where clients are walking
	Do they know where they are going?
	Are they aware of steps, and the salon layout?
	Is their behaviour suitable for the salon, or are they using threatening behaviour?
	Is there a risk that they could steal something?

Identifying people hazards

Reporting hazards

Hazards can and do happen and everyone should be aware of the safety implications. As part of your personal responsibility, you will need to know which hazards you can deal with yourself immediately, or when help may be needed, and the hazard should be reported to a supervisor/lecturer/technician/manager.

Type of hazard	Ways to avoid	When referral may be necessary
Breaches of security	Shut windows, lock cupboards and doors	When something is found open or something is believed to be missing. Full stock check required
Faulty/damaged products, tools, equipment, fixtures, fittings	Correct handling, correct storage, treat with care, follow manufacturers' instructions	When something is found to be broken
Spillage	Take care when mixing, pouring and filling, etc. – try to do it over a sink or draining board to catch any spillage	When spillage material is corrosive or irritant. When it is in the main traffic area where people may slip
Slippery floors	Make others aware by blocking the area with a chair or cone to prevent an accident, sweep up powder spills, mop up spills of liquid, refer to COSHH sheets for correct method	When acid, grease or polish is spilt
Obstruction to access and exit	Move large equipment away from doorways if able to do so, put bags and coats on a rack or shelving	When object is too heavy to be moved

Examples of hazards that should be reported

These hazards should be reported to a manager or the health and safety officer within your workplace, but there are hazards that will need to be reported to the local health officer or the HSE (see **You, your client and the law**, page 67).

ACCIDENT / ILLNESS REPORT FORM

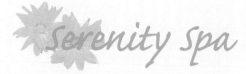
Serenity Spa

This form is to be completed by the injured party. If this is not possible, the form should be completed by the person making the report. If more than one person was injured, please comploto **a separate form for each person.**

Completing and signing this form does not constitute an admission of liability of any kind, either by the person making the report or any other person.

This form should be completed immediately and forwarded to the Health and Safety Officer and Salon Manager.

If it is possible that an accident has been caused by a defect in machinery, equipment or a process, isolate / fence off the area and contact the Health and Safety Officer or Manager immediately.

SECTION 1 PERSONAL DETAILS

Surname: _Fabrizio_ (Mr/(Mrs)/Ms/Miss) Forename(s): _Julia_

Date of birth: _29/01/57_ Address: _27 Ash Grove, Birmingham_

STAFF ☐   CONTRACTOR ☐   VISITOR ☐   GENERAL PUBLIC ☑

SECTION 2 ACCIDENT / INCIDENT / ILLNESS DETAILS

Accident (Injury) ☑   Illness ☐   Date: _19/04/04_   Time: _13:07_   (24-hour clock)

Location: _Salon room 4_

Nature of injury or condition and the part of the body affected:

Slipped on floor, hit elbow on trolley, possible dislocation

Account

Describe what happened and how. In the case of an accident state clearly what the injured person was doing. _Small patch of water on the floor – client got off couch and slipped on it._

Name and address of adult witness(es): _Camilla Neal, Serenity Spa_

Details of action taken

Ambulance summoned ☑   Taken to hospital ☐   Sent to hospital ☐
First aid given ☐   Taken home ☐   Sent home ☐   Returned to work ☐

SECTION 3 PREVENTATIVE ACTION

Recommended: _to ensure that all spillages are mopped up straight away_

Implemented: (Yes)/ No   Date: _19/04/04_

Report raised by

Name: _Willena Simons_

Position: _Therapist_

Signature: _W Simons_   Date: _19/04/04_

FOR OFFICE USE ONLY	
Copy sent to: Salon Manager	☐
Health and Safety Officer	☐

An accident report form

Dealing with hazards

Low-risk hazards

This is largely common sense. If the risk is low and you can deal with it straight away, then do so, and prevent an incident occurring. It could be something as simple as a client's handbag causing a minor obstruction where someone might trip over it. Pick it up off the floor, asking the client's permission where necessary, put it under the trolley out of the way and carry on with what you were doing. While this low-risk hazard does not need reporting, it still requires prompt action to prevent it becoming a more serious problem.

Always act within the policy of your workplace, so if there is a policy on where clients' handbags and coats may be stored to prevent congestion in the salon, then use the correct place.

Check it out

- What would you consider to be a low-risk hazard in your salon? Find out your salon procedure for dealing with this type of hazard.
- What do you consider to be a high-risk hazard? Write down how you would deal with this type of hazard and keep it as supplementary evidence in your portfolio.
- Where is your accident report book? What is the last entry? Fill out a sample page for a spillage incident.

High-risk hazards

You will need to be aware of the high-risk hazards associated with using electrical equipment. They are shown in the table below.

Identify the hazard	What is the risk? becoming a risk?	What should I do to prevent the hazard from
Frayed leads, cracked plugs, live wires showing	Electric shock/electrocution	DO NOT USE Remove appliance from general use Label it as faulty Report it to the designated person
Trailing leads	Tripping over Electrocution Pulling the appliance over on top of the therapist or client Pulling the plug out of the socket	Use a socket nearer to you, to avoid overstretching the lead Use an extension lead and keep the flex around the perimeter of the working area
Equipment/appliances left on after use, e.g. facial steamer or infrared lamp	Heater may burn dry Steam may scald Equipment may be an obstruction	Turn off the appliance and remove plug from socket Insulate the heated area by putting a towel over it, to show others it is hot Allow to cool and store safely

Electrical equipment hazards

Using electrical equipment

As a Level 3 student, you will be using a large number of electrical appliances during your working day, including:

- high frequency unit
- galvanic unit
- faradic unit
- microcurrent unit
- gyrator massager
- vacuum suction unit
- infrared lamp
- audio-sonic unit
- sunbeds
- spa, steam cabinet and sauna
- showers.

You will need to carry out sensible risk control at all times. Here are the general safety rules for all electrical appliances (for more specific ones for each individual piece of equipment, refer to the relevant unit – facial or body treatments). Remember always follow the manufacturer's guidelines.

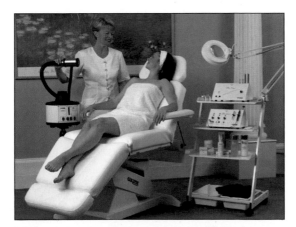

Make sure your equipment is in a safe position in relation to your client

Keys to good practice

General electrical safety rules

- Only use equipment you have been trained and insured to use – do not 'have a go' with a piece of equipment, just because you have seen someone else do a treatment with it.
- Always follow manufacturers' instructions for treatment use, appropriate products used and storage and cleaning.
- If your salon policy for a piece of equipment varies from the manufacturers' instructions, then you must notify the designated person immediately, as there could be significant risk attached.
- Inspect equipment regularly in accordance with the Electricity at Work Regulations, keep a safety check book and never use equipment you suspect may be faulty.
- Visually check the equipment prior to use – plugs and sockets should not be cracked or broken, no bare wires should be visible.
- Always carry out a full consultation and contra-indication checklist on the client prior to treatment.
- Always carry out a thermal and sensitivity test on the area to be treated.
- Always test on yourself before using the equipment on the client.
- When you have finished with equipment return all dials and settings back to '0' and leave it clean, sterile and ready for use.
- Do not overload plugs or extensions.
- Buy equipment from a reputable manufacturer who can offer after-sales and repair facilities, provide the accompanying correct products and regular updates for training.
- Store equipment safely to prolong its life and reduce fire risk. Never stack equipment on top of each other as this may break dials and knobs, reduce the effectiveness of the machine and ultimately endanger the client if the dials are not functioning correctly.
- Be careful to avoid trailing leads, which may trip people up, and moving equipment that is still plugged in.
- Always use the correct fuse in the plug – some galvanic machines, for example, require a 13-amp fuse, while some small equipment only needs a five-amp fuse.
- Never allow the client to interfere with your settings or dials – keep the controls out or reach.
- Remove all jewellery and metal objects from yourself and the client to prevent the current being attracted to the metal and causing a burn.
- Do not apply any electrical current over an open wound or broken skin, as the current will be attracted to the moisture content in the wound and cause a concentration of current to the area or a burn.
- Never exceed the client's tolerance to the intensity of the current – turn up the dials slowly and watch the client's reaction all the time. Ask for feedback on the comfort of the sensation.
- Always time the treatment and never exceed the recommended treatment time.

Reduce the risks to health and safety in your workplace

G1.2

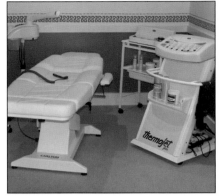

Minimise risks by keeping work area clean and tidy

In this outcome you will learn about

- minimising risk by taking action
- ensuring personal presentation minimises risk
- reducing workplace risks
- use of materials and hazardous substances
- smoking, eating, drinking and drugs

This outcome looks at ways of reducing or minimising the risks for the hazards you identified in Element G1.1. You will need to know how to carry out risky tasks safely, following both manufacturers' instructions and your workplace requirements. You must also have a thorough understanding of the health and safety policies within your salon that affect your working day. Part of this is your conduct and your personal presentation, which will ensure the health and safety of yourself, clients and colleagues.

Minimising risk by taking action

In Element G1.1 you looked at the various hazards and what to check for. Now you will look again at those hazards and see how to minimise those risks by taking the appropriate actions. The following tables contain ideas on minimising general risks in the workplace, risks from equipment and products, and from people.

Hazard	Minimise risk by taking the following actions
The working environment (the building)	Property owner's liability insurance, often known as buildings insurance, guards against claims relating to damage to the outside of the salon building, roof repairs, wall repairs, etc. Internal major fittings such as toilet facilities and kitchens are also often covered. Regularly maintain and check the outside of the property and repair minor damage before it becomes a major hazard.
Floors	Only use the correct products for floor cleaning and allow plenty of time to dry. Major stripping and recovering of the floor surface can be done outside of normal salon times. Repair or avoid carpets and rugs with frayed edges and those not easily kept clean. Pay for professional cleaning companies to chemically clean carpets outside of normal salon hours.
Doorways and hallways	Have a regular inspection from your local fire safety officer who will advise the salon on the correct exit route in case of fire. Keep corridors tidy and clutter free.
Windows and curtains	Keep all electrical equipment away from the window area. Employ a tradesperson to ensure the windows open, are hinged properly and are safe and secure. Invest in double-glazing if possible, or carefully maintain older-style windows. Loose windows are the ideal entry for a potential thief.
General décor and facilities	Invest in safe decorating products bought from a reputable DIY store. Regularly check and maintain the utility services – many of them provide a regular service agreement for a yearly maintenance of gas and electricity parts (boilers and central heating, etc.).

Minimising risks in the workplace

Hazard	Minimise risk by taking the following actions
Couch	Buy from professional suppliers only, with guarantees and maintenance and repair agreements. Ensure the couch is the correct height to avoid back problems and buy an adjustable one where possible. Use protective coverings, which are washable, and minimise the risk of cross-infection by regularly disinfecting the couch and covering.
Chairs	As above. The recommended chair for use by professionals is the five-castor movable chair with adjustable height and backrest, often called the 'super secretarial chair'. Test out whether the height of the chair is suitable for you by sitting squarely with your bottom at the back of the chair, and your feet firmly flat on the floor. Regularly maintain the chair and lubricate the castors.
Trolleys	Ensure that all legs are secure and that castors are properly fixed. Never use a glass-topped trolley for equipment that becomes hot. Never overload a trolley. Evenly distribute the weight of equipment. Never push a trolley containing hot equipment – if you drag it, you will have more control. Always remember that a trolley can move – never use it as a work surface.
Electrical appliances	As above. Always buy from a reputable manufacturer who provides training, suitable products, an after-sales service, repairs and servicing. Have the equipment tested by a competent person, keep a log book of testing, dated and signed, with a system of labelling and for removing faulty equipment from use. Regular training updates for all staff as well as fire-fighting training, use of an extinguisher, and knowledge of who to report to in case of an electrical fire.
Disposal of waste products	Clinical waste (waste which consists wholly or partly of animal or human tissue, blood or other bodily fluids, swabs, dressings, syringes or needles) to be kept apart from the general waste and be disposed of to a licensed incineration or landfill site by a licensed company. Subcontract the disposal of waste to a local firm, who will take away yellow bins with contaminated waste and replace them either daily or weekly. This can be expensive, but is a good service.
Products	Keep manufacturers' data sheets and ensure that their products are used in accordance with the manufacturers' recommendations. COSHH sheets have a space for the recommended first aid treatments if the product comes in contact with the skin, is ingested or spits into the eye. Learn these and be prepared for any eventuality. Ensure caustic ingredients are stored in clearly labelled and easily identifiable bottles or tubs. Keep thorough and up-to-date record cards for clients' treatments and products, especially if there has already been a reaction or allergy to a particular product, or if the client has a severe allergy to a specific substance such as nuts. Regularly attend commercial training courses to keep abreast of new products, and never guess a product use or equipment usage.

Minimising equipment and product risks

Hazard	Minimise risk by taking the following actions
Visitors	Be informed about visitors to the salon. Many salons employ a badge system to identify visitors, sales reps, tradespeople, delivery drivers, and so on. Do not be intimidated by a person shouting or abusive behaviour. Firmly ask them to leave, or consult with the manager/salon owner, and if necessary, call the police. Minimise the risk of client harm by asking tradespeople to carry out repairs in the quieter part of the day or when the salon is closed. Major repairs would necessitate the salon being closed, as the clients' safety must not be compromised.

Minimising risks from people visiting the salon

You should now begin to see that you can minimise the risk of harm, by following some basic steps, being responsible and thinking about your actions.

Ensuring personal presentation minimises risk

Look again at your personal presentation, but this time with safety in mind. Your presentation contributes to you being safe in the salon.

Hazard	Minimise risk by taking the following actions
You – the therapist	Be professional at all times. Wear the correct uniform – remember cleanliness and hygiene, short nails, no jewellery, safe shoes. Follow the Health and Safety at Work etc. Act and be responsible for both yourself and others. Regularly attend training courses to be safe and competent. Be knowledgeable and use your knowledge – know the correct person to inform in case of an accident, who to contact for a first aider, and the salon policies on health and safety. Be as hygienic and as thorough as possible when protecting the client. Fill out a full consultation card and carry out a contra-indication check prior to every treatment. Never knowingly endanger others.

If the therapist does not have a sense of personal safety and respect for the safety of others, accidents will occur.

Keys to good practice

- Take care of your personal appearance – always combine safety with professionalism. If an establishment provides a uniform as part of a corporate image, then wear it!
- Wear smart, comfortable shoes. Avoid wearing high-heeled shoes, which are not only uncomfortable but also unstable to walk on, and open-toe sandals, which will not protect the toes from spillage or impact injury.
- Avoid stooping and slouching – to prevent back problems.
- Have good posture and evenly distribute body weight by standing correctly with feet slightly apart. This will prevent accidents and injury.
- Always wear the correct protective clothing provided to shield your uniform.
- Always wear gloves when using chemicals or if there is a possibility of coming into contact with body fluids.
- Always follow the correct disposal regulations for gloves and waste materials.
- Hair should be tidy and not loose enough to fall into the eyes and cause eye problems.
- Regularly take part in training for equipment use, first aid and manual handling courses.
- Know how to safely use and move equipment.

Remember

Any unsafe behaviour has consequences. Not only will you be negligent under your legal obligations to both the client and your employer, you could be personally liable should the client prove that as a direct result of your unsafe behaviour, bodily harm was a result. It could cost you a lot more than just your job.

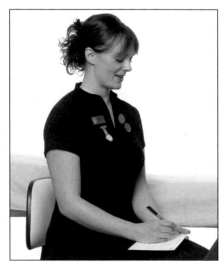
A high standard of personal presentation is essential at all times

A high standard of cleanliness will ensure no cross-infection can occur:

- Wash hands between clients.
- Wear your nails short.
- Cover cuts or open wounds.
- Do not attend work with an infectious disease.
- Do not spread germs with a cold or flu.
- Do not wear dangling jewellery, which may be a hazard.

Good conduct cuts down any risks.

- Do not run or rush about the salon.
- Use equipment properly.
- Follow manufacturers' instructions at all times.
- Take no short cuts when cleaning the salon and equipment.
- Always leave the equipment ready to use by the next person.
- Do not deliberately block a fire exit for any reason.
- Do not deliberately endanger anyone – even as a joke.
- Do not behave in a negligent way.
- Always use proper lifting procedures.
- Do take responsibility for yourself, machinery and problems such as spillage that may occur – do not expect someone else to clean up after you!

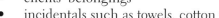

An essential part of good conduct is maintaining high standards of personal hygiene

Reducing workplace risks

There are so many areas to keep secure in a business and possible risk areas include:

- the premises
- stock and products
- equipment
- money
- display materials
- personal safety
- clients' belongings
- incidentals such as towels, cotton wool, etc.

The premises

For insurance and mortgage applications, the salon owner must have adequate security measures in place. It is advisable to consult the local crime prevention officer who will come and survey the premises and give advice regarding the most vulnerable areas and the most common forms of entry by a burglar.

Externally

- Deadlocks on all doors and windows will make it more difficult for a burglar to enter the premises.
- Double-glazing is expensive but is more difficult to break into – the older the window and frame, the easier the entry.
- A burglar alarm, or even a dummy box on the wall, often deters a burglar.
- Closed circuit television (CCTV) may be available if the premises are in a shopping area with other stores.
- Premises with metal shop-front shutters offer the most effective deterrent to a burglar.

Internally

- Internal doors can be locked at night to prevent an intruder moving from room to room.
- Fire doors and emergency exits should be locked at night and re-opened by the first person in at the start of business every morning.
- A light left on in reception may also deter would-be burglars who might feel that well-lit premises will make them more visible.
- Stock and money should be locked away or put in the bank. Nothing should be visible to entice a burglar to break in in the first place!
- Expensive equipment should be locked away in treatment rooms or in the stock cupboard.

Remember

Occupational accidents kill over 300 people and injure over one million every year. Over two million people suffer illnesses caused, or made worse, by their work. Preventing accidents and ill health caused by work is a key priority for everyone at work. Competent employees are valuable.

Very large businesses often employ security guards to patrol their premises at night, but along with alarmed infrared beams, these are not affordable for the average small salon owner. If, however, the salon is situated within a shopping centre or business park, night patrols *may* be included in the lease or purchase agreement or be offered for a set fee per year. Costs would need to be considered, but it may be an investment and save money in the long term.

The local police station can be contacted and police patrol vans will regularly check the building as part of their normal evening beat.

Stock and products

This includes products on display and those used in the treatment rooms. Of all the temptations to the thief, these smaller items may prove irresistible – they are small enough for a pocket, and are very accessible. Unfortunately, this form of shoplifting costs many businesses a great deal of money, as stock can be expensive to replace and can be a big part of the capital outlay of a salon.

Another sad fact is that the average 'thief' may be rather closer to home than is comfortable. Staff may 'borrow' an item of stock for home use, and think that this behaviour is acceptable. Also, some clients may like the look of a lipstick and 'forget' to pay for it!

Whether items are shoplifted or pilfered, either way it means the salon has bought an item of stock from the wholesaler that it has not been paid for by its customer, so it has to absorb that financial loss. If left unchecked, this could eventually bankrupt the business.

Tight precautions are called for, including the following.

- Make one member of staff, usually a senior therapist or senior receptionist, responsible for stock control – she should be the only one with keys and access to stock.
- Carry out a regular stock check – daily for loss of stock and weekly for stock ordering and rotation.
- Use empty containers for displays, or ask the suppliers if they can provide dummy stock – this will also save the product deteriorating while on display.
- Encourage staff and customers to keep handbags away from the stock area, usually reception, to stop products 'dropping' into open bags.
- Have one member of staff responsible for topping up the treatment products from the wholesale-sized tubs.
- Hold regular staff training on security and let staff know what the losses are and how it may affect them – some companies offer bonus schemes for reaching targets of both sales and minimising pilfering. Heavy losses may affect potential salary increases.
- Carry out banking of money in the till at different times of the day and do not keep too much money in the till at any one time.

Reducing risks to staff safety

See **You – the therapist**, pages 14 and 15 for information on personal security and safety.

Use of materials and hazardous substances

There are numerous substances within the salon which are considered to be hazardous to health, from caustic cleaning products and dishwasher tablets, to beauty products used in Level 3 treatments.

For your own and others' safety, follow these safety rules.

- Always follow manufacturers' instructions.
- Always read instructions and mixing labels carefully, to get the correct and safe recipe.
- Report any differences between the manufacturers' instructions and your salon guidelines.
- Be informed and knowledgeable on COSHH regulations and read the COSHH sheets for your particular area of work.
- Use personal protective equipment (PPE) where possible – it should be provided for you.
- Never use products or chemicals on a broken skin.
- Provide eye pads for the client (cotton wool rounds) when using products on the face, especially exfoliants and brush cleansing, or when carrying out treatments such as direct high frequency, and goggles for ultraviolet and infrared treatments.
- Be trained and be safe!

Keys to good practice

- If there is any doubt about the client's tolerance to a product, do a skin test 24 hours prior to the treatment. Some galvanic gels, for example, are quite strong, and may cause reactions on more sensitive skins. Check for any reaction, erythema, itchiness or stinging and burning sensations on the area of the patch test.
- Store products correctly to stop them deteriorating and reacting. A cool dark place is essential, in containers with tight lids. Those products which react to temperature changes or to heat will need to be kept in a fridge.
- Decant products with a spatula into a smaller bowl or dish, and never pour used products back into the main jar – the contamination will ruin the whole lot. Never use your fingers in products for the same reason.
- Never use a product past its use-by date or one that has started to deteriorate or react, has an unpleasant odour or has lost its natural consistency. If a product starts to separate and become watery, then it is not useable and may cause a reaction.
- Do not guess quantities or measurements, or substitute chemicals if what you require is unavailable.

Smoking, eating, drinking and drugs

Smoking

Many companies have declared their workplace a no-smoking zone, as cigarette smoking is recognised as a potential health risk, and there are safety risks attached to the use of chemicals and products. Not only has smoking been proven to be dangerous to the health of the smoker, it also has implications for the passive smoker, the person inhaling the smoke just by being in the area.

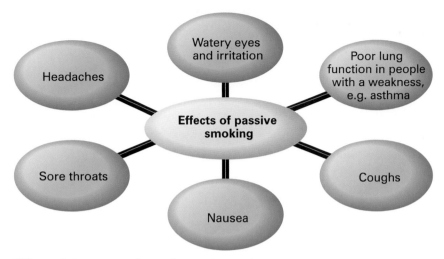

Effects of cigarette smoke on the passive smoker

In a beauty salon, it would be unusual to allow smoking, both for staff and for clientele, not only for the health and safety risks but also for hygiene reasons and the lingering odour of cigarette smoke. A beauty salon is all about cleansing and nourishing the body, relaxing the mind and replenishing the soul – a smoky atmosphere would be in direct conflict with this ethos.

From the therapist's point of view, it is unprofessional to smoke at work – it leaves an unpleasant odour on clothing, hair and on the breath. A client having a body massage or facial would certainly not appreciate the essence of smoke oozing from the therapist's every pore! A salon owner or manager might recommend to employees who smoke that the risks are too great at work, but they cannot dictate what the therapist does during her spare time.

For the client, smoking may undo all the good work carried out by the therapist and act against the treatment. Smoking robs the skin of vital oxygen; it causes dehydration, and can prematurely age the skin on the face. The therapist can only strongly recommend to the client that, like a healthy diet, moderate exercise and drinking lots of water, giving up smoking would greatly improve the client's health and sense of well-being.

Your employer has a duty under the Health and Safety at Work etc. Act 1974 to protect non-smoking employees from the hazards of tobacco smoke. Their duty of care also extends to clients and others who enter the salon (see **You, your client and the law**, page 67).

Eating

Eating in the salon is very unprofessional, and is a potential health risk for germs, with the added risk of spillage, causing slippery floors.

Therapists should have an eating area and proper storage facilities for food, such as a fridge and cupboards, but it needs careful management to prevent stale food accumulating and causing a health risk. One staff member needs to be in charge of kitchen duties, cleaning out the fridge weekly and replenishing tea, coffee, milk, and so on. Some salons offer drinks and light refreshments to clients, and care must be taken to minimise the risk of infection, by thoroughly washing all glasses, cups and cutlery, ideally on a hot cycle in a dishwasher.

Check it out

If you smoke, how much time have you needed to take off work or college for smoking-related illnesses, such as chest infections? How much money do you spend a week on buying cigarettes? How do you feel about the possible health risks you are taking? How fit do you think you are? Could you give up if you wanted to?

Remember

Discarded, still-alight cigarettes and accidentally dropped cigarettes on furniture or in a paper bin, are among the most common causes of fire, certainly domestic fires. A smoke detector which is in full working order can and does save lives.

Drinking

Providing drinks in the salon for clients has a high risk factor for spillage and infection from dirty cups and glasses. A hot drink may be split onto a client, causing scalds, and drinks may easily be spilt on the floor, causing a hazard. There should be a staff member in charge of the drinks arrangements, as electric kettles and coffee percolators also have an electrical risk factor, and need to be regularly maintained and replenished when necessary.

Alcoholic drinks are less frequently consumed in business. Many companies are alcohol-free and expect staff not to consume alcohol during the working day. Alcohol lowers concentration levels, relaxes the body and lowers the reflexes, which is a considerable risk to the client, salon and therapist, especially when using electrical equipment. The traditional cheese and wine opening of a salon has largely been replaced with soft drinks and demonstrations, which also discourages the client from drinking and then driving home. Certainly, no machinery should be operated under even the smallest influence of alcohol.

Too much alcohol can have health effects which may act against salon treatments. Going over the recommended 14 units for per week for a female or 21 units for a male (a unit being half a pint of lager, or a small glass of wine) can affect the absorption of vitamins, dull the hair and skin, dehydrate the skin, and stop the liver from functionally properly. Moderation should be the advice to clients, so that their salon treatments give the body maximum advantage.

Drugs

If you have to take medication prescribed by a doctor, ask about all the possible side-effects. For example, hay fever tablets can leave you feeling drowsy and tired, affecting concentration levels – this is a possible risk. If you combine those with a mild sleeping tablet, or an over-the-counter preparation to calm you down, the effects are doubled, as they are both sedatives, and you should not be driving, let alone operating electrical equipment on a client. If in doubt, do not mix medicines, and ask your local pharmacist about possible side-effects. You should always inform your employer about any medication you are taking, and your workload may have to be adjusted for the duration of the treatment.

Using recreational drugs while working in the salon is just not safe. All recreational drugs are hazardous as they stay in the system for up to 48 hours, which can lead to accidents, errors in judgement and poor performance. There is a strong possibility of absenteeism, which affects every member of staff and inconveniences clients, through cancellations and late appointments, and it is not good for the reputation of any business. Drug-taking affects the personality, producing mood swings, hyperactivity, depression, and manic episodes – none of which create the right customer care environment to enhance and develop a business.

Remember

A hangover from the previous night out can mean you are still over the drink-driving limit in the morning, and may seriously affect your capacity to work correctly.

Remember

The use of recreational (non-prescription) drugs is illegal in the UK. The classification of cannabis has recently been downgraded, and the police may now use their discretion whether or not to prosecute if a person is found to be in possession of a small amount. The long-term effects of these drugs have yet to be conclusively studied, although potential brain damage and personality disorders have not been ruled out as a possible side-effect. Stronger recreation drugs such as ecstasy have caused death.

Promote additional products or services to clients

Unit G6

Level 3 treatments offer a vast range of additional products and services for the benefit of the client. It is essential for the growth of the business to keep the client knowledgeable and informed about all the possible treatments and products available within the salon. It is not only helpful for the client, allowing him or her to made informed choices, it is also essential if the business is to survive in a very competitive market place.

This unit looks at the promotional side of the beauty therapy business. Think of it as 'prescribing' quality products for the benefit of the client to enhance salon treatments and ensure the maximum benefit from the range of treatments. Often salon-supplied products are specifically made to reinforce salon treatments and usually have higher active ingredients than those purchased over the counter in the high street. Generally, the salon offers exclusive products that cannot be purchased elsewhere and clients will be happy to pay more for quality products.

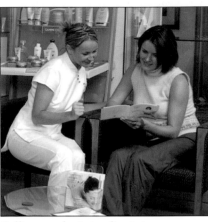

Selling products to clients is an essential part of the business

Often more money is made for both the salon, and yourself, from selling products to clients than for doing the treatment, *and* the client walks away with good quality products.

Within this unit you will cover the following outcomes:

G6.1 **Identify additional products or services that are available**
G6.2 **Inform clients about additional products or services**
G6.3 **Gain client commitment to using additional products or services.**

Identify additional products or services that are available

G6.1

In this outcome you will learn about

- working with others for up-to-date information
- checking with others when you are unsure
- matching products to clients' needs
- identifying opportunities to offer additional treatments.

It is vital that you have a complete knowledge of the services and product ranges offered by the salon in order to guide clients towards the most beneficial choices.

Working with others for up-to-date information

There are two key ways to ensure you have the latest information about products and services:

- knowledge
- regular training.

Communication with colleagues is also very important (for information on methods of communication, see **You and your client**, page 28).

Knowledge

Knowledge is empowering! When you join an established salon there will be a large pool of knowledge from which you can draw – the owner, senior therapists, junior therapists (who may have done specialised training), trade magazines and suppliers, and product or equipment suppliers.

Be open to new ideas and techniques – there is always more than one way to carry out a treatment and manufacturers normally employ beauty therapists on their development team, ensuring techniques and procedures are going to be workable in a commercial salon. Try to avoid thinking that the way you learned at college is the only right way! As you gain experience, and see new techniques for both massage and equipment use, your own style will emerge and should keep on developing. The most successful therapists continue to take training courses and introduce new equipment, techniques and products. Otherwise the business would not keep up with trends, and would not grow.

The general public is more aware than ever before about treatments available. The media will cover the latest trends, and clients will not be afraid to take their business elsewhere if their usual salon has not kept up to date.

Knowledge allows you to fulfil your entire professional obligation to your client.

Training

Training can be:

- in-house (within the salon)
- external.

In-house training

This should be a regular event. Senior therapists should demonstrate or impart their knowledge of the existing treatments and products on the price list to all staff. So, although the receptionist may not be a trained therapist, she will have seen a demonstration of a treatment and have the self-assurance to describe its benefits and effects to the client. Junior therapists are often given samples of products to try or given treatments so that they, too, can talk about them with confidence to clients. Another way to gain knowledge of all salon treatments and their benefits is to study the price list and promotional leaflets.

External training

External training, that is from an outside supplier, can either be offsite or onsite with the salon owner closing a treatment room for a day, or holding a training session on a day when the salon is closed.

There is a trade-off here – the salon owner invests in the cost of training and the therapist is then qualified and insured to carry out that particular treatment. In return, the therapist is expected to stay with the salon (usually called a loyalty clause) for a set period of time, which could be six months or a year. This is something that you will need to discuss at interview stage because you will be expected to sign, as part of your contract of employment, to say you agree with this.

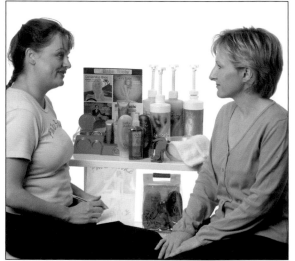

Use your product knowledge and training to help your client during the consultation

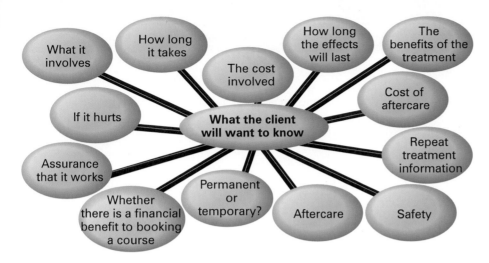

Useful information for the client

Checking with others when you are unsure

Always check with others when you are unsure of a new product or service. Find the right person to advise the client, even if it means making a separate appointment with the senior therapist or specialist within the salon. It will be seen as an investment in time, rather than a waste of time.

In the beauty therapy industry it is considered your responsibility to ensure you have sufficient knowledge to recommend all salon treatments and products, even though you may not yet be qualified to carry them out and are therefore uninsured. You will be generating new business for the salon and the senior therapist who will be carrying out the treatment. A commission structure will most likely be in place to act as an incentive and motivate all therapists to ensure the growth of the business. So the more you sell, in terms of treatments and products, the more you earn! (See Unit G11, Contribute to the financial effectiveness of the business.)

Be pro-active in your learning about the services and products offered by your salon. See the table on the next page for learning opportunities.

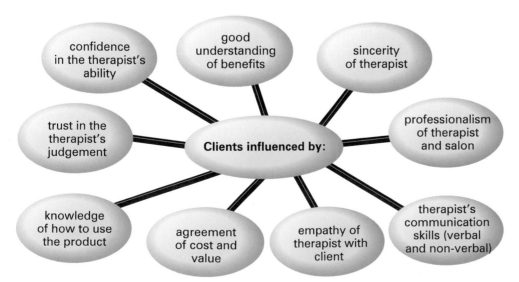

Factors influencing clients to use the salon's products or services

At work	Learning opportunities
Within the job	Attending staff meetings
	Attending training sessions
	Project work – design a course of treatments suitable for a wedding, summer holiday, etc.
	Making a presentation
	Acting as a spokesperson for the salon
	Writing a report on benefits of a treatment
	Learning or designing a price list
	Visiting a supplier
	Spending the day with the salesperson
	Showing people around
	Stock taking
	Visiting exhibitions/attending lectures
	Role play
Extending your job role	Standing in for a receptionist/senior therapist
	Shadowing/work experience
	Job sharing
	Job rotation
	Modelling for treatments at demonstrations
	Attending open evenings
	Watching the experts in action
	Applying for extra training courses

Finding learning opportunities at work

Matching products to clients' needs

With experience, and product and salon treatment knowledge, you will be able to match clients' needs with the correct product or service.

Having empathy with the client when discussing additional treatments or products is essential. Because Level 3 offers such a diverse range of mechanical and electrical treatments, you will need experience to be able to narrow down the choices to meet individual clients' needs. Develop an insight on what to mention and which treatment or product would be most beneficial to the client. If the choice is too varied, the client may become confused, alarmed at the costs or the time involved. Too much information is often overpowering.

Be aware of the clients' constraints – time, finances and the level of aftercare that they will be able to carry out. These will help you to make an informed choice about what to recommend.

Remember

Seeking help and asking questions of others with more experience than you currently have is a strength, not a weakness. Within the salon, there is a wealth of experience and knowledge, and checking with others will ensure your information is correct, and give you knowledge which, in turn, you will be able to pass on to others.

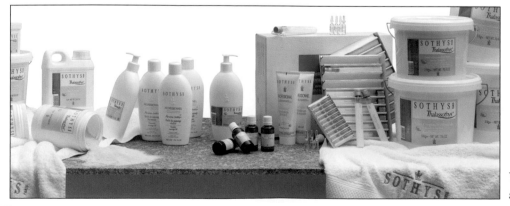

You will need to match the product to suit the client's needs

Identifying opportunities to offer additional treatments

Below are some natural links for products and services which complement the treatment the client is having.

Basic treatment	Related mechanical or electrical treatment	Aftercare sale
Facial treatments Electrical facial Steam treatment Eyebrow shaping Make-up or make-up lesson Eyelash perming Eyelash tinting Application of false lashes Facial waxing	Audio-sonic facial massage Steaming Infrared Galvanic facial High frequency Microcurrent Vacuum suction Faradic Epilation	Exfoliation products/peels, cleanser, toner, moisturiser, ampoules, masque, night creams, eye products, make-up, sun protection factor (SPF) products, soothing gels, after-shave balm and shaving products and other specialised aftercare products relating to a particular treatment, e.g. application of witch hazel after epilation
Body treatments Waxing Manicure Pedicure Body massage	Faradic Galvanic Vacuum suction High frequency Hydrotherapy Body wraps G5 Microcurrent	Moisturisers, artificial tanning, exfoliation products, shower and bath products, anti-cellulite products, specialised SPF products, lifting/circulatory stimulating products, breast-firming creams

Opportunities/links for promotion

In the salon

In the salon many products available for sale to the customer can be multi-purpose. During an epilation treatment, the client mentions she is going on holiday. This gives an additional opportunity to make a sale unrelated to the treatment being carried out.

What do you say?

- Have a nice holiday!

or

- May I recommend Sterex Aloe Vera soothing gel, containing 95 per cent aloe. This is wonderfully soothing after epilation, yet can be used in a number of ways and for very differing reasons. For example, as an after-sun soothing product. Aloe vera is well known for its benefits for soothing and healing sunburn and if you keep it in a fridge, the pain relief is instantaneous. Can you afford not to take this with you?

The client has already provided the lead, you just have to follow. This scenario also illustrates how versatile products can be.

Remember

Giving the client good aftercare advice and recommending the correct products to use at home will reinforce the benefits of salon treatments and continue your good work!

If you discuss the benefits and possible drawbacks of each treatment, as you are performing, say, an epilation treatment, that makes the whole approach more of a conversation than a sales pitch.

Other opportunities may arise if:

- the client is looking at a product stand in reception
- the client asks about a particular product that he or she has heard about or seen in the media
- the client observes another treatment as she is walking through the salon, e.g. nail extensions
- the client asks for a price list
- the client's friend has recommended a particular treatment
- an open evening/promotional demonstration creates interest
- a commercial company holds a training day and you request your favourite clients to model.

All these openings can be used as a chance to inform, educate and offer clients the best products and services for their needs.

Features and benefits of products and services

The key is to know and understand the features and benefits of the products and services that the salon offers in order to be able to promote them effectively. Everything you offer has a feature and a benefit.

A product's attributes or characteristics are its features. The advantages to the client of the product are its benefits.

The features and benefits of a facial cleanser are shown in the table below, as an example.

Features	Benefits
Unbreakable packaging	Cleanses the skin
Pump action convenience and control	Prevents facial blemishes
Variety of sizes	Removes make-up
Economical when purchased in larger sizes	Helps exfoliate
Exclusive products unavailable on high street	Helps regulate the acid mantle

Features and benefits of a facial cleanser

Inform clients about additional products or services

G6.2

| In this outcome you will learn about | |

In this outcome you will learn about

- introducing products and services
- giving clients accurate information
- giving the client time
- salon and legal requirements.

Introducing products and services

Spotting opportunities for offering clients additional products or services is easy if you are receptive and aware. A client will often ask, as he or she may have heard about a treatment from a friend, or have seen treatments avertised on a website and wish to know more. A special day or occasion will trigger extra interest – weddings, parties, holidays and Christmas functions always generate attention in extra treatments and products for the client.

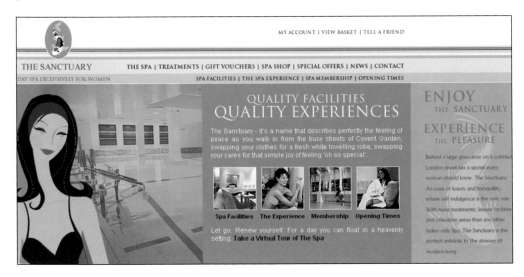

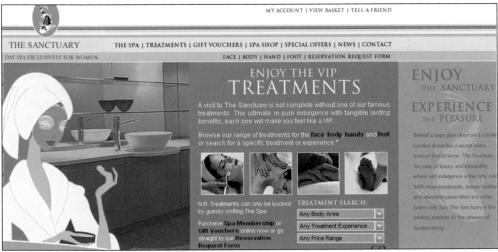

Salon websites are an effective way of introducing products and services

Pick your moment! It is important to choose the appropriate time in which to mention additional products and services. The prime time is when you have the client's full attention prior to and after the treatment. For example:

- in reception – as the client arrives, he or she could be offered a sample of a new product while the therapist outlines the features and benefits of the product
- during consultation
- upon skin diagnosis
- when considering and recommending the relevant products suitable for the client
- following treatment, during aftercare discussion.

Since you should avoid conversation when the client is relaxing during treatment, this is not the best time to sell products or services.

Remember

Capitalise on the previous sales of products by asking clients if they were happy with the product and whether they would like to buy more. Check the clients' record card before they come into the salon to see what items they have bought.

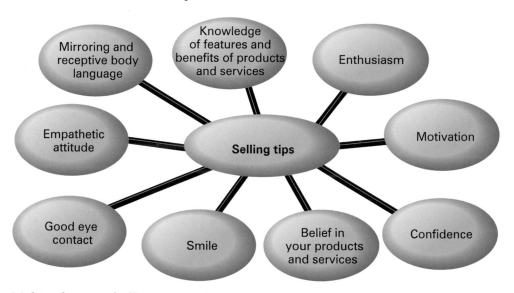

Making the most of selling opportunities

(See **You and your client**, pages 30–1 for questioning techniques to use during the consultation.)

Giving clients accurate information

Try to be as accurate as you can when giving information, as not only is your professional reputation at stake, you also have a legal obligation not to give any false or misleading information to clients. As consumers, clients have legal rights to protect them. You or your salon will be liable for prosecution if found to be in breach of the law. Not only that, you will lose clients very quickly if they have no faith in the information you are giving them – and if the products or services you recommend are unsuitable for their needs.

Giving the client time

Silence is a wonderful selling tool. Give clients time to take in the information you have given them and do not be afraid to allow them time to reflect and consider their options. Try to avoid the common mistake of jumping in through embarrassment in moments of silence. Clients may view this as harassment and leave empty-handed. Allow clients time to ask questions, which should be answered openly, accurately and honestly.

Remember

By describing the features and benefits of a product or service, you are giving clients accurate and sufficient information to enable them to make a decision.

By providing the link between additional treatments available and the current one, you can make the conversation seamless and you are not introducing lots of differing topics all at once. The client will be pleased to receive any suggestions, and will be delighted you are taking such an interest rather than viewing it as an intrusion, or a hard selling technique.

Salon and legal requirements

Underpinning all the product knowledge and treatment skills you have to pass on to clients are the legal aspects of selling and clients' and consumer rights.

The specific laws relating to this unit are:

- Health and Safety at Work etc. Act 1974
- Consumer Protection Act 1987
- Consumer Protection (Distance Selling) Regulations 2000
- Cosmetic Products (Safety) Regulations 2004
- Trade Descriptions Act 1968
- Sale of Goods Act 1979 (amended)
- Sale and Supply of Goods Act 1994
- Supply of Goods and Services Act 1982
- Supply of Goods (Implied Terms) Act 1973
- Unfair Contract Terms Act 1977.

(See **You, your client and the law**, pages 67, 75–8 for information on the above legislation.)

It is essential that you do not give misleading information, directly or by implication. This will protect the client, yourself and the salon's reputation in all your promotional activities.

As a professional therapist, you will need to work within your industry code of practice and salon guidelines (see **You, your client and the law**, page 81).

> ### Remember
>
>
> Clients may have entered into a contractual agreement with the salon if they have paid in advance for a course of treatments. Often an incentive of a free or additional treatment encourages clients to pay in full. Careful record keeping of the number of treatments taken will honour the agreement.

Gain client commitment to using additional products or services

G6.3

In this outcome you will learn about

- closing the discussion when the client shows no interest
- moving forward when the client shows interest
- sales targets and recording sales
- promotion of existing and new products
- obtaining client feedback
- checking client understanding of product use
- prompt delivery of products
- referring clients to alternative sources.

Closing the discussion when the client shows no interest

Just as important as giving time and enthusiasm to the client's enquiries is knowing when to stop if the client shows no interest. If the feedback from the client is minimal, or he or she says 'No thanks', then take your cue and stop. Nothing is more irritating to the client than an unwanted sales pitch; you will lose clients altogether if you come over as pushy and forceful.

If you experience a rejection, do not take it personally. There may be an objection that you can overcome and still secure the sale or part of it. Otherwise continue to advise positively and concentrate on building your relationship with the client. When you have sold the client some products, suggest other things that may be required on the next visit. Always book the next appointment before the client leaves the salon.

As a double check, ask yourself the following questions.

- Am I giving information relevant to the client's particular needs?
- Am I explaining myself clearly, or am I confusing the client?
- Am I being too technical in my explanation?
- Have I chosen a good time to give advice?
- Did I use the tool of silence effectively?
- Did I allow time for the client to ask questions?

Review your techniques in the light of your answers to the above questions.

- Try to make the sale relevant to the client's needs.
- Use role play with a senior therapist for hints with technique.
- Make your explanation of the treatment or product crystal clear.
- Avoid being too technical – give the benefits of the product, not the method or how it works.
- Stop the conversation when appropriate, and choose a better time to discuss the client's needs, e.g. when the client is not in a hurry.
- Give the client a sample and allow him or her to walk away with a 'goody bag'.

The way to close the discussion is to offer some literature, a price list, or leaflet on the subject and allow the client to read it at leisure. It may be that the client just does not have time to discuss it, or it could be a financial consideration, or the treatment just does not appeal – knowing when to step back and stop giving information is essential to maintaining good communication.

Moving forward when the client shows interest

There are several ways clients will give you feedback that they are in agreement with you regarding your recommendations. They may:

- book an appointment for the recommended treatments
- purchase the suggested products
- book a consultation for advanced treatments
- order the delivery of the product if not in stock
- put a deposit on a course of treatments
- buy a gift voucher to give as a present.

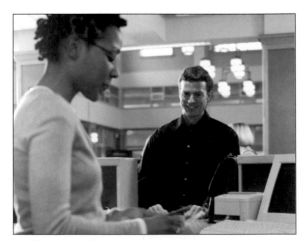

Making the sale

Once clients have made up their minds, they will clearly indicate the route you should take:

- escort the client to the till to purchase the product
- ask the receptionist to book the client a follow-up appointment
- fill out a purchase order for the chosen product and services while the client watches.

If the item is not in stock, make it quite clear to the client at the beginning – this will avoid disappointment and the client will keep his or her faith in you. Try not to enthuse about a product and then backtrack once you realise that you do not have the item in stock, only to suggest an alternative. That is not fair to the client and will put you in a bad light – it looks as though you are only after the client's money and not providing the best possible product.

Remember

It is common practice to have a sales record book as well as stock control data sheets on which any sale should be registered. This not only keeps a record of an individual's success rate in selling (upon which commission can be based) but also when the two records are tallied at the end of each day/week/month, they provide an accurate assessment of the stock control and stock levels at the salon.

Sales targets and recording sales

Salons improve their business through analysis of turnover and improvement in movement of items that are slow to sell. Most salons set targets, in both sales and treatments, and it is important, through regular meetings and agreed personal goals, that you understand what is expected of you.

It should be agreed at your interview what your personal goals are, what incentives there are for achieving them and what support there is to assist you to reach those goals.

Below are some of the possible implications for the salon if targets are not met.

- Profits drop.
- Less training is undertaken – to save money.
- Fewer products are offered.
- Staff are made redundant.
- Machinery is not replaced.
- No new treatments are offered.
- Current products and treatments become stale.
- Decoration and repairs are not carried out.
- There is less money for advertising and promotional activity.
- Senior therapists leave, so there is a drop in skill levels within the salon.
- Staff become demotivated.
- The goodwill and good name of the salon are lost.
- Clients go elsewhere.
- Eventually, the business closes.

See Unit G11, Contribute to the financial effectiveness of the business, for information on personal goal setting, how to work with your manager and how to develop your job role for personal satisfaction.

Promotion of exisiting and new products

Existing treatments and products
New treatments and products are always easy to recommend to the client. You have had your training, the products are new to you, you have had the treatment yourself, seen the excellent results and are brimming over with enthusiasm! It becomes infectious and soon the new buzz created means the cash registers are ringing and stock is moving very quickly.

But what about existing services and products? They may be seen as old hat and boring, and your excitement for all the new products only reinforces that. There is a danger that the standard, but still very trustworthy and beneficial, treatments will be overlooked. To avoid this, consider revisiting the price list, services and treatments you offer in order to give them a fresh new appeal. Rebranding a treatment or product with a new angle and fresh approach combined with promotional activity will bring additional sales.

Promotional activity enables you to:

- let your customers try treatments or products they have not experienced before
- retain customer loyalty
- convey an impression of activity and change within the salon
- attract new clients
- improve customer satisfaction
- improve the salon's public relations.

Displaying products

The way products are displayed is key to your success in selling them. Anything behind glass will not be picked up and will not be bought. The feel of a product and what is written upon it is as important as its appearance.

Display materials within the salon environment should do the following:

- attract **attention** – be eye catching
- create **interest** – once the client's attention has been gained, interest must be maintained
- stimulate **desire** to have the treatment or buy the product
- stimulate **action** on the part of the client to book an appointment or make a purchase.

A good display is one that catches the interest of clients and motivates them to buy your products and services. It should be neat and tidy so clients can see what is available. Place displays strategically around the salon, at eye level if possible to enhance visibility.

Have a space near the reception area where you stock *all* leaflets about *everything* you do. Do not photocopy leaflets – this looks cheap and unprofessional. Be careful of 'menu fatigue' in salon point-of-sale displays, where clients become so used to seeing the same thing in the same position every time they visit, that they no longer notice anything at all. Small changes every month or so can make a huge difference, with larger-scale changes on an annual basis.

Re-order your point-of-sale material from time to time so that it always looks pristine, and throw out display material that has become faded, curled up or dog-eared. Displays in the window should be changed regularly as the sun will fade the colours, and there is nothing enticing about a tired display.

Obtaining client feedback

Client feedback is an excellent way of collecting information about clients' needs and acts as a good monitor for the way the business should be developing. Verbal feedback will take place, and the client may comment on leaving reception: 'I really enjoyed

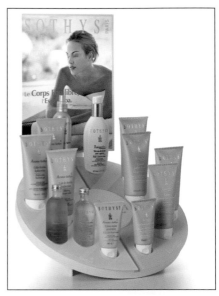

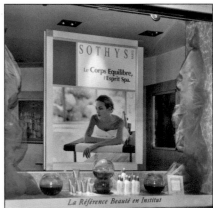

Eye-catching product displays

that head and face massage – Janine really does have healing hands. I drifted right off to sleep'. A good manager will remember this and relay the client's comments to the therapist (if she did not hear them) as positive reinforcement of a job well done.

On the other hand, a negative comment, even made in passing, should not be ignored. If the client says, 'I don't want to buy another of those cleansers, it really stung when I put it on my face', the comment needs further investigation to prevent you losing the client altogether. Spend five minutes, in private, talking through the product choice. Is she using the right one for her skin type? Is she using it correctly? Offer an alternative, for sensitive skin, as a replacement, so that you show the client you care and value her custom.

A more formal method of gaining client feedback is a short, simple questionnaire, with tick boxes (clients will not have time for anything more than this). The way to ensure that the questionnaire is returned is to add an incentive of a small free treatment such as a complimentary eyebrow shape with the next electrical facial, or a sample or goody bag as the form is handed in at reception.

Remember

Remember the hierarchy of your salon management, and do not start a promotional activity without seeking approval from the salon manager or owner. Should you exceed the limits of your own authority, and reduce prices or offer promotions without permission, there will be consequences. You may lose the salon money, and your line manager will certainly not see you as a team player.

Please mark ✓ for yes and ✗ for no in the boxes.

◆ Have you purchased anything from the salon in the past month? ☐

◆ Have you tried the new range of products yet? ☐

◆ Have you had an electrical treatment in the past month? ☐

◆ Were you kept waiting today? ☐

◆ Were you offered refreshment? ☐

◆ Was any query you had dealt with efficiently and quickly? ☐

◆ Did you feel your therapist acted professionally? ☐

◆ Was your future booking handled efficiently? ☐

◆ Did you feel the staff were informative and knowledgeable about treatments and products we offer? ☐

◆ Did the salon feel friendly and welcoming? ☐

A simple client questionnaire will enable the salon to obtain useful feedback

Checking client understanding of product use

To get the best from the product, the client should fully understand how to use it, or when to apply it, and its benefits and advantages. Refer back to **Professional basics**, pages 22-4, to refresh your memory on discussing the application of products, using your communication skills to reinforce clients' understanding, and how to follow up on product purchases.

Prompt delivery of products

If, following your advice, clients wish to purchase either a product or treatments, you will need to ensure that they understand the time constraints or delivery expectations (see **You – the therapist, Professional basics**, page 24). When a product has to be ordered, make sure that clients are kept informed about delivery dates to avoid any misunderstanding.

Referring clients to alternative sources

There are times when you will not be able to offer the client what he or she needs, either because you are not yet trained in the particular treatment or your salon does not offer it. If the salon cannot provide the treatment, you may recommend an alternative therapist. Refer back to **Professional basics**, page 24, for information on this.

Remember

Always take responsibility for your actions:
- Ensure you know how to order the correct goods, or give it to someone who does.
- Make an effort to juggle the appointment system to suit everyone.
- A little effort and thought goes a long way, and is always appreciated

Contribute to the financial effectiveness of the business

Unit G11

The key to a successful business is making and maintaining a profit. A profit is simply the amount of money left after all the outgoings of a business have been paid, including stock and wages. To be able to make a profit, a business must monitor its outgoings very closely, and a small business is only as good as its resources management. A sad truth is that regardless of how good skills are – you may be a very competent therapist – the business may fail if resource administration is poor.

A beauty therapy salon is a great user of resources – people, stock, tools, equipment and time. All have to be managed and coordinated so that the business grows and flourishes, and a healthy balance is maintained through vigilant supervision, with all members of staff appreciating their responsibilities for resources.

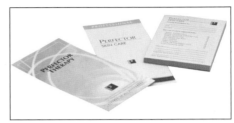

Selling complete skill care regimes benefits the client and is profitable for the salon

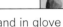

Remember

Maximum profit goes hand in glove with minimum waste.

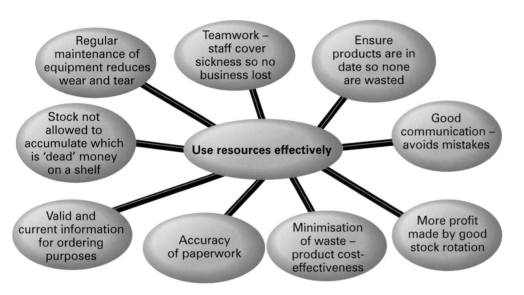

Regular maintenance of equipment reduces wear and tear

Teamwork – staff cover sickness so no business lost

Ensure products are in date so none are wasted

Stock not allowed to accumulate which is 'dead' money on a shelf

Use resources effectively

Good communication – avoids mistakes

Valid and current information for ordering purposes

Accuracy of paperwork

Minimisation of waste – product cost-effectiveness

More profit made by good stock rotation

The effective use of resources contributes to profitability

Within this unit you will cover the following outcomes:

G11.1 Contribute to the effective use and monitoring of resources
G11.2 Meet productivity and development targets.

Contribute to the effective use and monitoring of resources

G11.1

In this outcome you will learn about

- following salon and legal procedures
- types of resources
- the principles of stock control
- deliveries and checking stock
- resolving resource problems
- managing people.

The principle of keeping a track of what comes in and what goes out is the same, regardless of whether your eventual aim is to become a salon owner, or whether you are happy to stay an employee, or even if you intend to become a mobile therapist. Your role in monitoring resources may vary, as a salon manager has more resource responsibility than a junior therapist, but all staff should avoid wasting materials and try to be cost-effective, even if their job role does not include stock taking or ordering the required goods. Every staff member should contribute to the effective use and monitoring of resources.

Following salon and legal procedures

There are numerous legal requirements relating to safe working practices:

- Health and Safety at Work etc. Act 1974
- Manual Handling Operations Regulations 1992
- Reporting of Injuries, Diseases and Dangerous Occurrences Regulations (RIDDOR) 1995
- Electricity at Work Regulations 1989
- Cosmetic Products (Safety) Regulations 2004
- Control of Substances Hazardous to Health (COSHH) Regulations 2003

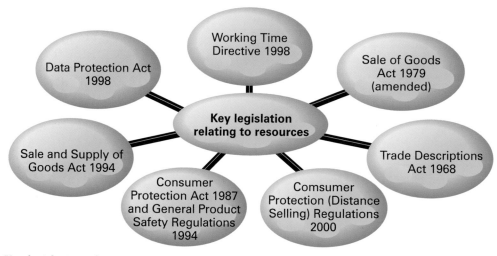

Key legislation relating to consumer protection and working conditions

(See **You, your client and the law**, pages 67–76, for information on the above legislation.)

Remember

What comes in and what goes out has to be accounted for.

Salon procedures

Salon procedures for managing resources will vary according to the size of the salon, the type of business and services it offers, the level of staffing and the efficiency of its management. There are no hard and fast rules for organisation of resources but large national corporations and beauty groups will have policies in place so that all their salons use universal paperwork regardless of who is in charge of the individual salon. The self-employed therapist will need a smaller-scale method of resource management, but the principle of the system is the same.

Types of resources

Resources in a busy salon include:

* stock
* tools and equipment
* people
* time.

Stock

Stock is both:

* the second largest investment of money – the first is people
* the lifeblood of the business, as no stock to perform treatments equals no clients.

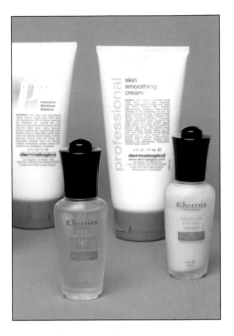

Controlling stock is often seen as tedious and boring, and the relevance is rarely appreciated by the younger therapist who is often given the job of checking all stock held, the arrival of deliveries and for damaged or broken goods. However, the importance of this should not be underestimated. Running out of best-selling stock through poor stock control is lost revenue, which may be reflected in lower commission for sales for individual therapists.

The first thing a salon has to decide is the level of stock to be held. This will, of course, depend upon the treatment ranges that are to be offered, the number of therapists using the products and the product suppliers. It is common practice to open an account with your choice of supplier and, initially, many of the larger suppliers have a minimum ordering level of either monetary value or stock level – a £2,000 investment in stock is not unreasonable. They will supply in bulk for larger salons, but once you are a proven reliable customer, smaller orders will be accepted, albeit with a higher delivery charge. The advantage of going to a larger company is once you have made the investment, it will advise you on best selling lines and give you a guide to the most popular retail products. For the smaller business of a single therapist, it is often a matter of trial and error and experience with the client base which will reveal the fast-moving product lines and those that gather dust.

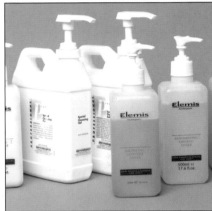

Trade and retail sizes of products

Stock is not just the retail products kept in reception for sales, it also includes the bulk purchase of products used at the workstations, which are often purchased in litres and then decanted into convenient sizes. Many suppliers will provide both trade and retail size products and new therapists soon learn it is far more cost-effective to order trade sizes for treatments while keeping a smaller level of retail stock for sale.

For promotion of products and services and profit margin in retail sales, see Unit G6, Promote additional products or services to clients.

The principles of stock control

Small salons will perform a manual stock take; larger salons with computerised tills will electronically count stock, rather like a supermarket, and automatically adjust stock levels according to the bar code of the product when scanned through the till. Whichever method is used, the principle is the same.

1 Count existing stock, including displays, retail, samples and in treatment rooms.
2 Compare that to the minimum stock level set and if it is below, reorder as required to keep up levels.
3 Coordinate this information with the salon ordering system so that minimum levels do not drop so low that an item goes out of stock.

4 Liaise with colleagues using clear communication to ensure accuracy.

Points 1–4 should be carried out sequentially on a regular basis – small salons may do this at the end of the working day, others weekly and larger salons as a monthly or bi-monthly operation.

Date: 13 October 2004

Code	Description	Size	Minimum stock level	In stock	Sold	On order	Date ordered
	Retail skin care						
1000	Cleanser	200 ml	14	2	12	12	15/10/04
1010	Toner	200 ml	14	5	9	9	
1020	Moisturiser	200 ml	14	6	8	8	
	Salon skin care						
1001	Cleanser	400 ml	14	4	10	10	
1011	Toner	400 ml	14	3	11	11	
1021	Moisturiser	400 ml	14	3	11	11	
	Aftercare pack						
2050	BioSkinJetting 1 and 2	Pack	20	8	12	12	
	Retail camouflage						
3100	Cover Crème Coffee	10 g	6	4	2	2	
3101	Cover Crème Apricot	10 g	6	7	0		
3102	Cover Crème Brown	10 g	6	2	4	4	
3103	Cover Crème Tan	10 g	6	4	2	2	
3104	Cover Crème Barley	10 g	6	4	2	2	
3105	Cover Crème Natural Tan	10 g	6	1	5	5	
	Salon accessories						
4010	Wand holder	Each	1	2	0		
4011	Wands	Each	20	28	0		
4012	Surgical hand piece	Each	1	2	0		
4013	Smoothing ball	20 units	1	2	0		
4014	Sharps box	Each	1	2	0		
4015	Foot switch	Each	1	1	0		
4016	Wand holder spare cable	Each	2	2	0		
	Promotional items						
9000	Client leaflets	50 leaflets	50	20	30	50	
9001	Aftercare leaflet pads	50 leaflets	100	50	50	50	
9002	Consultation cards	25 cards	50	25	25	25	
9003	Badge	Each	4	2	2	2	
9004	Hanging poster (720 x 260mm)	Each	3	2	1	1	

Stock control sheet

Ordering

Stock can be ordered in a variety of ways:

- by post – the top copy of the duplicated stock sheet can be sent off to the supplier
- by telephone – which is the quickest method but can prove unreliable if you are misheard, and if making a big order can prove expensive
- by fax (if available) – the drawback of using this method is that the copy is not always clear, so write in black pen as pencil or light pen does not copy well
- by e-mail (if available)
- in person – give your order to a visiting representative of the supplier.

Deliveries and checking stock

The method of delivery will vary depending on the size of the order. Small items will come through the post in a padded envelope; large orders will arrive in boxes via specialist companies dealing in deliveries; local suppliers will have a delivery van that brings the stock to your door. If your supplier is local, it is possible to pop in personally and pick up stock on the way to work.

Quantity	Description	Sterex initial	Customer initial
1	Salon BioSkinJetting Lotion Size 1	EFS	JH
1	Salon BioSkinJetting Lotion Size 2	EFS	JH
1	Salon BioSkinJetting Cleanser (400 ml)	EFS	JH
1	Salon BioSkinJetting Toner (400 ml)	EFS	JH
1	Salon BioSkinJetting Moisturiser (400 ml)	EFS	JH
3	Retail BioSkinJetting Cleanser (200 ml)	EFS	JH
3	Retail BioSkinJetting Toner (200 ml)	EFS	JH
3	Retail BioSkinJetting Moisturiser (200 ml)	EFS	JH
18	Assorted BioSkinJetting Retail Cover Crème 10 g	EFS	JH
5	BioSkinJetting Finishing Dust 35 g	EFS	JH
1	Surgical Hand Piece	EFS	JH
25	Microprobes (15 x 3s and 10 x 4s)	EFS	JH
1	BioSkinJetting Cover Crème Palette x 18 shades	EFS	JH
5	Client Aftercare Kits	EFS	JH
10	Client Information Leaflets	EFS	JH
1	Sharps Box	EFS	JH
1	BioSkinJetting Badge	EFS	JH
1 pack (25)	Consultation Cards	EFS	JH
1 pack (50)	Aftercare Leaflets	EFS	JH
1	Smoothing Ice Ball	EFS	JH

Date: **9.6.2004**   Checked by: **E F Stoddart**

BioSkinJetting package checklist

Checking stock on arrival

It is important that all deliveries are checked accurately and completed against the order documentation, with any inaccuracies or damage immediately reported to the relevant person. The supplier must be notified immediately and will usually despatch a replacement the same day. Depending on the company's policy and how much the supplier values your custom, this may be free of charge. If the goods are hand delivered, damaged goods will be taken back to the supplier by the delivery person; otherwise you will need to post them.

Resolving resource problems

The working therapist may spot a potential resource problem that the stock controller is unaware of, for example the therapist may notice a seasonal increase in a treatment or publicity in a magazine that may generate interest in a particular product. At the weekly staff meeting, there should be an opportunity for the therapist to recommend increasing stock levels of the particular item. This should not be viewed as challenging the authority of the stock controller, but rather as a positive contribution to the financial effectiveness of the business. The therapist will need to show clearly the benefits to the business and if agreed, implementation may well be immediate. It may be as simple as increasing the basic stockholding, or reinforcing the promotion with displays and demonstrations.

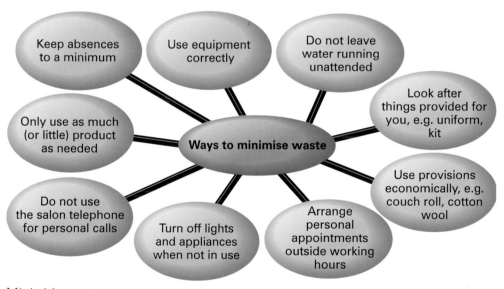

Minimising waste

Check it out

- Who in your salon is responsible for stock control?
- How often is stock ordered?
- How is it delivered?
- What happens if something goes missing?

Remember

You must always remember the limits of your authority when dealing with any stock problems. For example, it may not be your job to complain to the supplier. You might lose goodwill and upset a good working relationship if you interfere when it is not your place to do so.

Remember

Records for which you are responsible should be accurate, legible and up to date.

In the salon

Fiona was expecting a client for a body massage and in her eagerness to prepare she decanted the massage oil into a warmed bowl in readiness. Unfortunately, during the consultation Fiona discovered the client was only having a back massage.

Once decanted, oil cannot be poured back into the original container and so there was considerable wastage. Even though Fiona gave the client the remaining oil for home use, the cost was borne by the salon – which equalled the profit margin from the back massage.

Managing people

Managing people is probably one of the most difficult tasks, but good staff are essential for a growing business. The key to success is to employ the right people in the first place – those who are enthusiastic, show commitment and a willingness to work as part of a team. Once the right team is in place, it will need nurturing. Staff need:

- a professional environment in which to work (see Unit G1, Ensure your own actions reduce risks to health and safety, and **You, your client and the law,** pages 67–8
- a sense of self-esteem through a defined job role, incentives and good staff training
- respect from peers and management as a professional
- financial recognition, e.g. a fair wage for a skilled professional
- appreciation from clients, colleagues and management.

(See **You – the therapist** on pages 10 – 29 for further information on managing resources, tools and equipment, dealing with others, how to cope with conflict and personal time management.)

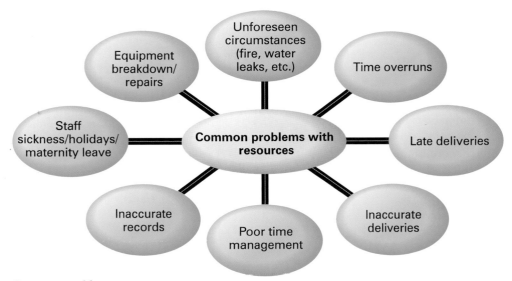

Resource problems

Resolving common problems

Most common problems can be resolved with a calm approach, a little thought and contingency planning. There should be plans in place for a number of unforeseeable difficulties such as staff sickness. Regular staff meetings will allow all staff to be informed of the procedure if a member of staff phones in sick. This may include rearranging appointments by phoning the clients, or drawing upon a bank of part-time staff, who may be available on the day, with minimum disruption to the client. Good quality, professional and efficient staff training will ensure that accurate records are kept, deliveries are accurate, equipment repairs are carried out in good time and time is well managed. For unforeseen circumstances, ensure you know health and safety procedures.

Meet productivity and development targets

G11.2

In most salons, productivity and development targets are set for retail sales, technical services and the staff's personal learning. These three key areas are all essential for the growth and development of the business.

In this outcome you will learn about
• setting and agreeing productivity and development targets   • reviewing and recording your progress   • promotions and opportunities to achieve targets.

Setting and agreeing productivity and development targets

We all react well to praise. By having goals to work towards, you will feel you have achieved something, knowing that your efforts will be recognised.

A keen therapist will want to increase her client base and/or product turnover if she knows that not only is her work to be rewarded with praise but there is an extra incentive to do so. Targets should be realistic and achievable. They should be mutually agreed between you and your manager, with a set target over a defined period of time. It could be monthly, every other month or every three months, depending on your terms of employment. Short-term goals are often a good idea too – they feel more achievable and reinforce the work ethic when reached.

Target setting will be both personal, for your own growth and development, and commercial for the salon, including sales targets, treatments per day, and so on.

It is important that you try to achieve your targets – doing so will not only keep you employed, it will also make you very commercial and give you invaluable experience should you decide to run your own salon or develop a mobile business.

The setting of targets is part of your action plan to improve your performance at work, which is incorporated within the appraisal system of monitoring your performance. You will find it easier to set achievable targets if you make sure they are SMART:

S = Specific. Have particular targets, or aims, in mind rather than too grand an idea. Set a goal specific to you, e.g. I want to complete two assessments each week.

M = Measurable. Make sure you are able to measure your aims with a start and a finish. Assessments can be measured against the NVQ performance criteria and ranges. Targets could be related to sales. You must know what you sell at present, and how much you want to improve, e.g. product sales might be on average £50 per day now, and a 10 per cent increase would raise them to £55 per day.

A = Achievable. Do not set a target that cannot be realised. A short-term target may be to complete an NVQ Level 3 unit by a set date.

R = Realistic. Doing ten treatments an hour is not realistic – be sensible with your aims. How long realistically will it take you to cover all the performance criteria and ranges in one unit?

> **Remember**
>
> Rather than view targets as a negative aspect of work, most therapists look forward to the challenge – knowing that they can only benefit by trying their hardest to achieve. A large salon incentive can be anything from free products or treatments, to a weekend break, shopping vouchers or even a trip abroad. If you read the trade magazines, you will find some fabulous prizes given by commercial companies, rewarding a therapist who has become therapist of the year, or salesperson of the year.

T = Timed. For the target to be achieved there should be a time scale for you to aim towards, e.g. by next month I will improve my timekeeping by 50 per cent or by Christmas I am going to have my portfolio for Unit G6, Promote additional products or services to clients, ready to be signed off by my assessor.

Retail sales

Retail sales are an important part of generating income for the salon as sales are not labour intensive and are very cost-effective. Being successful in selling requires sufficient stock, knowledge of the products and confidence to be able to sell. Retail sales are a major part of your profit and an integral part of your overall treatment and aftercare.

Successful retail selling:

- higher sales brings profits without taking up treatment time
- complements treatments, leading to increased client satisfaction
- helps clients keep up the good work between appointments
- encourages repeat buying when clients like a product
- adds to your exclusivity with professional-only products.

(See also G6, Promote additional products or services to clients.)

Technical services

These refer to your skill areas and how much income you generate for the salon by giving the clients treatments. The appointments page is a good indicator of success in this area. The manager will be looking at the number of clients returning to the same therapist, new clients drawn to her and her treatment portfolio. There is a danger of the therapist favouring certain clients and offloading others, perhaps because they are not as generous. Some therapists like to stay in their comfort zone and ignore those treatments that require greater skills or more time to perform. The appointments pages will reflect this pattern should it emerge. Therefore, in your productivity goals agreed with your line manager, your treatment repertoire will be analysed and targets set for development and increasing your skills base.

Personal learning

Personal learning is your individual development within the existing salon structure and includes:

- selling
- treatments
- identifying gaps in the market
- new training
- working with others
- identifying your strengths and weakness and working to improve them

- responsibility for training others
- taking on more responsibility
- time management
- planning and rescheduling your own work.

Check it out

To improve sales of the salon's aftercare products and gifts, you will need to create a space that people want to be in. The next time you go into the salon, forget that you work there! Think of yourself as if you were a client or even a competitor. Take an objective approach and note what detracts from the environment you are in, what looks poor and what looks interesting. Where is your eye drawn to and why? Be your own worst critic and work out how to improve your space and your service.

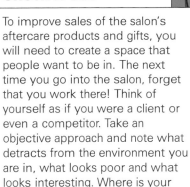

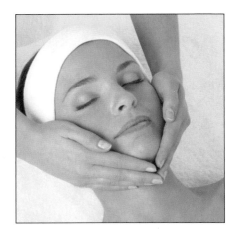

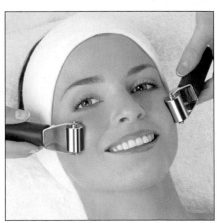

Some therapists enjoy performing hands-on treatments, while others may prefer electrical treatments

Remember

When working with others, always give clear, accurate and timely instructions to those who may be assisting you.

Agreeing targets

Agreeing targets for productivity and development with your line manager requires good communication, preparation and a willingness to accept the process and the feedback as constructive. (For detailed communication skills, see **You and your client**, pages 28–31.)

A good manager will set realistic targets in discussion with you, and you should feel able to negotiate an achievable goal. If targets set are unachievable, staff become demotivated, relations become strained, the business is affected and a no-win situation results. It is important to regularly review targets to consolidate and to keep them SMART (see pages 124–5).

When achievable targets are not met, there will also be consequences for the business.

Improving your performance

Your performance will develop alongside your experiences in the salon, but you will also need to set a target for improvement.

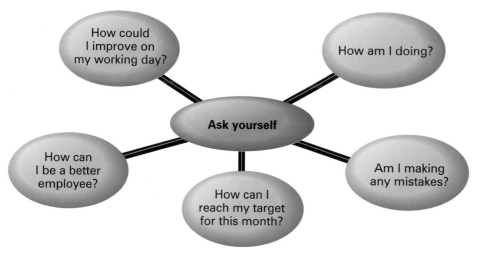

Improving yourself requires self-analysis

Self-analysis is essential for growth and maturity of the therapist within a salon environment. This is often referred to as professional development, and some companies provide a commercial professional development folder – rather like a record of achievement at school! All your training certificates and qualifications may be put in there, and it helps you spot where there are gaps in your training.

Identifying training needs

If a therapist keeps making the same mistakes over and over, and clients complain or stop coming to the salon altogether, this indicates that something is wrong! Often, with age, it is easier to be reflective and spot our own mistakes and then make changes to put things right. Sometimes it is not so easy to be inward looking, and this is where a good manager will help by giving regular work-related reviews. This is called an appraisal.

Targets not met

Unhappy and demoralised therapist

Pressure from superiors and peers

Stress/illness/time off sick resulting in worsening figures

Ineffectual/seen as not being team player

Costs to the business financially

Loss of job

Loss of business

Failure to achieve targets will affect the business

Many large companies provide both self-assessment sheets for the employee to fill in, throughout a set period, and then a joint review sheet with the manager, to help improve performance.

A self-assessment appraisal is not just about achievement within the job role, and how many sales have been completed – that is really only a part of being a therapist. (However, it is an important aspect of remaining profitable.) It is also about short-term plans and development of the individual and it opens up many areas for discussion between a manager and an employee. It should highlight how well the individual is coping within his or her job role, whether the salon is asking too much of an employee, and provides an opportunity for the therapist to offer opinions on improvement.

The diagram below shows the benefits of keeping within treatment times, as an example of good performance.

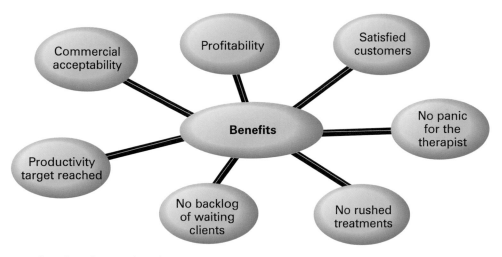

Benefits of working within the treatment time

An appraisal or team review should happen on a regular basis, perhaps once a month, or every three months.

- It should be at a mutually agreeable time.
- It should be constructive and open, not conducted in fear of job loss.
- It should be objective and as non-personal as possible.
- It should be a review for both parties, not just a performance judgement.
- It should be constructive and positive.
- It should leave the employee feeling enthusiastic, not depressed!

Reviewing and recording your progress

A self-assessment form can contain whatever the employer/manager feels is relevant to the job role. On the next page is an example of a common format.

Remember

Appraisal will give you the opportunity to learn, progress in personal growth and maintain good working relationships. It is important to react positively to any feedback or review. Nobody likes criticism, but it is important to listen carefully to what is said and take on board the suggestions and advice being offered to you. Appraisal should be viewed very much as a two-way discussion, not a reprimand.

Remember

When negotiating targets with your line manager there should be a mutual respect. Avoid confrontation and try to appreciate the greater experience and wealth of knowledge your manager has. Consider the bigger picture – look, listen and learn. Your manager may be pressurising you because he or she is confident in your abilities to deliver, and also has greater responsibilities to ensure steady growth within the business.

A self-assessment form

Salon: Blissed Out

Date: 5 July 2004

Position held: Beauty Therapist

Therapist: Yocilida Jones

Please add comments on how you feel you are progressing in each area listed. Thank you.

Appearance — Good. I do try to look professional every day.

Absences — Room for improvement as I have had 5 working days ill with flu this month. However, no other absences this year.

Time keeping — Could be better. I have been late twice this month as I have been relying on public transport. I have now organised a car share system with a colleague to ensure this will not be a problem in the future.

Job performance — Good. My regular clients always ask for me, and I have worked hard this month to attract new ones.

Sales targets — Good, as above. My sales are from my regulars but with the help of our recent sales meetings I am developing additional sales with other clients. My sales figure this month is in excess of target to date. My annual figures are well on target.

Treatment targets — In light of our recent training, I am not content to stay in my comfort zone and am actively encouraging my existing clients to try new treatments. This month I have had 3 clients book in for the new body-wrap treatment we have launched.

Strengths — I am confident with my treatments and I especially enjoy facial electrical treatments.

Weaknesses — Time management. Treatment can over-run because of time spent on sales at reception, therefore I need one of the juniors to prepare my working area ready for the next client. I am happy to train whichever junior is designated to this task and will communicate my requirements daily.

Any areas of change — I have organised for Joanna to assist in the wet area – putting clients in the sauna – this month, as Carol seems to have the flu bug that I had and is still off sick.

Staff development request — I would like to go on a BioSkinJetting training day if possible, as we have been asked for the treatment by several regular clients.

Action plan for next review — To improve on time management and complete my course.

Feedback

It is important to get feedback on your performance, both good and bad, to help you grow into a commercial therapist and enable you to develop your skills and maturity. It also helps you become more employable, opening up new exciting avenues of opportunity in your career.

In the salon

Sarah and Caroline have both been working at Escape for the same amount of time, and are each due to have a review of their job role and performance by their manager.

Sarah is a hard worker, reliable, punctual and enthusiastic, and thinks of her review as an opportunity for further development. Caroline is not as reliable as Sarah, particularly her time keeping and punctuality, and she is not always motivated. Caroline is not looking forward to her appraisal – she feels threatened and feels sure she is going to get a reprimand.

- Who needs the appraisal the most? Why do you think that?
- How can both employees get the most from their appraisal?
- If you were the manager, how would you handle each review?

Promotions and opportunities to achieve targets

As well as carrying out treatments to the very best of your ability, you must keep abreast of trends and innovations within the beauty industry. Beauty editors are sent hundreds of samples and given treatments to promote the latest innovative developments, as a favourable report generates free publicity in newspapers and magazines. Advertisements in both men's and women's magazines keep clients aware of the latest treatments, so expect your clients to ask for them.

You should find out how your salon keeps up with the latest trends, for example visiting major trade shows is an excellent way of seeing demonstrations of new equipment and products. Entering national competitions is also a good way to meet like-minded professionals and share good practice. This can help to raise the standard of skill levels in the industry, and motivate and enthuse all who take part.

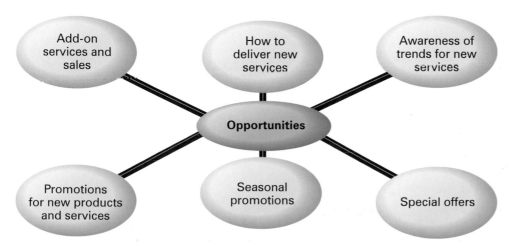

Opportunities to achieve productivity and development targets

Promotion

The first step is to allocate a percentage of the business's income to promotion and to use some of the profits generated by sales to help generate future sales and drive the business forward. Promotions are about perception – how your existing and potential clients see you and your business. It is about steady and maintained business growth and increased profitability.

Objectives

Marketing needs careful planning, for example a salon might set an annual budget and then plan advertising and promotions on a monthly basis. It can be as little as £50 per month or it could be set as a percentage of turnover, but it is essential to think ahead to maximise the return on the business's investment. The first thing to consider is the business's unique selling points (USPs).

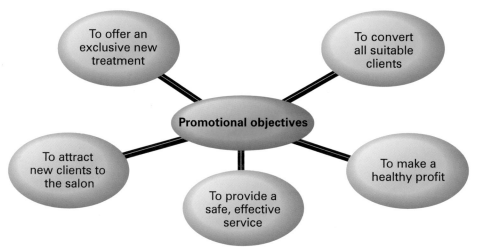

The salon's promotional objectives

Proactive promotion

A perfect way to boost sales, increase bookings and attract new clients is through sales promotion. It is important to put together a calendar of promotional activity at the beginning of the year so that you endeavour to promote your business throughout the year. Highlight quiet periods or the times when you are introducing something new. Ensure that there is always something happening within the salon.

Promotional activity enables you to:

- allow clients to try treatments or products they have not experienced before
- retain customer loyalty
- convey an impression of activity and change within the salon
- attract new clients
- improve customer satisfaction
- improve your public relations.

Newspaper advertising

Local advertising tips

- Use suppliers' or manufacturers' additional marketing support information and packages whenever possible.

- Make sure you have a chance to see your completed advert before it is printed and keep a copy of the proof.
- Request a good position in the paper. If you advertise regularly, the paper will probably do this for no extra charge.
- If you have a choice of publications, find out which one best covers your area, and suits your needs.
- If you pre-book a number of issues, ask for a discount – just as clients do when they book a course with you.

One other method is to advertise in the local Yellow Pages. This is a measurable way of reaching potential clients in your area.

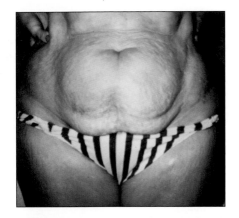

Journalists

Invite a local reporter to visit your salon for a treatment. This may result in a feature article written about the salon and the treatment given. The following tips may help when dealing directly with the media.

- Avoid answering questions with a simple 'yes' or 'no'. Provide as much relevant information as possible, which will allow the journalist to write an interesting article full of useful information.
- Try to anticipate what the journalist will ask; you will then be able to prepare answers to likely questions.
- Remember to be positive. Tell the journalist what you do offer, not what you don't.
- Keep your communication suitable for the consumer – avoid jargon. Use language that everyone will be able to understand.

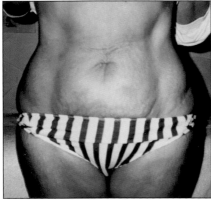

Showing before and after photographs of clients is an effective way of promoting treatments

Press releases

Use simple statements with a strong headline. Always cover the key facts, avoid using jargon and include a quote.

If you are successful, your information may be included in the editional content of a local publication.

- Editorial is more effective than advertising.
- Two to three days after sending your press release to the beauty editor, phone and check that it has been received. Invite the editor for a complimentary service at the same time and start to build a relationship.
- If you are prepared to offer a competition prize, let the editor know. Newspapers love to offer prizes to their readers.
- If a journalist comes to see you, make sure your salon looks at its best and that you make his or her time as enjoyable as possible.
- If you are holding an event at your salon, let the local paper know in advance.

Radio advertising

There are numerous local radio stations operating from town or city centres and hospitals. The radio station may wish to cover a beauty therapy topic and this would be a good opportunity for you to participate and lend your expertise. This will often attract clients and is good experience for you.

Mailings

There are many different types of mailings, including:

- distributing leaflets through letterboxes
- negotiating an 'insert' of your leaflet within the local newspaper

- approaching local businesses who may consider supplying leaflets to their employees.

Leaflet drops could be questionnaires which, when completed, the prospective client could drop into the salon in return for a gift. This will give you invaluable information for future marketing strategies and possibly gain a new client.

If you concentrate distribution of leaflets in small controlled areas, you will be able to assess the feedback quite easily, and this will allow you to work out a systematic method for future mailings.

Newsletters

In the run-up to Christmas, a newsletter detailing special offers and Christmas gift vouchers should help to increase sales. It does not have to be professionally produced – you could produce your own leaflet on a computer – but it does need to look professional and be spell checked!

Clients love to know everything that is going on in 'their' salon. Suggestions for news might be:

- a treatment new to the salon
- a new therapist joining the salon
- a therapist leaving
- news of special offers or promotions
- advance information regarding an open evening
- review of a previous open evening
- reminder to book early for Christmas, the summer holiday season, etc.

How often should you send newsletters? The answer is as often as is profitable. Analyse the results, and if sales go up, you have it right, so keep doing what you are doing!

Local clubs and groups

Local clubs and societies often struggle to find interesting speakers. You could offer to give a talk for the local women's groups and other groups, or give demonstrations of various treatments your salon offers, to tempt members into the salon.

Promoting the business locally

Local shop owners and workers will be more willing to help you with promotion (and more enthusiastic about your services) if you offer them a complimentary service or two.

Give leaflets to all salon clients. Offer them a discount or a complimentary treatment when they introduce a friend.

Open evenings are an excellent way to attract new clients to the salon. To make sure the evening goes well, you may like to try some of these tips.

- Advertise the evening well in advance.
- Have enough staff on hand to talk to the clients.
- Run a competition to win free treatments, or give special offers on products or services, to encourage prospective clients.
- Offer good quality, complimentary refreshments.
- Timing is everything – capitalise upon an occasion (e.g. Summer holidays), try to have a theme and encourage sales by selling gifts and offering free gift-wrapping.
- Dare to be different – organise a male-only night.
- Offer loyalty schemes and bonus-points incentives.

You could also try marketing ideas such as vouchers. For example, when clients make a purchase they will be given three or four vouchers with offers relating to their next visit or possibly money-off vouchers to try a new treatment. Alternatively, a customer loyalty scheme, where clients are rewarded under a bonus-point system, could increase their loyalty and number of purchases. This way you encourage the clients to try things they may not have considered before. These schemes have been tremendously successful and encourage both brand and salon loyalty.

Capitalising on celebrations

Father's Day, Mother's Day, Easter, Valentine's Day, birthdays, Christmas, Yom Kippur, New Year and New Year's resolutions – the list of special occasions when clients may be encouraged to bring you extra business is endless!

Testimonials

Written recommendations, known as testimonials, are the best advertising you could ever achieve as long as plenty of people get to read them. Ask your happy, satisfied clients to write a comment on the treatment and how pleased they are with the salon and its services.

A makeover is a special treat to celebrate a milestone birthday

E-mail

Record e-mail addresses whenever available. E-mail is a rapidly growing form of communication, and the great thing about using it in marketing is the low cost. It costs very little to send an e-mail, so you can send details of special offers or promotions to all your clients for no more than the cost of the telephone connection. Alternatively, if you use an external marketing company, it is now possible to send full-colour e-mail bulletins or 'e-bulletins', including full-colour photographs, for less than the price of a first-class stamp.

> **Remember**
>
> Sending too many e-mails, and e-mails that take too long to download, are annoying, and can cost the client extra money. You will put the client off by sending SPAM e-mails.

Dynamic displays

Displays must be eye catching and attractive, regularly updated, topical and spotlessly clean. Think about what you want to say about your salon and yourself – does your window display do you justice? (For more information, see Unit G6, Promote additional products or services to clients, page 114.)

Using and converting existing clients

A large number of customers will be existing salon clients. It is therefore important to find out which treatments and products your clients would be willing to purchase. Identify your target market by asking yourself the following questions.

- What are my client profiles?
- Who are my ideal clients?
- What methods am I using to target clients, and are these achievable?
- What percentage of my business consists of existing clients?
- Do I keep my old clients?
- Do I know if my clients are satisfied?
- Do I have an updated database, and if so, how frequently do I use it?
- Am I making the best possible use of the resources available (including media resources, the local community and financial services)?
- Are my opening hours suitable for the people I am trying to attract?

- Am I aware of current plans for the local area that might affect my business?
- Am I making the best use of the local community?
- Am I involved and aware of local activities that could be of benefit to the salon?
- What is the public view of the salon in the local community?
- Where are my main competitors located? Realistically, how much of a threat are they to my business?
- How do I differentiate products and services from competitor salons?
- Do I know my best-selling product and treatment?
- Do I have an adequate stock system in place?
- Am I cross-selling products?
- Do I display products effectively?
- Are there any niche markets that I could reach and attract to the salon?

Knowledge check

1   Why should you not wear jewellery when carrying out electrical treatments?

2   List five ways you can ensure your personal safety.

3   Why is good posture essential when carrying out body massage treatments?

4   Carry out a risk assessment for your own work and list five factors which contribute to the safety of yourself and your clients.

5   Give five essential safety rules for using electrical equipment.

6   Give examples of what you consider to be safe salon conduct.

7   Give one example of possible conflict in the salon and how you would deal with it.

8   List four duties in the salon that you are responsible for.

9   List four duties you are not responsible for, and should not attempt to do.

10   Why is it important to care for your tools?

11   Why should the client have full understanding of product use?

12   What should a good display of the salon's products achieve?

13   When might you need to refer clients to alternative sources for treatments?

14   What do you understand by time management? Give three examples.

15   Give three important things to remember when sharing equipment.

related anatomy and
PHYSIOLOGY

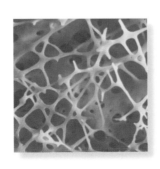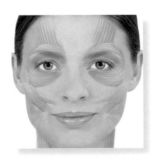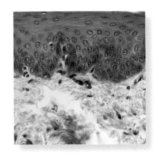

Related anatomy and physiology

As a beauty therapist you will perform a range of manual, mechanical and electrical body and facial treatments, and each of these treatments will have specific benefits for and effects on the client. It is your responsibility to assess the suitability of each client for treatment through consultation, making sure clients do not have any **contra-indications** which could result in adverse reactions.

Another of your responsibilities is to understand how the treatments work, on a physical and physiological level, and to relate the effects to the client. In order to fulfil your responsibilities as a beauty therapist, it is essential that you have a sound knowledge of how the body works; its structure, or anatomy, and its functions, or physiology.

This section of the book will help you to explore the structures and functions of the human body, from cells and skin to muscles and bones, as well as all the body's internal systems, such as circulatory and lymphatic systems. You will learn how the various parts of the body work together to keep us living, breathing and working. Many students struggle at first to understand the science aspects of beauty therapy, but these pages provide an introduction and you will continue to learn about how the body works and relate this essential knowledge to your developing expertise in beauty therapy.

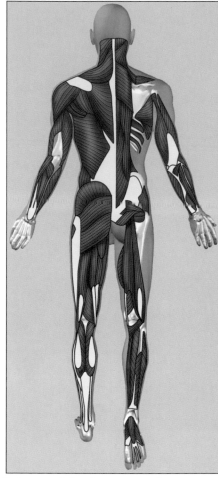

It is essential to have a sound knowledge of the underlying structures of the human body

Cells and tissues

You will learn about

- biological organisation
- cells
- tissues
- organs and organ systems.

Biological organisation

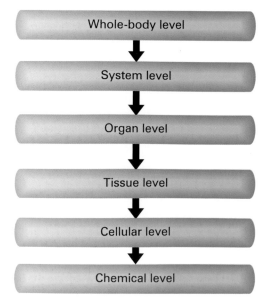

Hierarchy of biological structures

In order to understand how the human body functions, the different levels of biological organisation need to be explored. These are arranged in a hierarchy of structures. The smallest biological structure which can exist independently is the **cell**. A cell consists of structures called **organelles**, meaning 'little organs'. Many different types of cell make up the human body and each group of cells has its own distinct structure and function. For example, cells called **melanocytes**, which are found in the deepest layers of the skin, are responsible for producing the colour pigment **melanin**. Groups of cells with a shared structure and function are called **tissues**, and the human body contains many examples – muscular tissue builds muscle, connective tissue holds everything together and blood is an example of a fluid tissue.

An **organ**, such as the heart, kidneys or skin, is a specialised structure which consists of different types of tissues organised in a specific way. Each organ has a particular and unique function. For example, the heart and kidneys are important organs. The heart pumps blood around the body and to the lungs while the kidneys filter the blood to remove harmful waste substances.

The uppermost level of organisation is the **organ system**. This term is used to refer to a group of organs which work together. In the circulatory (or cardiovascular) system, for example, the heart works in conjunction with the vast network of blood vessels to pump blood all around the body. So the hierarchy of biological organisation, from the basic cell to the complex organ system, makes up the human body to produce a living, breathing, eating, reproducing and fully functioning person.

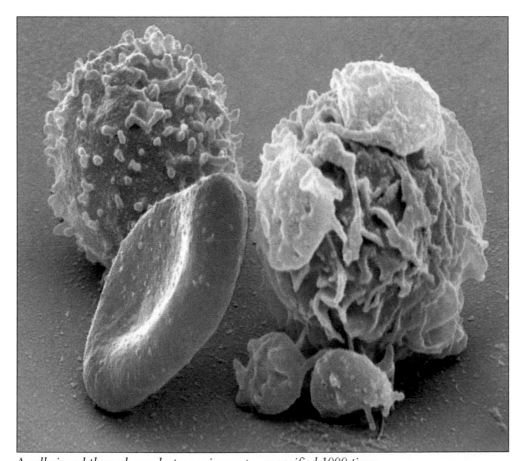

A cell viewed through an electron microscope, magnified 1000 times

Cells

The cell is the basic building block of all life forms. There are many types of cell in the human body which vary in size, structure and function and as such there is no such thing as a 'typical cell'. However, cells do have certain structural characteristics in common.

Structure of cells

Cells are minute structures which can only be studied using specialist viewing equipment called microscopes. The structure of cells viewed through electron microscopes is sometimes called the ultra-structure to emphasise the high levels of magnification required. Different parts of the ultra-structure are known collectively as **organelles**.

Structure	Function
Plasma/cell membrane	Outer or cell membrane – layer of lipids sandwiched between two layers of larger protein molecules allows selective permeability, passive transport of fat soluble substances, active transport of charged particles.
Mitochondria	Often referred to as the power-houses of the cell, these rod-shaped structures consist of a double membrane. The inner membrane is folded into ridges which contain enzymes that break down glucose to form a compound rich in energy called adenosine triphosphate (ATP).
Ribosomes	Some are attached to rough ER (see below); some remain free in cytoplasm. Contain ribonucleic acid (RNA). Manufacture enzymes and proteins both for export and for use within the cell.
Endoplastic reticulum (ER)	A network of branches with similar structure to and continuous with plasma membrane. Rough ER is studded with ribosomes which contribute to cell support, and channel transport materials within the cell. Rough ER produces proteins and enzymes; smooth ER produces phospholipids and steroids.
Gogli apparatus	Similar to smooth ER with vesicles that contain proteins and enzymes, lipids, collagen and mucus. Produces collagen and mucus, keeps all secretions away from cytoplasm, is best developed in secretory cells such as those in the pancreas and salivary glands.
Lysosomes	Powerful enzymes produced as vesicles from the Gogli apparatus. Break down bacteria and destroy damaged cell structures and extracellular matter, e.g. osteoclasts in bone formation.
Nucleus	Largest cell structure, containing a double-layered membrane continuous with the ER. Contains a tangle mass of chromatins made up of DNA (deoxyribonucleic acid) and protein. Controls all cellular activities, genetic material and nucleic acids (DNA and RNA).

Structure and function of cell organelles

Tissues

A group of cells which all perform the same function is called a **tissue**. Some cells have more than one function and can therefore be classified as more than one type of tissue, for example some cells of the immune system are also blood cells. Tissues can be classified into four main groups:

- epithelial
- connective
- muscular
- nervous.

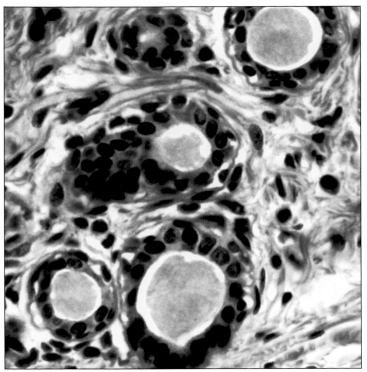

Human tissues

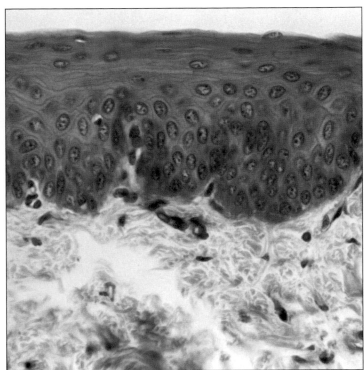

Types of epithelial tissue

Epithelial tissue

Epithelial tissue (epithelium) provides the lining for surfaces inside and outside the body, protecting it from wear and tear and continually renewing itself as required. Epithelial tissue is also the tissue from which glands are developed. Lining epithelia can be subdivided according to its structure. The various types are shown in the table below.

Type	Structure	Location
Simple pavement	Simple flat cells form a smooth lining	Lining blood vessel walls
Simple cuboidal epithelium	Simple cube-shaped cells	Covering the ovaries
Simple columnar epithelium	Tall, column-shaped cells on a basement membrane providing greater protection against wear and tear	Lining the stomach and intestines
Ciliated columnar epithelium	Tall, column-shaped cells with hair-like projections which move mucus and other substances	Lining the respiratory tract
Stratified epithelium	Many layers of cells with flattened surface	Skin
Transitional epithelium	Similar to stratified epithelium but with rounded surface cells which adapt to expansion	Waterproof organs, e.g. bladder

Types of epithelial tissue

Glands

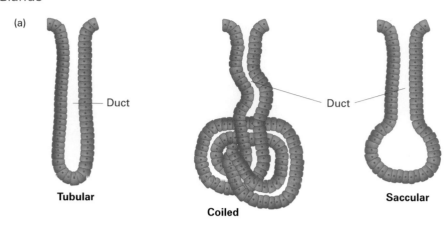

(a)

Tubular

Coiled

Saccular

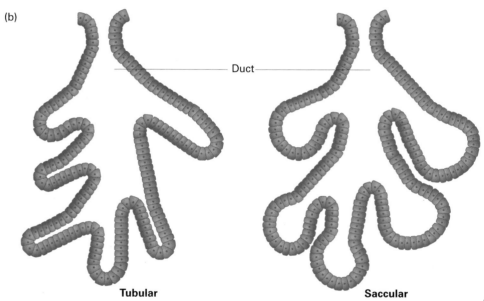

(b)

Tubular

Saccular

Simple and compound glands

Glands develop from epithelial tissue and can be classified as **exocrine** or **endocrine**. Endocrine glands secrete hormones directly into the bloodstream (see page 168). Exocrine glands pass their secretions through a single duct (simple glands) or through several secretory ducts (compound glands). Many of these secretions contain enzymes which produce chemical changes in specific substances but remain unchanged by the reaction. The types of exocrine glands are shown in the table below.

Type	Location in the body	Secretions
Simple tubular glands	Walls of small intestine, stomach	Substances which aid digestion
Simple coiled glands	Sweat glands in skin	Sweat to control body temperature
Simple saccular glands	Sebaceous glands in skin	Sebum which lubricates skin and hair
Compound tubular glands	Duodenum	Substances which aid digestion
Compound saccular glands	Salivary glands in mouth	Substances which aid digestion

Types of exocrine glands

Connective tissue

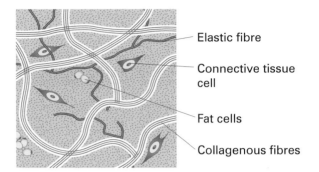

Connective tissue

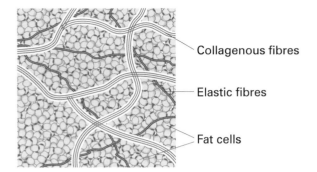

Adipose tissue

As the name suggests, connective tissue connects and supports all other types of tissue. It consists of living cells as well as non-living matrix and fibres. There are two types of fibres.

- Collagenous fibres develop from cells called fibroblasts which secrete **collagen**, the main supporting cells of the body. These form coarse fibres which are grouped into bundles.
- Elastic fibres allow for the stretchy or elastic properties required in some areas of the body such as tendons and internal organs.

There are five types of connective tissue, as shown in the table below.

Type	Structure	Location in the body
Loose connective tissue or areolar tissue	Loose network of collagen and elastic fibres, few blood cells and nerves, some fat cells	Forms tough transparent lining between and within organs
Fatty tissue or **adipose** tissue	Similar to areolar tissue but with network of fat cells which provides food reserves for the body and insulates against heat loss	Protects delicate organs such as the kidneys
Dense connective tissue or fibrons tissue	Bundles of strong collagenous fibres and fibroblasts arranged regularly or irregularly	Regular bundles in tendons, ligaments, irregular arrangement in fascia surrounding muscles
Cartilage	Cells called chondrocytes separated by fibres, no blood vessels, tough and elastic	Intervertebral discs
Bone tissue	Specialised type of cartilage which has undergone ossification, collagenous fibres provide strength and mineral salts provide rigidity, has a rich blood supply	Bones of the human skeleton

Types of connective tissue

Muscle tissue

Muscle cells are long and thin, and often called muscle fibres. Muscle contraction produces skeletal movement. Muscle tissue can contract without first being stretched, unlike elastic connective tissue fibres. There are three types of muscle tissue, which are shown in the table below.

Type	Structure	Function
Skeletal muscle or voluntary muscle or striped muscle	Long muscle cells/fibres containing striped myofibrils of actin and myosin bound together by connective tissue, with rich blood supply provided by capillaries running between muscle cells	Contracts strongly when stimulated to provide voluntary movement
Smooth muscle or unstriped muscle	Spindle-shaped cells bound together by connective tissue, supplied by automatic nerves	Contracts automatically without conscious contractions over long periods of time
Cardiac muscle	Short, cylindrical branched fibres bound together by connective tissue which allows nerve impulses to spread from one to another and along the muscle. Involuntary and irregularly striped	Contractions are controlled by nerves, occur automatically throughout life in the heart wall only

Types of muscle tissue

Nervous tissue

Nervous tissue consists of nerve calls called **neurones**. Neurones have a large cell body containing a nucleus as well as several short projections called **dendrites** and one long projection called an **axon**. The function of nervous tissue is to transmit messages or nervous impulses from inside or outside the body to other tissues in a process of communication. The dendrites import nervous impulses from other cells and tissues while the axon exports nervous impulses away from the cell body to other structures. You could think of dendrites as taking incoming calls and axons as making outgoing calls from a single neurone!

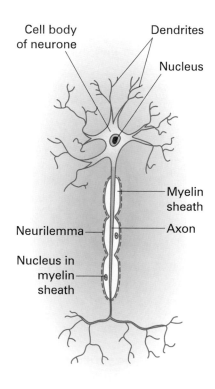

A neurone

Organs and organ systems

A group of tissues functioning together is called an organ. The skin is an example of an organ which consists of epithelial tissue, connective tissue and muscular tissue. Organs can be classified as tubular or compact and while each type shares some common structures, none are identical. All organs contain a blood supply.

Type	Structure	Example
Tubular	Three common layers – outer epithelium, middle muscular layer, inner endothelium – plus unique layers associated with its individual function and a space called a lumen	Heart, small intestine
Compact	Superficial layers called the cortex; deeper layers called the medulla; no lumen	Liver, kidney

Types of organ

One or more organs functioning together is called an **organ system**. The structure and function of each organ system is shown in the table below.

System	Structure	Function
Circulatory	Blood, heart and blood vessels – arteries, veins, arterioles, venules and capillaries	Transports oxygen and nutrients to the tissues in blood and carries waste away
Respiratory	Mouth, nasal cavities, trachea, bronchii, bronchioles, lungs	Facilitates gaseous exchange (oxygen and carbon dioxide) between body and environment
Lymphatic	Lymph, lymphatic vessels, lymph nodes, spleen	Filters and eliminates harmful bacteria and waste, produces lymphocytes which fight infection
Digestive	Mouth, oesophagus, pancreas, liver, gall bladder, stomach, small and large intestines	Breaks down food and facilitates the absorption of nutrients and elimination of waste
Urinary	Kidneys, bladder, ureter, urethra	Main excretory system, storage and elimination of urine
Nervous	Central nervous system – brain and spinal cord, peripheral nervous system and sense organs	System of communication within body and between the body and the environment
Endocrine	Endocrine glands – hypothalamus, pituitary, thyroid, adrenals, gonads and pancreas	Produces hormones which control many functions and facilitate homeostatic regulation
Skeletal	Axial and appendicular skeleton, joints, cartilage and tendons	Supporting framework which provides protection and facilitates movement
Muscular	Skeletal muscles	Facilitates movement in conjunction with skeletal system
Reproductive	Male – penis, testis, epididymis, scrotum, sperm duct; female – ovaries, uterus, vagina, mammary glands	Hormonal regulation, menstrual cycle, fertilisation, pregnancy, birth, lactation, continuation of the species

Organ systems

Skin

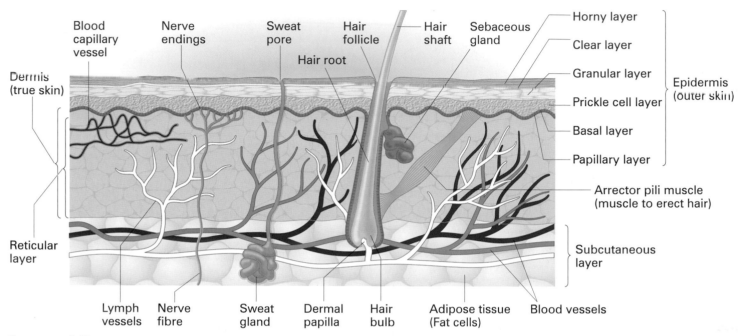

Structure of skin

The skin acts like a container to keep fluids inside as well as a barrier to keep certain substances out, such as harmful bacteria, dirt and excess moisture. We are able to feel sensations such as pain or heat because of sensors in the skin which transmit messages to the brain and our skin plays a major role in maintaining optimum body temperature and in protecting the body from harm.

The skin has many different surfaces. Some are smooth while others contain deep furrows. Some areas of skin are covered with fine, soft hair while other areas are covered with much thicker, coarser hairs which serve a different function. Some areas of skin are thicker than others and have a coarser texture. Some areas might feel more oily than others because of the larger number of oil-producing glands and larger pore size. Some areas of the skin are much more sensitive to heat or pain. Skin also comes in a variety of colours. As well as the effect of sunlight and the melanin content, the colour of skin is also affected by the amount and condition of blood vessels and by the thickness of skin. Even different areas of one person's face consist of a variety of colours and textures.

These are important considerations for beauty therapy treatments which involve the use of colour, such as the application of make-up, eyebrow tints or nail enamelling. Skin colour, as well as texture, can also determine such factors as skin sensitivity, dehydration and allergy, which together with any illness and fatigue will influence the analysis and diagnosis of clients for a variety of beauty therapy treatments.

The functions of skin

Skin has six main functions:

- sensation
- heat regulation
- absorption
- protection
- excretion
- secretion.

Sensation

The sense of touch is often thought of as the most important function of the skin. We touch ourselves a countless number of times each day when we wash, dress, apply products, rub an aching limb or scratch away an itch. Touch is also an important way in which we communicate our feelings with others and, of course, it is the basic technique of most, if not all, beauty and complementary therapy treatments. It is the underlying principle of manual or 'hands on' treatments.

In the same way that people transmit and receive messages through touch, the skin is involved in a communication process with the brain via sensory nerves which carry messages around the body. There are thousands of sensory nerve endings in the skin which send and receive messages to and from the brain. They recognise sensations of pain, pressure, touch, heat and cold on the skin and carry messages about these sensations to the brain, which sets off a reaction. For example, if the finger is pricked with a pin, the sensory nerve endings in that area will recognise the skin damage and send a message to the brain. The brain will send a message back to the finger which is recognised as pain and instructs the finger to move. Of course, this all happens very quickly! Some messages do not travel as far as the brain, but instead produce automatic and immediate reflex actions in response to the stimulation of the nerve endings. So, the skin's function of sensation is a two-way process of receiving and transmitting information between the external world and the internal systems.

Heat regulation

The skin plays an important role in helping to maintain the optimum body temperature for normal functioning of its systems. Normal body temperature, which is measured by a thermometer either under the tongue or in the axilla, is 36.8°C. Body temperature is slightly higher at night than in the morning and higher in younger than older people as they tend to be more active, but it fluctuates slightly as a response to internal or external factors. Extreme changes in body temperature can be dangerous, even fatal. Like sensation, temperature regulation is controlled as the brain stimulates specific nerve endings in the skin. Body temperature is regulated internally in two ways, by sweating and vasodilation.

Sweating

Sweat comprises water and waste products, and the amount excreted varies according to changes in temperature. The body is producing small amounts of sweat all the time, which we are usually unaware of, and this serves to maintain the temperature of the body. When body temperature increases, more sweat is produced in an attempt to lower the body's internal temperature through the process of evaporation. Body temperature can increase as a response to external or internal factors such as a hot climate, vigorous activity, stress or illness.

Vasodilation

The skin, like the entire body, contains a network of vessels which transport blood. The smallest and most superficial of these vessels are **capillaries**. Vasodilation of the capillaries causes them to expand, resulting in a larger superficial surface area. As more blood is brought closer to the surface of the skin, it can cool down more quickly, cooling the body at the same time. When the body feels cold the opposite happens. **Vasoconstriction** of the capillaries results in a smaller surface area and less blood volume close to the skin's surface, so less heat is lost. Another change that occurs on the surface of the skin when the body feels cold is the appearance of 'goose bumps' which make the little hairs on the skin stand up on end. These hairs trap warm air close to the skin's surface, providing insulation to help to maintain the body's normal temperature.

Absorption

One of the skin's most important properties is its ability to repel moisture and bacteria and, on the whole, act as a waterproof seal. To this end, the skin has the ability to absorb only a small amount of oily substances. The outermost layer of the **epidermis**, the stratum corneum (see pages 148-9), acts as a barrier against water, though a tiny amount can be absorbed, and oily substances can be absorbed via the hair follicles. Many molecules are simply too big to penetrate the skin at all. Manual massage and electrical current which is applied in some salon treatments such as galvanism or high frequency aids absorption by dissolving larger molecules and thus assisting their passage through the layers of the skin.

The varying thicknesses of the stratum corneum affect the absorption of substances. Where it is thickest, on the soles of the feet, there is limited absorption. Where it is thinner, on the face and neck, absorption is greatest. Absorption is further assisted by manual or mechanical exfoliation which helps to remove the outer keritinised layers of the stratum corneum.

Protection

The skin serves to protect the body and its internal structures in a number of ways. Physical sensation alerts the sensory receptors to environmental factors which may cause damage through the perception of heat, cold and pain. Skin is also a water-tight container. If it were not, the body would absorb the water it came into contact with whenever a person went swimming or took a shower, and also the water inside the body would escape. The stratum corneum, or horny layer, together with a layer of fatty tissue provide this water-tight seal. The fatty **adipose** tissue has a further protective quality. It cushions the body against knocks and blows, protecting the bones and internal organs from injury.

Ultraviolet light is a well-documented enemy of the skin and exposure to it can cause severe, irreversible damage such as burning or skin cancer. When the skin is exposed to the sun, melanocytes are stimulated to produce increased levels of the colour pigment melanin. This darkens the outer layers of the epidermis and slows down penetration by ultraviolet rays to the deeper layers of the **dermis**. Melanin production protects the skin by blocking out some of the harmful effects of UV.

The skin and sunlight also work together to benefit the body. Exposure to ultraviolet rays stimulates the production of vitamin D by the skin, which is necessary to promote healthy bone tissue. The skin requires protection from harmful bacteria and other disease-forming micro-organisms. The stratum corneum blocks the invasion of foreign bodies, while sebum has a mild antiseptic quality and so can destroy some bacteria. Sweat and sebum combine to form the **acid mantle** which helps to prevent invasion by bacteria and fungi.

The acid mantle

The skin has the ability to balance acid and alkaline factors and maintain a **pH** of 4.5 to 5.5. This is what is known as the acid mantle.

The acid mantle plays a part in the function of protection as it prevents the invasion of harmful micro-organisms which could cause infection. Because of the alkaline content of cleansing products, excessive or incorrect use will have the effect of stripping the skin of its natural oils. As sebum has an antibacterial effect, the disturbance of the pH balance combined with the drying effect can leave skin prone to infection and irritation.

Nourishing products	
pH	Similar acidic pH to skin (4.5–5.5)
Examples	Moisturisers, cuticle conditioners, massage mediums, nourishing masks, hair conditioners
Precautions	Use correct product for skin/hair type to avoid over-nourishment
Cleansing products	
pH	Alkaline pH
Examples	Cleansers, exfoliators, cleansing masks, soap, shampoo
Precautions	Overuse can have a drying effect

pH of nourishing and cleansing products

Excretion

The skin eliminates waste products by excretion. The sweat glands excrete sweat which contains salt, urea and other impurities which would be hazardous to the body if not expelled. Excretion of sweat is minimal under normal circumstances.

Secretion

The skin secretes substances from specialised cells and glands which are beneficial to the health of the skin. For example, the sebaceous gland secretes sebum which is an oily substance made up of fatty acids and waxes. Sebum serves the purpose of nourishing the skin and hair and also plays a part in protecting against infection.

The structure of skin

Some of the skin's structures such as sweat and sebaceous glands and blood vessels and nerves have been discussed above.

Remember

The letters pH stand for 'percentage Hydrogen'. The pH value given to a substance identifies whether the substance is acid or alkaline; pH is measured on a scale of 1–14, where 1 is a strong acid, 7 is neutral and 14 is a strong alkali.

The skin can be divided into three distinct layers.

- The outer layer is the epidermis.
- Beneath it is the dermis. The epidermis and dermis are 'glued' together by the **basement membrane**.
- Deepest of all is the subcutaneous or fatty layer which consists of adipose tissue.

Structure of the epidermis

The epidermis consists of five layers:

1 stratum corneum (the surface or horny layer)
2 stratum lucidum (the clear layer)
3 stratum granulosum (the granular cell layer)
4 stratum spinosum (the prickle cell layer)
5 stratum germinativum (the deepest or basal cell layer).

Stratum means layer and the second part of the name refers to its structure or function.

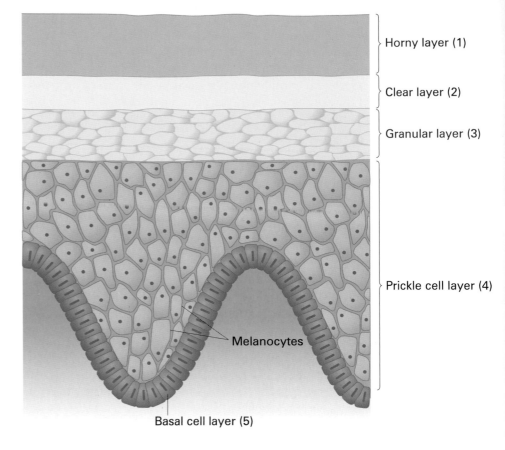

Structure of epidermis

Stratum corneum / horny layer

The stratum corneum is a layer of cornified cells which forms the surface of the epidermis. It is the visible part of skin and the area where skin is shed. Here the cells are flattened, consist mainly of keratin and overlap to protect the skin from damage. The stratum corneum is sometimes called the horny layer because of the thickness of the dead skin cells. Darker skins have a thicker stratum corneum than paler ones and therefore have greater protection from the damaging effects of ultra violet light. The stratum corneum is thickest on the soles of the feet and thinner on the face, which affects the absorption of applied substances.

Stratum lucidum / clear layer

Lucid means clear and the stratum lucidum is a layer of dead, transparent cells. It is thickest on the soles of the feet and the palms of the hands which are subject to more wear and tear than other areas of the body. The thicker layer provides added protection.

Stratum granulosum / granular layer

This granular layer contains living cells which are beginning to wear down. The cells are much flatter than those in the deeper layers and contain less fluid.

Stratum spinosum / prickle cell layer

The stratum spinosum consists of living cells which are plump and filled with fluid. This is also known as the **prickle cell** layer because of the way the cells look. They are shaped like spines or spikes, which allows them to attach to other cells.

Stratum germinativum / basal cell layer

The deepest layer of the epidermis is the stratum germinativum, also known as the **basal cell layer** because of its position at the base of the epidermis. This layer consists of living 'parent' cells which reproduce by continually dividing to make new cells called **keratinocytes**. Keratinocytes produce the protein keratin, the main building block of skin, hair and nails.

Keratinisation

Skin is continually making new cells in the stratum germinativum and shedding them from the stratum corneum in a process called keratinisation. The three lower layers of the epidermis contain living cells which are fed by the dermis, while in the two uppermost layers the cells start to die. A new cell is formed when a parent cell divides. It moves up through the layers and changes in shape and structure to become flatter and more horny. By the time the cell reaches the stratum corneum, it is no more than a flat, empty shell which is shed away. This natural shedding process is called **desquamation**.

The process of keratinisation, which carries a new cell on its journey from the stratum germinativum to the stratum corneum, takes approximately 28 days. As a person ages, the process of keratinisation slows down. This explains why older people seem to keep a suntan for longer – they retain their dying skin cells so that there is a build-up of old skin cells in the stratum corneum as they wait for new ones to push through.

Beauty therapists use techniques to manually slough off dead skin cells, such as facial and body scrubs, or electrotherapy such as galvanism, which makes the skin look brighter and fresher.

Structure and function of the dermis

The dermis contains many fewer cells than the epidermis and more connective tissue. The dermis is divided into two layers as well as a number of appendages such as sweat and sebaceous glands, hair follicles and nails.

The uppermost layer of the dermis is rich in nerves and blood supply, which exist to feed the lower, living layers of the epidermis. Blood carries nutrients and oxygen to the cells and carries away waste products. The deepest layer of the dermis is made up of two types of protein fibres – **collagen** and **elastin**. These fibres are tangled together and form the connective tissue of the dermis. Each has a separate structure and function.

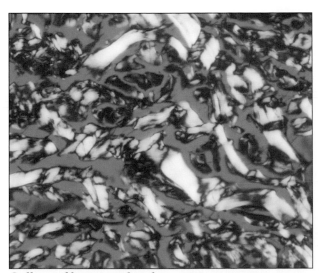

Collagen fibres viewed under a microscope

Collagen fibres are thick strands of protein which provide skin with structure and strength. Collagen fibres exist in bundles which run in different directions in different parts of the body.

Elastin is present in the dermis in tight bundles of fibres. These, along with collagen fibres, provide skin with its characteristic elasticity – the ability to stretch and return to its natural state. Renewal of elastin fibres slows down with age and the skin loses its elastic quality, appearing looser. A decline in the regeneration of collagen and elastin fibres of the dermis is the cause of lines, wrinkles and the less pronounced facial contours characteristic of mature skins.

Sweat glands

There are two types of sweat gland:

- **Eccrine** glands are found all over the body, but there are more of them in the palms of the hands and the soles of the feet. They are constantly excreting small amounts of sweat in order to maintain optimum body temperature.
- **Apocrine** glands are attached to hair follicles under the arms, in the groin and around the nipples. They are the larger of the two glands and are activated when we are excited, stressed or anxious. Apocrine sweat also contains pheromones which are the hormones thought to play a role in sexual attraction.

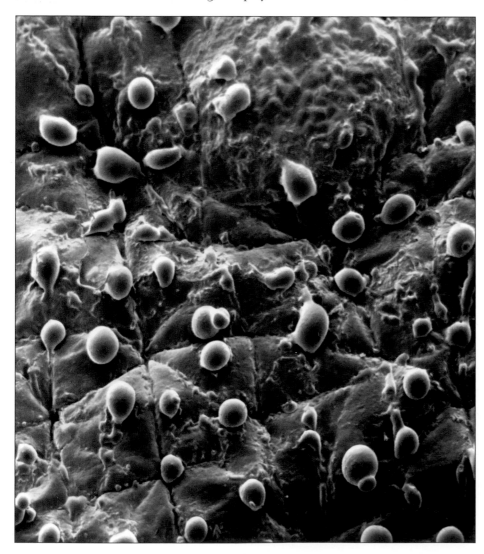

Sweat droplets emerging from eccrine glands

When sweat comes into contact with bacteria it causes an unpleasant smell which we recognise as body odour. Deodorants contain an antiseptic which decreases the activity of bacteria while anti-perspirants contain an astringent which reduces the pore size, as with a toner, and so less sweat reaches the surface of the skin. Both products commonly contain a perfume which masks body odour.

Factors which increase sweat production	Factors which decrease sweat production
Warm external climate or warm clothing	Temperatures lower than 36.8°C, which result in
Vigorous activity which increases muscle temperature	vasoconstriction
Hot, spicy foods and alcohol which can cause vasodilation of	Limited activity, which results in a lowering of body
the capillaries	temperature
Skin colour – black skin contains more sweat glands	Removing certain foods from the diet that cause vasodilation
Certain illnesses or medical conditions are accompanied by a	Skin colour – white skin contains fewer sweat glands
fever which results in a high temperature	Certain illnesses result in a decrease in sweat production,
Hot flushes and sweating are characteristic of the menopause	such as low blood pressure and diabetes
Certain forms of medication have side-effects which	As the body ages, circulation becomes sluggish and the
increase body temperature	body has a tendency to feel cold
Hormonal activity caused by an emotional response to	With age the sweat glands eventually become redundant
fear or excitement, which causes vasolidation in all areas of	due to inactivity
the body	

Factors which affect sweat production

Sebaceous glands

Sebaceous glands secrete sebum, a natural oily substance, which moisturises the skin and helps protect against infection due to its antibacterial quality. There are no sebaceous glands on the palms of the hands, the soles of the feet or the surface of the lips. Areas containing the most sebaceous glands are the scalp, the back and the chest. There are more sebaceous glands in a man's body than in a woman's and more in black skins than in white. This explains why male clients and black skins are more likely than females and white skins to have an oily skin type.

Structure and functions of the subcutaneous layer

The subcutaneous layer separates the dermis from muscles. The subcutaneous layer is therefore underneath the main layers of skin (the dermis and the epidermis). The subcutaneous layer functions as a storage area for fat. This layer of fat serves to protect the body against knocks and bangs by cushioning the blow. It protects the internal organs, the bones, the blood vessels and nerves. There is an abundance of nerves and blood vessels throughout the dermis and they are protected by fat cells.

The subcutaneous layer has another important function. As fat is a poor conductor of heat, it insulates the body by preventing heat loss – the same way that draught insulation works in the home when it is fitted around doors and windows. It keeps the cold on one side and the heat on the other. Female skin tends to retain more fluid than male skin and the subcutaneous layer is thicker, giving it a 'softer' appearance.

The skeleton

You will learn about

- the functions of the skeleton
- bones and bone tissue
- the structure of the skeleton
- movement at joints.

The functions of the skeleton

The human skeleton is a mobile, bony framework consisting of approximately 206 bones, which establish its characteristic shape. As well as providing shape, the skeleton has other important functions linked to its structure which are shown in the table below.

Function	Description
Support	Without a skeleton we would be a wobbly, floppy mass of cells and tissue, unable to stand, move or support ourselves
Protection	The various parts of the skeleton protect the underlying structures, e.g. the cranium protects the brain and the thoracic cage protects the heart and lungs
Attachment for skeletal muscles and leverage	Muscles attach to the bones of the skeleton and pull them into different positions so that the bones act like levers. This allows many types of movement at joints
Source of blood cells	Many bones are hollow and consist of spongy bone tissue which is filled with red marrow. Red marrow is the site for the production of blood cells in adults
Store of calcium	Calcium makes bone hard and is used to maintain the compact tissue of bones. Its release into the bloodstream, initiated by **parathyroid hormone**, is required to maintain heart rate, respiration and muscle contraction

Functions of the skeleton

Bones and bone tissue

The skeleton of a human embryo consists of a flexible tissue called **cartilage** which is made of strong collagen and stretchy elastin fibres. Nearly all cartilage is gradually replaced by hard bone tissue in a process called **ossification**, although some remains on the joint surfaces of most bones in the form of articular cartilage. Development of the skeleton continues until about the age of 25, by which time the final size and shape of the skeleton has been established. However, growth, destruction and repair of bone tissue continues throughout life to maintain the strength and health of the skeletal system.

Bone formation and growth

Bone tissue is rigid and non-elastic and consists of about 67 per cent calcium and 33 per cent organic matter, mainly collagen. The process of ossification depends on a delicate balance between the construction and destruction of bone tissue. This is maintained by specialist cells, as described on the next page.

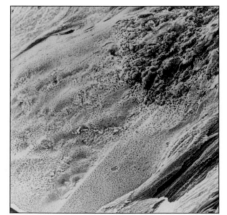

Ossification and growth of bone

- **Osteoblasts** make new bone tissue. They secrete collagen which forms a strong yet flexible framework. Mineral salts, especially calcium, are then deposited within this framework to provide hardness in a process called **calcification**. Osteoblasts become trapped in the framework of bone tissue and develop into osteocytes which release further calcium ions that become part of the bone tissue.
- **Osteoclasts** contain **lysosomes** which are enzymes that digest protein and also break down minerals in bone because of their acidic quality.

In this way the skeleton is maintained, as oscteoclasts destroy old bone tissue while osteoblasts construct new bone. The process also allows bone tissue to act as a storage medium for calcium.

Cancellous bone

Structure of bone

There are two types of bone tissue:

- **compact**
- **cancellous.**

Type of bone tissue	Characteristics
Compact	Hard, strong and relatively heavy. Forms the tough outer shell of most bones in the human skeleton.
Cancellous	Spongy texture (also known as spongy bone tissue). Spaces in the tissue contain red bone marrow where blood cells are formed. Lightweight.

Characteristics of compact and cancellous bone tissues

Classifications of bones

There are five types of bone:

- long
- short
- flat
- sesamoid
- irregular.

They have structures suited to their function and position in the human body.

Type of bone	Structure	Examples
Long	Consists of a shaft of compact bone tissue and two spongy extremities called **epiphyses** made of cancellous bone tissue	Femur (thigh) Humerus (upper arm)
Short	Short, irregular bones consisting of cancellous bone tissue surrounded by a thin layer of compact bone tissue; lightweight	Carpals (8 wrist bones) Tarsals (7 ankle bones)
Flat	Plate-like layers of compact and cancellous bone tissue make these bones strong yet lightweight	Frontal (forehead)
Sesamoid	Oval-shaped bone located in tendons	Patella kneecap)
Irregular	Mass of cancellous bone tissue surrounded by a thin layer of compact bone tissue	Vertebrae (spine)

Classifications of bones

Effects of ageing on bone tissue

One of the greatest influences on skeletal development in infancy is nutrition. Vitamin A influences osteoblast and osteoclast activity, which is needed to maintain a homeostatic balance, and vitamin D is required to aid the absorption of calcium from the intestine. Vitamins C and B12 are also essential to bone growth.

Age-associated changes in the digestive system can radically affect the condition of the skeleton. Less calcium is absorbed from the diet, which appears to affect post-menopausal women more than men of the same age, adding to the tendency towards **osteoporosis**. Changes in the digestive system also effect the absorption of vitamin D and changes in the skin slow down the production of vitamin D activated by natural sunlight. As the function of vitamin D is to transport calcium from the digestive system to the bones, a deficiency means that new bone tissue is produced at a slower rate than existing tissue is destroyed. During middle age and into old age, bones start to shrink and the skin can become saggy as it fits less snugly on the internal framework. Bones in the face diminish in the same way as bones in the body and this bone shrinkage is partly to blame for the lack of tautness which is noticeable in mature skins.

Hormone replacement therapy (HRT) is commonly prescribed to women to treat the effects of the menopause. Treatment with the hormone **oestrogen** has been found to have a positive effect on calcium metabolism, which in turn reduces loss of bone density and lowers the risk of osteoporosis. Additional advice would be to maintain regular gentle exercise, such as walking, which prevents bone mass loss and encourages the production of vitamin D in the skin via natural sunlight. Also, the diet should contain adequate amounts of calcium, which the body needs to produce new bone tissue. The recommended daily intake is about 700 mg or one pint of skimmed milk.

The structure of the skeleton

Axial and appendicular skeleton

The skeleton is divided into two parts:

- the axial skeleton
- the appendicular skeleton.

The axis of the body (axial skeleton) is made up of 80 bones of the skull, thoracic cage (rib cage) and vertebral (spinal) column. The appendicular skeleton consists of 126 bones found in the upper and lower limbs, the pelvic girdle and the shoulder girdle.

Axial skeleton			
1 frontal	4 nasal	7 cervical vertebrae	
2 parietal	1 vomer	12 thoracic vertebrae	
2 temporal	1 maxilla	5 lumbar vertebrae	
1 occipital	1 mandible	5 fused bones of sacrum	
1 ethmoid	2 zygomatic	4 fused bones of coccyx	
1 sphenoid	2 palatine	24 (12 pairs) ribs	
2 lacrimal	1 hyoid	1 sternum	**Total: 80 bones**

Bones of the axial skeleton

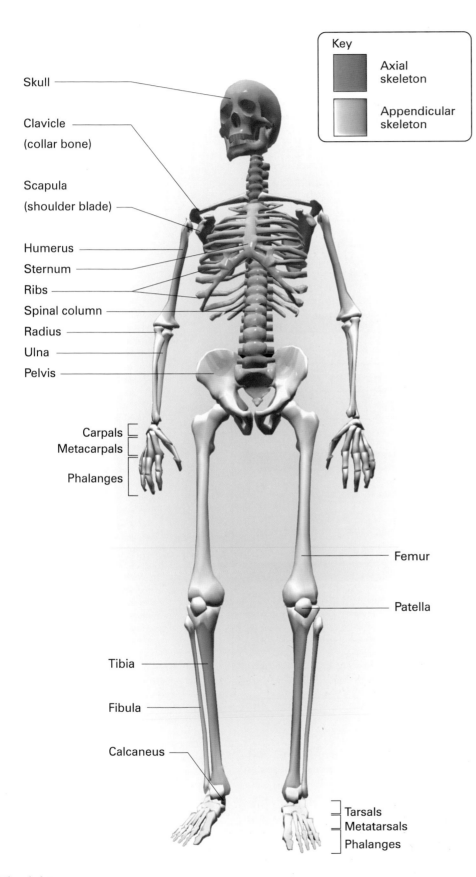

Skull

Clavicle
(collar bone)

Scapula
(shoulder blade)

Humerus

Sternum

Ribs

Spinal column

Radius

Ulna

Pelvis

Carpals
Metacarpals

Phalanges

Femur

Patella

Tibia

Fibula

Calcaneus

Tarsals
Metatarsals
Phalanges

Key

Axial skeleton

Appendicular skeleton

Appendicular skeleton
2 scapula
2 clavicle
2 humerus
2 radius
2 ulna
16 carpals
10 metacarpals
28 phalanges
2 pelvic bones
2 femur
2 patella
2 fibula
2 tibia
14 tarsals
10 metatarsals
28 phalanges
Total: 126 bones

Bones of the appendicular skeleton

The skeleton

Relation of bone structure and function

The axial skeleton has a central position in the structure of the body.

The skull has two parts, the cranium which forms the roof and back of the skull and contains the brain, and the face at the front of the skull which contains the eyes and teeth. The cranium forms a deep cavity to protect the brain and is constructed of flat bones which are strong yet lightweight. The facial bones are irregular and formed into peaks and furrows to protect the eyes, nasal cavities, teeth and tongue.

The vertebral column consists of 33 individual bones, though some are fused together. Between each vertebra is a pad of fibrous tissue called an intervertebral disc which acts as a shock absorber against gravity and injury. Each vertebra contains a hole in the centre and through this runs the spinal cord which forms part of the **central nervous system** (CNS).

The thoracic cage consists of 12 thoracic vertebrae and 12 pairs of ribs as well as one sternum. This cage protects the heart, lungs and major blood vessels and is a point of attachment for the diaphragm and intercostal muscles which assist respiration.

Functions of the skull
Cranium protects the brain
Base of the frontal bone and zygomatic bones form the eye sockets
Mandible forms the lower jaw and aids mastication (chewing)
Temporal bone protects the ear canal
Functions of the vertebral column
Protects spinal cord
Provides attachment for ribs
Provides attachment for muscles
Functions of the thoracic cage
Protects lungs
Protects heart and major blood vessels
Provides attachment for diaphragm
Provides attachment for intercostal muscles

Functions of the axial skeleton

The appendicular skeleton consists of the limbs, clavicles and scapulae. Together with muscles, the appendicular skeleton is responsible for voluntary movements. These can range from complex coordinations involving the whole body such as walking and jumping to small, specific movements such as writing or wriggling the toes. (Movement is investigated fully in 'Movements at joints' on page 158 and in **The muscular system**, page 160.)

Movement at joints

A joint is formed where two bones meet. Without them, the skeleton would be static and movement would be limited. The most obvious joints in the human body are found at the knees and elbows, which allow movement of the upper and lower limbs. But movement is also possible in the vertebral column, which enables us to twist and bend, in the hands and feet, enabling us to write, wave, pick things up, dance and walk, and in the thoracic cage for respiration.

You know that different areas of the body are capable of different movements and you can probably work out why. The size and structure of bones, type of joint and size, tone and structure of muscle all play a part in the movements possible. You can train your body to be more flexible and you can facilitate movement through massage and passive exercise, but still there are limitations to the movements possible at different joints.

Synovial joints are freely moving joints, though movements are limited by the shape of the articulating surfaces and the ligaments which hold the bones together. Three types of movement are possible at synovial joints:

- angular movements including flexion and extension, abduction and adduction
- rotary movements including rotation and circumduction
- gliding movements where one part slides on another.

As a beauty therapist you must be able to describe movements for the purpose of making accurate records, prescribing exercise and monitoring client progress, and you will therefore need to use anatomical terms to describe movements precisely.

Term	Description
Flexion	Reduces angle between two bones
Extension	Increases angle between two bones
Abduction	Moving away from midline of the body
Adduction	Moving towards midline of the body
Circumduction	Moving an extremity around in a circle
Rotation	Turning on an axis
Supination	Outward rotation
Pronation	Inward rotation
Inversion	Turning inwards
Eversion	Turning outwards
Elevation	Raising body part
Depression	Lowering body part

Anatomical terms

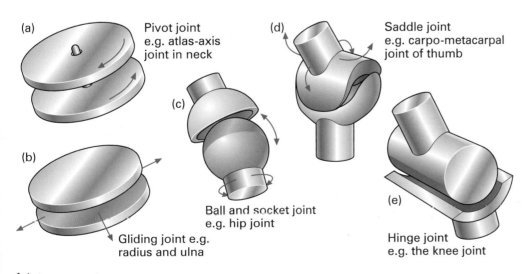

(a) Pivot joint e.g. atlas-axis joint in neck

(b) Gliding joint e.g. radius and ulna

(c) Ball and socket joint e.g. hip joint

(d) Saddle joint e.g. carpo-metacarpal joint of thumb

(e) Hinge joint e.g. the knee joint

Joint movements

Homeostatic disorders of joints

Joints undergo a lot of wear and tear in a lifetime and it is common for older clients to complain of stiff, swollen or aching joints. However, it is difficult to separate age-associated changes from mechanical strain or injury. Repetitive actions of joints due to occupation, sporting activities or strain caused by poor posture can certainly influence the stability of joints as we age. Cold weather and inactivity during sleep cause the body's circulatory system to slow down, which can lead to a build-up of fluid at the joints resulting in swelling or discomfort.

A further age-associated problem is the loss of water from cartilage. Think again about the intervertebral discs. These 'cushions' contain water which is squeezed out by the pressure of gravity over time which makes them less flexible and can cause problems with lifting and bearing heavy weight. As the discs lose water, they become flatter, which also explains why our height decreases with age.

Disorder	Description	Example
Arthritis	Inflammation of joints	Swollen, aching joints
Spondylosis	Degenerative disorder of intervertebral discs	Pain in cervical and lumbar region
Rheumatoid arthritis	Chronic, progressive disorder	Typically affects fingers, wrists, feet, ankles
Bursitis	Inflammation of bursae	Housemaid's knee
Torn cartilage	Damaged menisci	Footballing injuries to knee joint
Tendinitis	Inflammation of tendons	Caused by overuse, e.g. tennis elbow or repetitive strain
Sprain	Overstretched tendon, cartilage or muscle	Sporting injuries
Dislocation	Bones in joint become disconnected	Sudden or unnatural movements

Disorders of the joints

The muscular system

You will learn about	
• the functions of skeletal muscle • the structure of skeletal muscle • muscle tone • attachment of muscles to the skeleton	• origins, insertions and actions of chief muscles of the face and body.

There are three types of muscle tissue:

- cardiac muscle – forms the heart
- smooth muscle – forms the internal organs
- skeletal muscle – attached to bones.

While cardiac and smooth muscle activity is involuntary (we have no control over it) and responsible for functions such as heartbeat or the passage of food through the digestive system, some skeletal activity, such as movement, is under conscious control. However, all types of muscle tissue have some characteristics in common:

- muscle tissue is excitable – it responds to a stimulus
- muscle tissue has the ability to contract (shorten)
- muscle tissue has the ability to stretch (lengthen)
- muscle tissue is elastic – it returns to its original shape after contraction or stretching.

The functions of skeletal muscle

Skeletal muscle has four main functions.

- It facilitates movement.
- It raises body temperature.
- It maintains posture.
- It assists venous return.

The most obvious function of skeletal muscle is to facilitate movement at joints and thereby increase or decrease the angle between two bones. Muscle is attached to bones via tendons at the point of **origin** and the point of **insertion**. When a muscle contracts, the origin remains fixed while the insertion moves towards it, so reducing the angle of the joint. For example, sitting up from a lying down position shortens the angle between the trunk and the thighs as the abdominal muscles contract or shorten.

As well as enabling movement, skeletal muscle is responsible for maintaining posture, which is achieved by the same concept of contraction. Under normal, resting circumstances the muscles are in a state of partial contraction known as **muscle tone**. If our muscles were completely relaxed all the time, our bodies would not be able to hold themselves upright, as the weight of our bones and organs, particularly the skull and brain, would pull us over. Not surprisingly, the muscles with the greatest tonicity in humans are found in the neck and back. Postural muscles do not require conscious effort to carry out their function, although they can be affected by bad habits and improved through training.

The structure of skeletal muscle

Muscle tissue consists of large striped cells which are elongated and highly specialised. They are bound together in bundles by connective tissue which contains collagen and elastin fibres that give muscle its strength and elastic properties. Running the length of muscle cells are filaments of the proteins actin and myosin. It is these fibres of protein that give muscle its characteristic striped appearance. Within the bundles of muscle fibres there is also a rich supply of blood vessels and nerve attachments.

Muscle tone

Skeletal muscle is responsible for different types of contraction during dynamic or static activity. If the origin and insertion move closer together, the muscle is shortened or contracted and is said to be working **concentrically**. If the muscle tries to halt a movement during exertion, it is said to be working **eccentrically**. The muscle attempts to contract but is extended by external forces which force the origin and insertion apart. If the muscle has to contract to prevent movement, it is said to be working **statically**. Concentric and eccentric contractions are also known as **isotonic** contractions. Static muscle work is known as **isometric**. The term isometric means equal measures, as in a muscle working in equal measures with an external force to prevent movement. Isometric exercises are used to increase muscle strength by increasing tension without causing contraction, usually by pushing against a solid, immovable force. Isometric and isotonic contractions can be illustrated by considering the different types of muscle work involved in doing pull-ups on a high bar.

Muscle structure

Muscle comprises:

- 75 per cent water
- 20 per cent actin and myosin
- 5 per cent mineral salts, glycogen and fat.

Attachment of muscles to the skeleton

Skeletal muscles may be attached to bone, cartilage, ligaments or skin via **tendons** and **aponeuroses**. Tendons have the appearance of cords and consist of fibrous collagen tissues, while aponeuroses are a thin sheet of fibres which attach flat muscles, as in the abdomen. The most well-known tendon is the Achilles which connects the calf muscles to the heel. Fibrous tissue also forms a protective and supportive sheath of connective tissue around muscles known as fascia, which contains a rich supply of blood and nerve fibres. Where muscles attach to each other the fibres of one interlace with the fibres of the other. In the muscles of the abdominal wall the fibres of the aponeuroses interlace forming the linea alba, the shallow groove which leads from the umbilicus to the sternum.

Origins, insertions and actions of chief muscles of the face and body

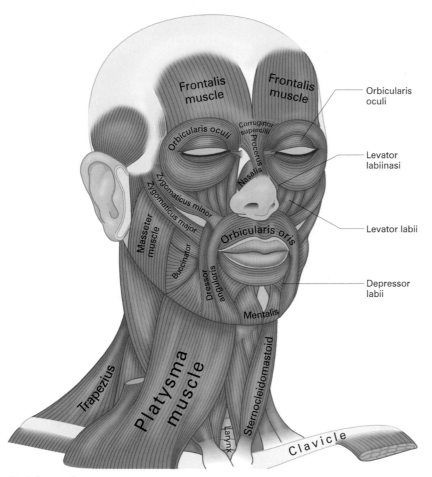

Facial muscles

Muscle	Origin	Insertion	Action
Frontalis	Epicranial aponeurosis	Behind eyebrow	Raises eyebrows, wrinkles forehead
Orbicularis oculi	Medial rim of orbit	Forms sphincter around eye area	Closes eyelid
Orbicularis oris	Sphincter muscle	Around mouth	Closes mouth
Buccinator	Maxilla and mandible	Angle of mouth	Compresses cheeks, aids mastication
Risorius	Maxilla and mandible	Angle of mouth	Retracts mouth
Masseter	Zygomatic arch	Mandible	Raises lower jaw, aids mastication
Temporalis	Temples	Mandible	Raises, retracts lower law, aids mastication
Platysma	Fascia over pectorals and deltoid	Mandible, lower face	Draws down lip and jaw in yawning, wrinkles neck
Sternocleidomastoid	Sternum and clavicle	Mastoid process	Flexion of neck

Chief muscles of the face and head

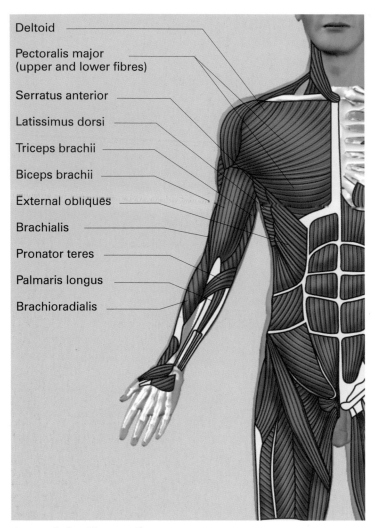

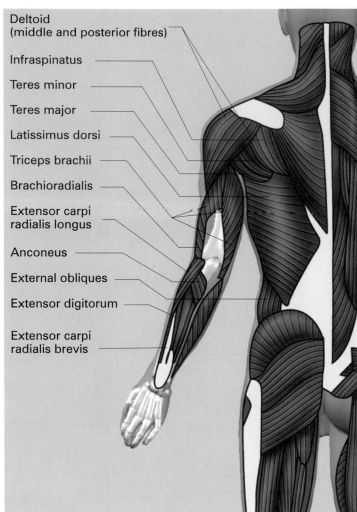

Deltoid

Pectoralis major
(upper and lower fibres)

Serratus anterior

Latissimus dorsi

Triceps brachii

Biceps brachii

External obliques

Brachialis

Pronator teres

Palmaris longus

Brachioradialis

Deltoid
(middle and posterior fibres)

Infraspinatus

Teres minor

Teres major

Latissimus dorsi

Triceps brachii

Brachioradialis

Extensor carpi
radialis longus

Anconeus

External obliques

Extensor digitorum

Extensor carpi
radialis brevis

Arm and shoulder muscles

Muscle	Origin	Insertion	Action
Biceps	Scapula	Tuberosity of radius	Flexion at elbow, supination of forearm
Brachialis	Shaft of humerus	Tuberosity of ulna	Flexion at elbow
Triceps	Scapula and humerus	Olecranon of ulna	Extension at elbow
Deltoid	Clavicle, spine of scapula	Tuberosity of humerus	Abduction of shoulder
Levator scapulae	Upper 4 cervical vertebrae	Vertebral border of scapulae	Elevate shoulder, rotate scapula
Superficial extensors	Lateral aspect of humerus	Metacarpals and phalanges	Extension of wrist and fingers
Superficial flexors	Medial aspect of humerus	Metacarpals, palmar aponeurosis, phalanges	Flexion of wrist and fingers

Chief muscles of the arm and shoulder

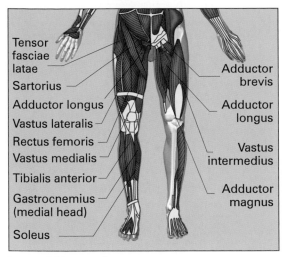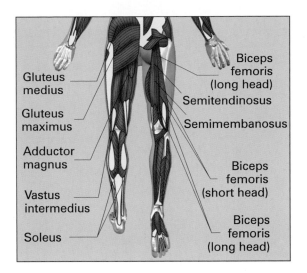

Leg and hip muscles

Muscle	Origin	Insertion	Action
Quadriceps femoris: rectus femoris, vastus lateralis, vastus intermedius, vastus medialis	Anterior inferior iliac spine, greater trochanter, shaft of femur	Through patella and ligament to tubercle of tibia	Together: extension of knee; rectus femoris: flexion of hip
Adductors	Pubis and ischium	Linea aspera	Adduction, lateral rotation of femur
Tensor fascia lata	Outer surface of iliac crest	Iliotibial tract	Abduction of thigh and hip, extension of knee, medial rotation of femur
Sartorius	Anterior superior iliac spine	Medial condyle of tibia	Flexion and abduction of hip, flexion of knee, lateral rotation of femur
Tibialis anterior	Upper tibia	Intermediate cuneform and first metatarsal	Dorsiflexion and supination of ankle, inversion
Gastrocnemius	Lateral and medial condyles of femur	Through Achilles on heel	Flexion of knee, plantarflexion of ankle
Soleus (beneath gastrocnemius)	Head of fibula	Through Achilles to heel	Plantarflexion
Adductors: brevis, longus, magnus	Pubic bone	Linea aspera	Adduction at hip, rotation out (adductor brevis) and inward rotation (adductor magnus)
Gluteus maximus	Posterior pelvis, sacrum, coccyx	Outer aspect of femur	Adducts hip, outward rotation of thigh, extension of knee
Hamstrings: biceps femoris, semitendonosis, semimembranosis	Ischial tuberosity	Tibia and fibula at either side of popliteal	Extension of hip, flexion of knee, lateral rotation of femur when semi-flexed
Gluteus medius	Back of femur	Greater trochanter	Abduction and rotation of hip
Gluteus minimus	Outer aspect of ilium, under and behind gluteus medius	Greater trochanter	Abduction and rotation of hip

Chief muscles of the leg and hip

Muscle	Origin	Insertion	Action
Pectoralis major	Clavicle, sternum and costal cartilage	Lateral aspect of bicipital groove	Adduction, inward rotation of arm, supports mammary glands
Pectoralis minor (beneath pectoralis major)	Ribs 3–5	Coracoid process	Depression of scapula
Diaphragm	Tip of sternum, lower ribs, first three lumbar vertebrae	Central aponeurosis of abdominal wall	Flattens to create more room in thorax during inhalation
Intercostals	Lower borders of ribs	Upper border of rib below	Pulls ribs up and out during inhalation, maintain shape of thorax
Rectus abdominus	Pubis	5th–7th costal cartilages	Ventral flexion of trunk
External obliques (form waist)	Lower eight ribs	Iliac crest, linea alba through abdominal aponeurosis	Flex trunk ventrally, rotation of trunk

Chief muscles of the chest and abdomen

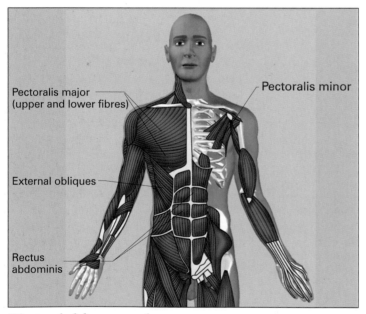

Chest and abdomen muscles

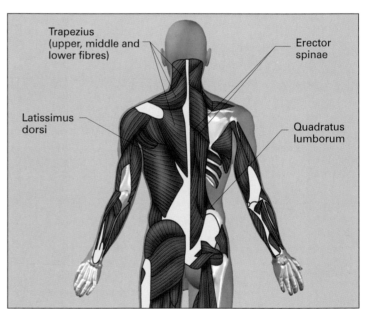

Back muscles

Muscle	Origin	Insertion	Action
Trapezius	Occipital bone, thoracic vertebrae	Clavicle, spine of scapula	Elevates and braces shoulder, rotates scapula
Erector spinae	Sacrum, iliac crest, ribs, lower vertebrae	Ribs, vertebrae, mastoid process	Extension of spine, lateral flexion of trunk, pulls head back, erect posture
Latissumus dorsi	Lower six thoracic vertebrae, lumbar vertebrae, iliac crest	Bicipital groove of humerus	Adduction of arm at shoulder, depression of shoulder
Quadratus lumborum	Iliac crest	12th rib, upper lumbar vertebrae	Extension and lateral flexion of trunk, steadies 12th rib

Chief muscles of the back

The cardiovascular system

You will learn about

- blood
- the structure of the heart
- the structure of the blood vessels
- the functions of the cardiovascular system.

The cardiovascular system consists of:

- a fluid – blood
- a pump – the heart
- a network of blood vessels, arteries, veins and capillaries.

Blood

Blood is a thick, alkaline fluid which appears bright red in the arteries and dark red in the veins, depending on the presence of more or less oxygen respectively. It makes up about 8 per cent of our body weight so that the average volume of blood in an adult is between 5 and 6 litres. Blood contains about 55 per cent fluid in the form of **plasma** and about 45 per cent solid in the form of blood cells.

Components of plasma	Function
Water = 90% of total volume	Renews cellular fluid
Minerals: chlorides, phosphates, carbonates	Maintain pH of blood at 7.4; maintain electrolyte balance for correct functioning of body tissues
Proteins: albumin, globulin, fibrinogen, heparin	Make blood viscous (sticky) which controls its flow and maintains blood pressure
Nutrients: glucose, amino acids, fatty acids, glycerol, vitamins	Required for energy, heat and raw materials
Gases: oxygen, carbon dioxide, nitrogen	Required for/produced by cellular respiration
Waste products: urea, uric acid, creatinine	By-products of metabolism
Antibodies and antitoxins	Protect against infection and neutralise some toxins which may enter the body
Hormones	See **The endocrine system**, page 175
Enzymes	Produce chemical reactions in other substances

Composition of plasma

Type of cell	Structure	Function
Erythrocytes (red blood cells)	Produced in red bone marrow of spongy bone, minute biconcave discs, about 5 million per cubic millimetre of blood. Contain the protein **haemoglobin** which attracts oxygen to form oxyhaemoglobin, which is bright red in colour	Carry oxygen to the tissues from the lungs and carry carbon dioxide away
Leucocytes (white blood cells)	Larger than red blood cells and less numerous. Three types: 75% **granulocytes** which can pass from bloodstream to site of infection; 20% **lymphocytes** made in the lymph nodes; 5% **monocytes**	Concerned with immunity. Granulocytes/phagocytes: ingest bacteria and cell debris (**phagocytosis**); lymphocytes: produce antibodies; monocytes: phagocytosis
Thrombocytes (platelets)	Made in the bone marrow and are even smaller than red blood cells	Concerned with clotting the blood (**haemostasis**) which has three stages – narrowing of lumen in blood vessels, formation of platelet plug, clotting and retraction of fibrin

Blood cells

The structure of the heart

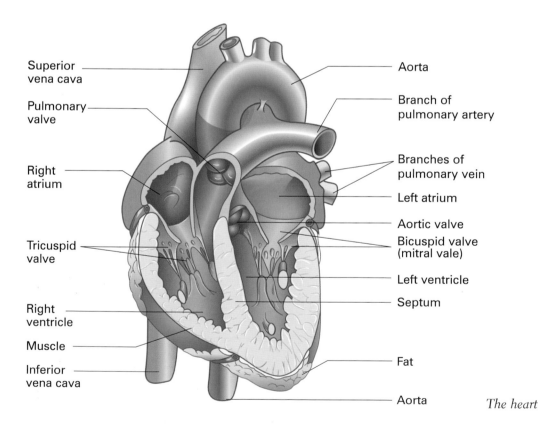

Superior vena cava
Pulmonary valve
Right atrium
Tricuspid valve
Right ventricle
Muscle
Inferior vena cava
Aorta
Branch of pulmonary artery
Branches of pulmonary vein
Left atrium
Aortic valve
Bicuspid valve (mitral vale)
Left ventricle
Septum
Fat
Aorta

The heart

The heart is a hollow, muscular, cone-shaped organ located behind the sternum, slightly to the left side of the body. It consists of four chambers: two upper chambers, called the left and right **atriums**, and the two lower chambers, called left and right **ventricles**. The heart also contains four main valves which are mechanisms to prevent blood from flowing in the wrong direction.

Structure	Location	Function
Left atrium/right atrium	Upper chambers	Receive blood flowing towards the heart from veins
Left ventricle/right ventricle	Lower chambers	Direct blood away from the heart through arteries
Right atrio-ventricular valve (tricuspid)	Between right atrium and right ventricle	Prevents backflow of blood into the right atrium during contraction of the right ventricle
Left atrio-ventricular valve (bicuspid)	Between left atrium and left ventricle	Prevents backflow of blood into the left atrium during contraction of the left ventricle
Aortic valve	Between the aorta and the left ventricle	Prevents backflow of blood into the left ventricle
Pulmonary valve	Between the pulmonary vein and the right ventricle	Prevents backflow of blood into the right ventricle

Structure and function of the heart

The structure of the blood vessels

Blood vessels are the tubes which form a network around the body for the transport of blood. When the ventricles of the heart contract, blood is pumped around the body via vessels called **arteries** which branch into smaller vessels called **arterioles** and then even smaller vessels called **capillaries**.

Capillaries form the link between arterioles and other tiny vessels called **venules**, which collect the blood from the capillaries. Venules then unite to form **veins** which carry blood on its journey back towards the heart. Arteries are thicker than veins and have larger lumen. With one exception, they carry oxygenated blood away from the heart. Veins carry deoxygenated blood towards the heart, with one exception. Unlike arteries, they contain valves which prevent the backflow of blood. The largest artery in the body is the **aorta** which carries oxygenated blood from the left ventricle to all parts of the body (except the lungs). The largest veins in the body are the superior and inferior vena cavae. The **superior vena cava** carries deoxygenated blood from the upper parts of the body and the **inferior vena cava** carries deoxygenated blood from the lower parts of the body to the right atrium.

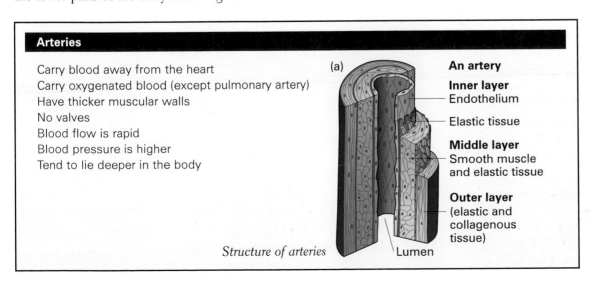

Arteries

Carry blood away from the heart
Carry oxygenated blood (except pulmonary artery)
Have thicker muscular walls
No valves
Blood flow is rapid
Blood pressure is higher
Tend to lie deeper in the body

(a) **An artery**
Inner layer Endothelium
Elastic tissue
Middle layer Smooth muscle and elastic tissue
Outer layer (elastic and collagenous tissue)

Structure of arteries Lumen

Veins

Carry blood towards the heart
Carry deoxygenated blood (except pulmonary vein)
Have thinner muscular walls
Have valves
Blood flow is slower
Blood pressure is lower
Tend to be more superficial in the body

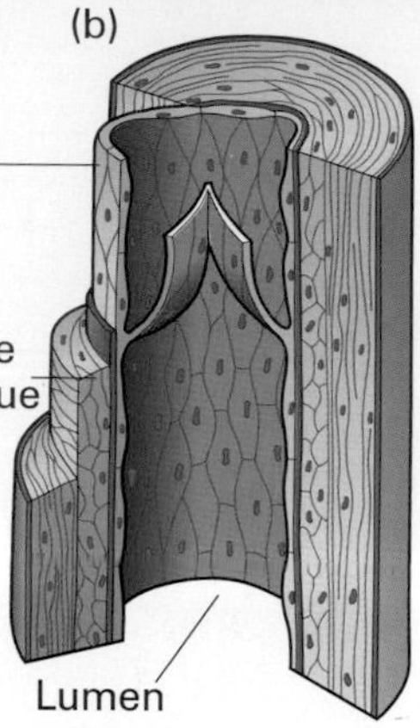
(b)
A vein
Inner layer
Endothelium
Middle layer
Smooth muscle
and elastic tissue
Outer layer
(elastic and
collagenous
tissue)
Lumen

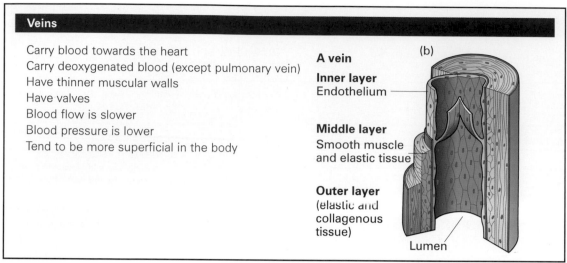

Structure of veins

The functions of the cardiovascular system

The cardiovascular system:

- transports nutrients to the tissues
- transports oxygen to the tissues in oxyhaemoglobin
- transports water to the tissues
- transports waste products to the organs of excretion
- transports hormones and enzymes
- has leucocytes and antibodies to help fight infection
- provides the raw materials from which glands produce secretions
- transports heat and regulates body temperature
- has a clotting mechanism which prevents haemorrhage.

Pulse

As blood is pumped from the left ventricle into the aorta, the aorta is already full of blood and so it becomes distended in order to accept more. The left ventricle contracts which causes vibrations along the arteries due to the expansion of the aorta. The expansion and contraction of the aorta causes a wave of similar movements throughout the arterial network which is known as the pulse. The average resting pulse rate is approx 72–75 pulses per minute.

Pulse rates are higher in women than men, higher in infancy than old age and higher in hot weather than cold.

Blood pressure

Blood pressure refers to the pressure exerted by blood on to the walls of the blood vessels. It is greatest in the large arteries leaving the heart, falls slightly in the arterioles and is hardly apparent at all in the capillaries. Blood pressure is even lower in the veins and in those veins entering the heart there is negative pressure, or suction, caused by the relaxation of the heart's chambers. Blood pressure fluctuates with each pumping action of the heart. It is highest when the ventricle contracts, forcing blood from the heart, and lowest when the ventricle relaxes. The maximum value is called **systolic pressure** and the lowest value is called **diastolic pressure**.

Blood pressure is measured by the weight of a column of mercury (Hg) it can support, calculated in millimetres. Normal arteriole pressure is 110–120 mm Hg systolic pressure and 65–75 mm Hg diastolic pressure. High blood pressure, known as **hypertension**, occurs when blood is forced through the arteries at abnormally high pressure which can damage the artery walls. Low blood pressure, known as **hypotension**, can occur after shock, haemorrhage or heart failure and is dangerous because there is an insufficient blood supply to the vital organs.

The lymphatic system

You will learn about

- lymphatic circulation.

The lymphatic system consists of lymphatic capillaries, vessels, nodes and ducts. The capillaries and vessels form a network around the body which act as tunnels for the transportation of lymph fluid, in the same way that blood vessels provide a network for the transport of blood.

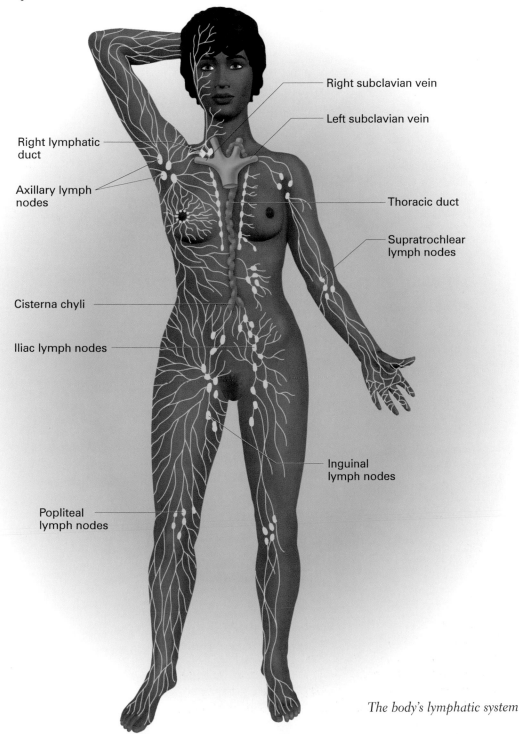

Right subclavian vein

Left subclavian vein

Right lymphatic duct

Axillary lymph nodes

Thoracic duct

Supratrochlear lymph nodes

Cisterna chyli

Iliac lymph nodes

Inguinal lymph nodes

Popliteal lymph nodes

The body's lymphatic system

Lymphatic circulation

As blood travels through the capillaries in the body's tissues, fluid oozes out through the porous walls to form tissue or **interstitial fluid**. Interstitial fluid circulates through the tissues transporting nutrients and oxygen to the cells and carrying waste back into the blood. Excess fluid which does not return to the blood is called **lymph** and it is collected and returned to the blood by the lymphatic system. Lymph travels from the **lymphatic capillaries** to the larger **lymphatic vessels**. Along its journey it passes through **lymphatic nodes** which are situated in areas of the body where there is a greater risk of infection. At these points, the lymph is filtered and cleaned and also **lymphocytes** are produced – these are antibodies that help prevent infection. Having passed through at least one lymph node, lymph fluid travels into **lymphatic ducts**. The ducts pass lymph back into the blood circulation where it becomes part of blood so that the cycle can begin once again.

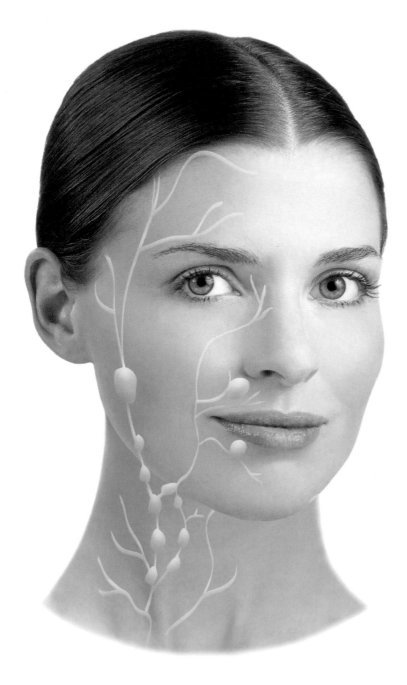

Location of lymphatic vessels in the face

Feature	Structure	Function
Lymph	Straw-coloured fluid	Carries more waste than nutrients
Lymphatic capillaries	One cell thick, hair-like structures which combine to form lymphatic vessels	Transport lymph from the tissues
Lymphatic vessels	Larger and thicker than capillaries, contain valves which prevent backflow of lymph	Transport lymph through one or more lymphatic nodes
Lymphatic nodes	Vary in size from a pin head to an almond	Filter lymph to remove bacteria so can become swollen and tender if infection is present. Produce some antibodies
Lymphatic ducts	Larger thoracic duct is about 45 cm long, has valves and is located at the back of the abdomen; smaller right lymphatic duct is about 1 cm long and formed by the joining of the vessels from the head, thorax and right limb	Collect lymph and return it to the bloodstream. Thoracic duct receives lymph from vessels in the abdomen and lower limbs and empties into the left subclavian vein; right lymphatic duct empties into the right subclavian vein

Structures and functions of the lymphatic system

Lymphatic circulation and beauty therapy

The circulation of both blood and lymph is increased by manual and electrical beauty therapy techniques. Effleurage movements gently stimulate lymphatic flow and have a draining effect, which helps rid the body of toxins and waste products, as well as reducing puffiness. Electrical vacuum suction is particularly stimulating to the lymphatic system, which is why it is important to always work in the direction of lymphatic flow, towards the nearest lymphatic duct.

The digestive system

You will learn about

- the structure of the digestive system
- the process of digestion
- excretion
- regulation of blood glucose.

The digestive system is made up of a number of organs and glands which facilitate the chewing, swallowing, digestion, absorption and elimination of food. It runs from the mouth, where food is ingested (taken in), to the rectum, where waste is expelled. Food is passed from one structure to another in a process which breaks it down into its component parts, ensuring that essential nutrients are absorbed into the bloodstream.

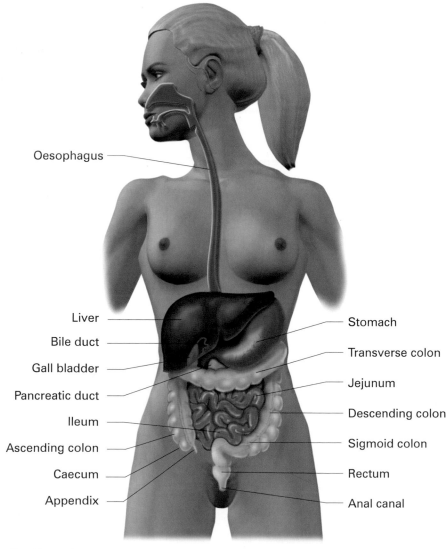

Oesophagus

Liver

Bile duct

Gall bladder

Pancreatic duct

Ileum

Ascending colon

Caecum

Appendix

Stomach

Transverse colon

Jejunum

Descending colon

Sigmoid colon

Rectum

Anal canal

The digestive system

The structure of the digestive system

Name	Structure and location
Mouth	Cavity bound by lips and cheeks consisting of the hard palate (palatine bones and maxillae) and soft palate. Contains the tongue and teeth which assist in mastication, and the salivary glands which produce saliva, the functions of which include softening food, digestion of carbohydrates and cleansing of the mouth and teeth
Pharynx	Muscular flap of skin which prevents food entering the windpipe
Oesophagus	Muscular canal which extends from the pharynx to the stomach, located behind the trachea and in front of the vertebral column
Stomach	J-shaped structure located below and to the left of the diaphragm. The upper opening from the oesophagus consists of a weak sphincter muscle, while the lower opening into the small intestine consists of a strong pyloric sphincter which prevents the regurgitation of food
Pancreas	A gland approx. 12–15 cm long which lies across the posterior abdominal wall behind the stomach
Liver	Largest gland in the body which is located in the upper right section of the abdominal cavity, beneath the diaphragm
Gall bladder	A pear-shaped organ located near the right lobe of the liver. The cystic duct of the gall bladder joins the hepatic duct of the liver to form the bile duct
Small intestine	Consists of the duodenum, jejunum and ileum and is a long tube (6 metres) extending from the pyloric sphincter to the large intestine, located in the central and lower abdominal cavity within the curves of the large intestine
Large intestine	A tube approximately 1.5 metres in length which extends from the ileum to the anus and consists of seven sections: caecum, ascending colon, transverse colon, descending colon, sigmoid colon, rectum, anal canal

Structure and location of the digestive system

The process of digestion

The journey of food begins in the mouth with the process of **ingestion**. Food is broken down and softened by chewing and becomes mixed with saliva. Mechanical digestion is the term given to the physical breakdown of food in the form of biting and chewing. The churning of food in the stomach is also an illustration of mechanical digestion – it works a bit like a food processor, mashing up food and mixing it with digestive juices. Chemical digestion involves the production of digestive juices which act on food and break it down into smaller molecules. During the process of digestion, nutrients are broken down into small, soluble molecules which can be easily absorbed into the bloodstream and later used as raw materials for cells and tissues or as energy for respiration.

Excretion

The final part of food's journey is elimination, which takes place when 'food' passes from the colon to the rectum. In fact, the material which enters the large intestine contains very little food at all, as it has mostly been absorbed before it arrives. The material entering the large intestine contains water, salt, indigestible cellulose and bacteria. Most of the water and salts are absorbed by the colon, which causes the bacteria to die, leaving only cellulose and dead bacteria which form a paste. This paste forms the faeces, which consist of a little water and a solid part which is about 50 per cent dead bacteria and 50 per cent cellulose. The brown colour of faeces comes from the breakdown of old red blood cells.

Regulation of blood glucose

The typical blood glucose level is about 80–90 mg per 100 ml of blood. Glucose is present in higher levels after meals, particularly but not necessarily meals rich in carbohydrates. This is known as the **absorptive state**, when blood glucose levels rise to a maximum of 140 mg per 100 ml of blood. If glucose were transported immediately from the digestive system to other parts of the body, there would be a shortage of glucose between meals and blood sugar levels would fall dramatically. Glucose that is not immediately required for energy is converted into glycogen and triacylglycerols (fat) and stored in the liver, skeletal muscle and adipose tissue. Blood glucose levels typically return to normal within two and a half hours after eating, even though digestion continues for longer.

During the **post-absorptive state**, when glucose is not entering the bloodstream from the digestive system, it is obtained from supplies built up in the liver, adipose tissue and skeletal muscle during the absorptive state, and also from the catabolism of proteins. The use of glucose is reduced to maintain stores and fatty acids are instead metabolised to provide energy.

The pancreas also plays an important role in the regulation of blood glucose (see **The endocrine system**, page 175). Alpha cells secrete the hormone **glucagon** in response to a *fall* in blood glucose levels, which stimulates the conversion of glycogen to glucose. Beta cells secrete the hormone **insulin** in response to a *rise* in blood glucose levels, stimulating the conversion of glucose to glycogen for storage.

A deficiency in insulin results in high levels of blood glucose, and this is characteristic of the condition **diabetes mellitus**. The diet for a diabetic should be the same as the recommended balanced diet for all adults – regular meals based on starchy foods which contain less sugar and fat. People suffering from diabetes might require more snacks in their diet to help maintain blood glucose levels, and they should make sure that these are of nutritional value.

The endocrine system

You will learn about

- the functions of the endocrine system
- the pituitary gland
- the thyroid gland
- the pancreas
- the adrenal glands
- gonads.

The endocrine system is often described as functioning like an orchestra, with the **hypothalamus** acting as band leader and the **pituitary gland** acting as the conductor. The pituitary is sometimes referred to as the 'master gland' because of its regulating function although, as in an orchestra, all the components must work together. If one gland is not working efficiently, the others must become more active to compensate and maintain harmony.

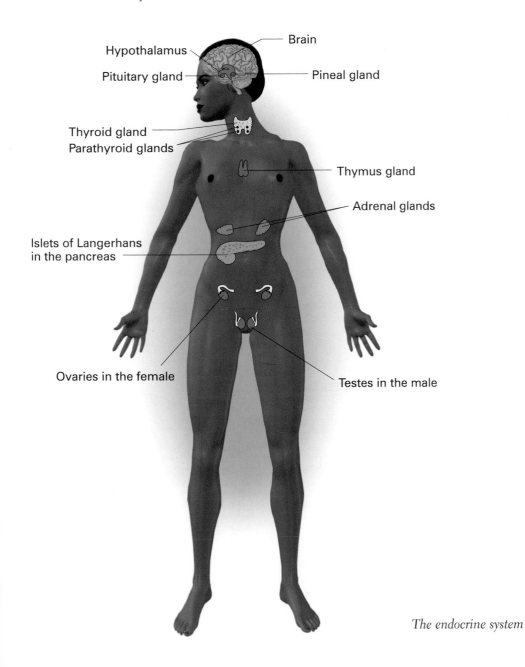

The endocrine system

The functions of the endocrine system

Endocrine glands could accurately be described as organs. They produce chemical compounds called **hormones** which are secreted directly into the bloodstream and carried to specific organs, glands or tissues in other parts of the body where they have a specific effect. Hormones are slow-acting chemical messengers which control many of the body's functions including growth, metabolism, sexual development and coordination. Endocrine glands continually secrete hormones although the level of secretion is altered to meet the body's needs. If glands over- or under-secrete hormones, the body reacts by displaying abnormal physical or physiological symptoms.

Disorders of the endocrine system are of concern to the beauty therapist as they can contra-indicate certain treatments, or a client's concerns, such as superfluous hair growth, may point to the presence of an endocrinological disorder.

The hypothalamus controls the endocrine and autonomic nervous systems and it therefore has an effect on many of the body's functions, including:

- emotion
- sexual activity
- secretion of pituitary hormones
- appetite

- autonomic nervous system
- body temperature
- metabolism
- water balance.

The pituitary gland

The pituitary gland is divided into two sections which have different functions and secretions, as shown in the tables below.

Hormone	Target	Function
Thyroid stimulating hormone (TSH)	Thyroid gland	Regulation of metabolism, breakdown of fat, control of water content
Somatrophic (growth) hormone	Hard tissues of the body	Increases rate of growth and maintains size in adulthood. Over-secretion in children can cause **gigantism**, under secretion can cause **dwarfism**
Follicle stimulating hormone (FSH)	Sexual organs	Controls maturation of ovarian follicles in females and sperm production in males
Lutenising hormone (LH)	Sexual organs	Formation of corpus luteum in ovaries, prepares breasts for lactation in pregnancy

Secretions of the anterior pituitary gland

Hormone	Target	Function
Oxytocin	Pregnant uterus, breasts	Contraction of smooth muscle
Antidiuretic hormone (ADH) or vasopressin	Kidneys	Increase in absorption of water so less urine is excreted. Under-secretion can cause **diabetes insipidus** which is characterised by excess excretion of dilute urine

Secretions of the posterior pituitary gland

The thyroid gland

Hormone	Target	Function
Thyroxine and tri-iodothyronine	Cells and tissues throughout the body	Regulates metabolism in tissues, increases urine production, breaks down protein and increases uptake of glucose by cells
Parathormone		Distribution and metabolism of calcium and phosphorus
Under-secretion		
Hypothyroidism – dry, coarse skin and hair, low metabolism, weight gain, low body temperature, cold Dry, brittle hair, muscle spasm (tetanus)		
Over-secretion		
Hyperthyroidism – anxiety, high pulse rate, increased metabolism, weight loss, heat intolerance Brittle, porous bones, kidney stones		

Secretions and disorders of the thyroid gland

The pancreas

The pancreas produces pancreatic enzymes which play a part in digestion and are described as an exocrine function of the pancreas. The pancreas also has an endocrine function. An area called **the islets of Langerhans** produces two hormones from alpha and beta cells. The alpha cells produce glucagon and the beta cells produce insulin.

Hormone	Target	Function
Insulin	Blood sugar	Controls metabolism of carbohydrates, lowers blood sugar levels
Glucagon	Blood sugar	Releases glycogen stored in the liver to raise blood sugar levels

Secretions of the pancreas

The adrenal glands

The adrenal glands consist of two separate endocrine glands:

- The **adrenal medulla** secretes mineralocorticoid, glucocorticoid and sex hormones.
- The **adrenal cortex** secretes adrenaline and noradrenaline.

Hormone	Target	Function
Mineralocorticoids, e.g. aldosterone	Water content of tissues	Regulate mineral content of body fluids, regulate salt and water balance
Glucocorticoids, e.g. cortisone, cortisol, hydrocortisone	Blood sugar, liver	Regulate metabolism of carbohydrates and proteins, conversion of protein to glycogen for storage in the liver, increase blood sugar level by decreasing use of glucose
Sex hormones (androgens and oestrogens) and steroids	Reproductive organs	Development and function of sex organs, physical characteristics in both sexes, psychological characteristics in both sexes

(continued on next page)

Hormone	Target	Function
Adrenaline	In conjunction with and stimulated by the sympathetic nervous system	Fight and flight mechanism increases heart rate and supply of glucose, blood and oxygen to muscles, digestion slows down
Noradrenaline	Circulation	Contracts blood vessels, raises blood pressure
Over-secretion		
Increased likelihood of ulcers, increased blood pressure **Cushing's syndrome** – excess fatty tissue on trunk, oedema, male pattern hair growth, raised pH of blood (**alkalosis**) An **adrenal tumour** in females produces male characteristics – male pattern hair growth, deepening of the voice		
Under-secretion		
Excess water loss from the body, lowered pH of blood (**acidosis**) **Addison's disease** – anaemia, low blood pressure, muscle wastage, hyperpigmentation		

Secretions and disorders of the adrenal glands

Gonads

Gonads are the **ovaries** which produce ova in females and the **testes** which produce sperm in males. They are controlled by follicle stimulating hormone (FSH) and lutonising hormone (LH). They produce the hormones oestrogen, progesterone and androgens.

Hormone	Target	Function
Oestrogen	Secondary sexual characteristics in females	Development of female reproductive system, development of external genitalia, uterus and breasts, regulation of menstrual cycle
Progesterone	Structures involved in pregnancy	Maintenance of pregnancy, development of placenta, prepares breasts for lactation
Androgens	Secondary sexual characteristics in males	Development of male reproductive system, male hair growth pattern, voice deepening, muscle bulk

Secretions of the gonads

Disorders of the ovaries

If the ovaries fail to respond to stimulation by the pituitary gland, the production of oestrogen and progesterone can be reduced or the secretion of androgens can increase. Such an imbalance is usually characterised by a masculine pattern of hair growth in females, which is known as **hirsutism**.

Primary hirsutism is caused by an increased sensitivity to normal levels of androgens in the blood, which usually begins during puberty and settles down during the thirties. Secondary, or true, hirsutism is caused by increased androgen production in the ovaries or adrenal glands and can begin just prior to or just after puberty.

The nervous system

You will learn about	
• the central nervous system	• sense organs.
• the autonomic nervous system	

The central nervous system

The nervous system provides a network of communication between different areas of the body and also acts as a receptor for information from the external environment. The **central nervous system** (CNS) consists of the brain and spinal cord. An example of the simplest circuit in the CNS involves communication between a single sensory nerve and a motor neurone in the brain or spinal cord. This then transmits an impulse to a muscle or gland causing a reaction. Some reflex actions involve several nerves, such as the knee-jerk reflex which is used to indicate the condition of the nervous system.

The autonomic nervous system

The **autonomic nervous system** (ANS), supplies the internal organs and is so called because these organs function without conscious effort – that is, their functions are *automatic*. There are two parts to the ANS.

- The **sympathetic** nervous system has nerves that supply the internal organs and run back to the spinal nerves, as well as nerves which supply the blood vessels, sweat and sebaceous glands and the arrector pili muscle in the dermis.
- The **parasympathetic** nervous system has branches which run to all of the internal organs.

Therefore each organ has a double nerve supply which provides opposing actions.

Sense organs

The sense organs are the eyes, ears, nose, mouth and skin and their function is to pass on the many impulses which are continually stimulating them. They receive sensory impulses from the external environment and transmit information to the CNS via nerves which stimulate a physical or a psychological reaction. Obvious illustrations of sensory impulses are those of sight, sound, smell, taste and touch – see the table on page 180.

Sensory impulse	Path from sense organ to CNS	Point of interpretation
Sight	Optic nerve (2nd cranial nerve)	Interpreted in the visual areas of the occipital lobes
Hearing	Vestibulococlear nerve (8th cranial nerve)	Interpreted in auditory areas of temporal lobes
Smell	Olfactory nerve (1st cranial nerve)	Interpreted in the temporal lobe
Taste	Facial nerve (7th cranial) and glossopharyngeal nerve (9th cranial)	Interpreted in the temporal lobe with the corresponding smell. Few tastes can be interpreted without corresponding sense of smell
Pain, heat and cold	Nerve endings that transmit pain and temperature changes	Sensory nerve fibres run in the spinal nerves to the posterior nerve roots in the spinal cord
Light touch	Nerve endings that transmit light touch	Sensory nerve fibres run in the spinal nerves to the posterior nerve roots in the spinal cord
Firm pressure	Nerve endings that transmit firm pressure	Sensory nerve fibres run in the spinal nerves to the posterior nerve roots in the spinal cord

Sensory impulses

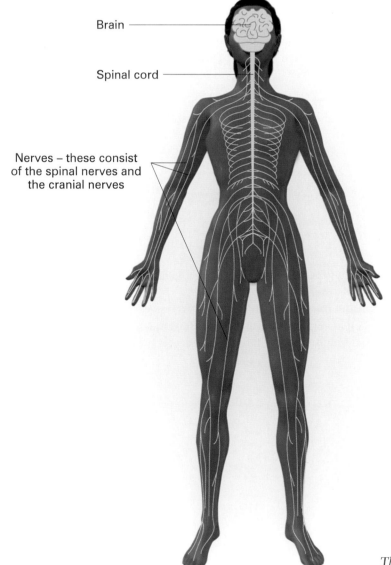

Brain

Spinal cord

Nerves – these consist of the spinal nerves and the cranial nerves

The nervous system

The respiratory system

The structure of the respiratory system

The respiratory system consists of the structures leading to the lungs and the structures within the lungs. Air is breathed in through the nose and/or mouth and travels along the respiratory tract to the lungs. As we breathe in, the chest expands, the diaphragm flattens and the intercostal muscles lift the ribs upwards and outwards. The lungs expand to fill the increased area and become filled with air. As we breathe out, the intercostal muscles relax and the diaphragm is dome-shaped. If the airways become blocked, accessory muscles assist the main muscles of respiration. The sternocleidomastoid raises the sternum while serratus anterior and pectoralis major pull the ribs outwards. During forced exhalation latissimus dorsi and the anterior abdominals help to compress the thoracic cavity.

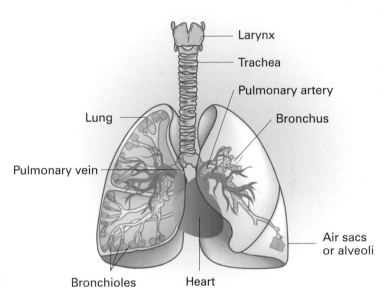

Cross section of the lungs

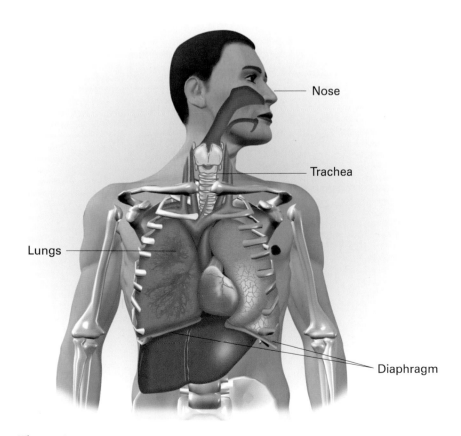

The respiratory system

Respiratory system	Structure	Function
Nose	Lined with mucous membranes which prevent the entry of foreign particles, nostrils lead into the nose and posterior nares lead out to the pharynx	Vascular mucous membranes warm air as it passes through the nose, mucus moistens air and traps dust particles
Pharynx	Leads from nasal cavity and is continuous with the oesophagus	Auditory tubes carry air to the middle ear. The pharynx is part of the respiratory and digestive systems but cannot be used simultaneously so breathing ceases momentarily during swallowing
Larynx	Continuous with the pharynx above and trachea below, consists of several cartilages including the **epiglottis**	During swallowing the larynx shifts upwards and forwards so that the epiglottis blocks its opening
Trachea	Below the larynx extending down the front of the neck and into the thoracic region between the lungs. Consists of muscle, fibrous tissue and rings of cartilage	Epithelium lining the trachea secretes mucous, which combines with dust particles and is swept upwards by the cilia away from the lungs
Bronchii	Two structures, one on either side, leading from the trachea to the lungs. Left bronchii are narrower to allow room for the heart. Similar structure to trachea	Carry air from the trachea into the bronchioles
Bronchioles	Bronchii divide progressively into smaller bronchii, the finest of which are the bronchioles, which consist of muscular fibrous tissue	Carry air from the bronchii towards the lungs
Alveoli	Bronchioles branch to form minute tubes called alveoli	Inhaled air reaches the alveoli via the respiratory tract
Capillary networks	Network of blood vessels surrounding the alveoli	Location of gaseous exchange between the air in the alveoli and the blood in the vessels

Structure of the respiratory system

The reproductive system

You will learn about	
• the female reproductive system	• menstruation and fertilisation.
• the male reproductive system	

The function of the reproductive system is to ensure the continuation of the species.

The female reproductive system

The female reproductive system consists of the ovaries, uterus, vagina, external genitalia and mammary glands.

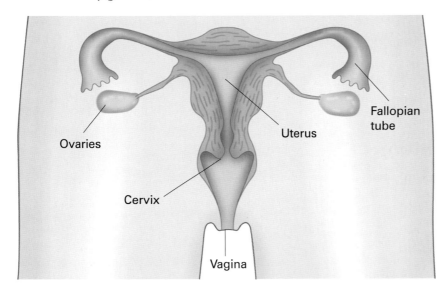

The female reproductive system

Female reproductive system	Structure	Function
Ovaries	Two small glands the size and shape of almonds located on either side of the uterus	Release ova at monthly intervals and secrete the female hormones responsible for sexual development
Uterus	Hollow, thick-walled organ located between the rectum and the bladder at 90° to the vagina. Lined by the **endometrium**	Receives fertilised ovum which grows to fill the uterus, then uterus grows with the foetus until birth
Vagina	Extends from uterus to labia, behind the bladder and urethra and in front of the rectum	Vaginal orifices secrete lubricating fluid to moisten the vulva and assist penetration during sexual intercourse
External genitalia	**Labia** – two fleshy folds covered with skin and hair; **mons pubis** – pad of fat covered with skin and hair over the pubis symphysis; **clitoris** – small, sensitive organ of erectile tissue	Mons pubis and labia protect the internal structures such as the clitoris
Mammary glands	Consists of 15–20 lobes of glandular tissue which, in turn, consists of several smaller lobes called lobules	Act as reservoirs and secrete milk during **lactation**

Structure and function of the female reproductive system

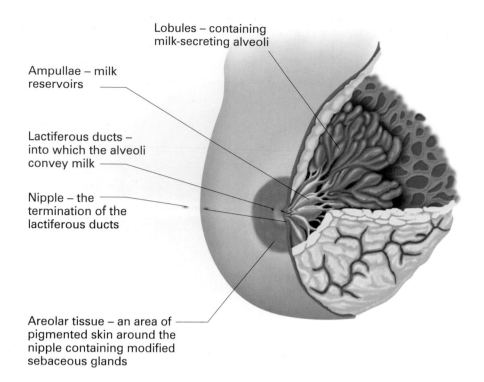

Lobules – containing
milk-secreting alveoli

Ampullae – milk
reservoirs

Lactiferous ducts –
into which the alveoli
convey milk

Nipple – the
termination of the
lactiferous ducts

Areolar tissue – an area of
pigmented skin around the
nipple containing modified
sebaceous glands

The mammary glands

The male reproductive system

The male reproductive system consists of the testes, epididymis, scrotum, sperm duct and penis.

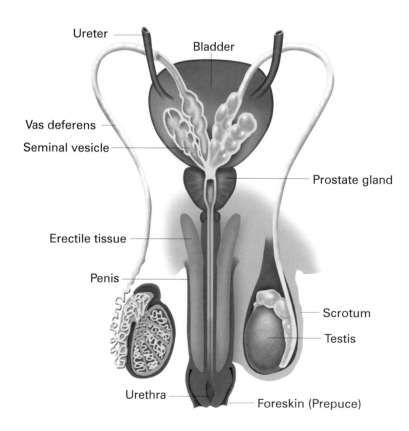

Ureter

Bladder

Vas deferens

Seminal vesicle

Prostate gland

Erectile tissue

Penis

Scrotum

Testis

Urethra

Foreskin (Prepuce)

The male reproductive system

Male reproductive system	Structure	Function
Testes	Reproductive glands which become suspended in the scrotum. Each testis contains 200–300 lobules which contain convoluted tubes called **seminiferous tubules**	Lining of seminiferous tubules develop into **spermatozoa**; interstitial cells in connective tissue secrete **testosterone**
Epididymis	Tightly coiled tubes attached to the back of the testes	Seminiferous tubules open into epididymis which leads to the deferent duct of the seminal vesicle
Scrotum	Sac-like structure which hangs outside of the body	Contains the testes
Sperm duct	Formed by the deferent ducts and seminal vesicles, leading from the base of the prostrate to the urethra	Passage for seminal fluid and sperm
Penis	Tubular organ with plentiful supply of venous sinuses and a tip called the glans penis covered with foreskin	Becomes engorged with blood to cause an erection which facilitates sexual intercourse

Structure and function of the male reproductive system

Menstruation and fertilisation

The female ova is one of the largest cells in the body, measuring about one tenth of a millimetre in diameter. You might think that the production of a single ovum takes one month, the period of the menstrual cycle. In fact, it is a continual process which begins even before birth and continues until the menopause. Following puberty, a few ova are reactivated every day so that there is a steady supply to ensure the release of a single egg each month. At the time of ovulation, the ova is at the surface of the follicle. Increased fluid pressure within causes it to pop and the ova is ejected into the fallopian tubes. If sperm are present, fertilisation can occur at this location.

The menstrual cycle

This describes the (approximately) 28-day reproductive cycle that occurs in most females. Day 1 refers to the first day of menstruation and day 14 is the day ovulation usually occurs. The menstrual cycle is controlled by the relative levels of the hormones oestrogen and progesterone which determine whether an egg is released. If the egg is not fertilised, progesterone levels drop, the endometrium is shed as menstrual blood and the cycle begins once again. Menstruation usually begins between the ages of 12 and 15 and continues until the menopause.

Fertilisation

This describes the process of bringing together the male and female gametes in the fallopian tubes. Natural fertilisation occurs following sexual intercourse when the male penis deposits seminal fluid in the vagina. The sperm are helped by a number of physiological factors. The cervix, which is usually blocked by mucus, becomes more permeable during ovulation. Secondly, cilia lining the entrance to the cervix waft the sperm through. Finally, sperm have a tendency to swim towards the tube containing the ovulated egg rather than the empty one due to their response to chemical signals.

At this stage, the membrane of one sperm fuses with that of an egg. Immediately, the sperm stops swimming and the composition of the egg membrane adjusts to prevent any other sperm from entering. Normal pregnancy in humans lasts 40 weeks and involves a series of changes in the mother as well as in the developing foetus.

Knowledge check

1   *Illustrate the main structures of a cell using a simple diagram.*

2   *Describe the main functions of the skin*

3   *Name the five layers of the epidermis.*

4   *Describe the process of keratinisation.*

5   *Name the main bones of the human skeleton.*

6   *Describe the main functions of the human skeleton.*

7   *Describe the different structures of compact and cancellous bone tissue.*

8   *Give examples in the body of a long bone, short bone, flat bone and irregular bone.*

9   *Name and describe three disorders of joints.*

10   *Define origin and insertion in relation to skeleton muscle.*

11   *Name the two proteins in muscle tissue.*

12   *Name the chief muscles of the face, arm, leg, abdomen and back.*

13   *Illustrate the main structures of the heart using a simple diagram.*

14   *Create a chart to illustrate the differences between arteries and veins.*

15   *Describe the functions of the lymphatic system.*

16   *Name the main structures of the digestive system.*

17   *Name four hormones and explain the function of each.*

18   *Describe the difference between the sympathetic and parasympathetic nervous systems.*

19   *Name the main structures of the respiratory system.*

20   *Describe the process of menstruation.*

you and the
SKIN

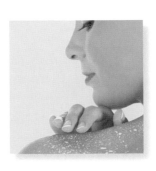 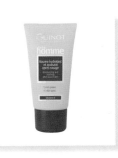 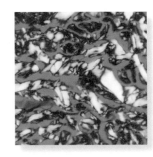

You and the skin

An in-depth knowledge of the skin is essential if you are going to offer clients the full range of mechanical and electrical treatments and manual massage techniques. You will already have an understanding of how the skin behaves, how it grows and what its problems or reactions may be. For Level 3, this knowledge needs to be built upon, to enable you to be confident in your treatment planning using more advanced techniques.

(For the structure of the skin, refer to **Related anatomy and physiology**, page 147; see also **Facial treatments**, page 220, for facial consultation techniques, and **Body treatments**, page 286, for body consultation techniques.)

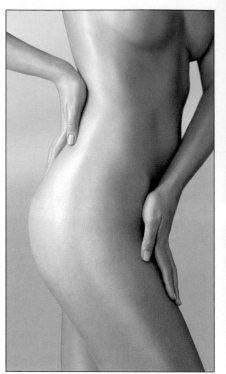

Skin is determined by both genetic and environmental factors

You will learn about

- individual skin characteristics
- how the environment affects skin
- free radicals
- skin colouring
- the pH of skin
- desquamation

- allergic reactions
- contra-indications to treatment
- recognising skin types
- ageing of the skin
- products and skin

Individual skin characteristics

Skin colour, and to a large degree, how it behaves and ages, is determined both genetically and environmentally.

Genetics

From each parent, we inherit a set of genes – an arrangement of codes, known as our DNA. The instructions within the genes will produce our own unique set of features – often called units of inheritance. These will determine our hair colour, eye colour, skin colouring, and so on.

A simple way to visualise this is to think of a gene as carrying a set of instructions for the manufacture of an enzyme (a building block). For example, if you have brown eyes, it is because you have the enzyme which helps in the production of the brown pigment. This enzyme can only be made if you have this gene. So, you are a product of your genes! (See also the section on skin colouring, page 195.)

Global origins

Skin colouring also has its origins in where your ancestors were born. People living close to the Equator, where the sun's rays are strongest, require more protection from the sun than those further north and south. Their bodies developed a natural defence against the intensity of the sun – a darker skin colouring. The darker the skin colouring, the more protection from the sun's rays.

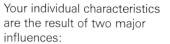

Remember

Your individual characteristics are the result of two major influences:

- the genes you inherit from your parents
- the environment in which you live.

How the environment affects skin

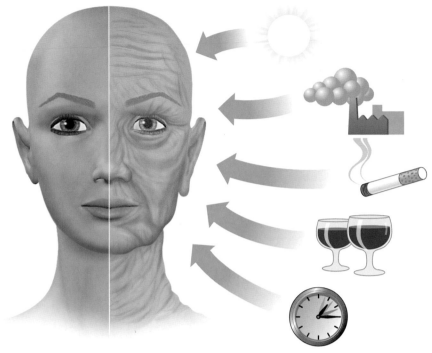

How the environment affects skin

After genetic influences, the second most powerful influence on the skin is the environment. Not only where you originate in the world affects your skin, but also the type of environment in which you live – exposure to smoking, wind, pollution and chemicals greatly affects the skin, as well as the ultraviolet (UV) radiation levels the skin is exposed to, from the sun. The quality of the environment, both external and internal, affects the health of skin.

Internal environment

Internal environment is affected by the lifestyle choices a person makes, including:

- sleeping patterns
- nutrition
- water consumption
- exercise
- alcohol consumption
- smoking
- drug taking – medicinal and recreational
- products used
- stress levels
- exposure to UV rays
- general neglect/bad skincare habits.

It is also affected by factors beyond our control:

- age and the influence of hormones
- the body's immune system and disease/illness.

Remember

A healthy lifestyle does not only apply to the client you are treating; it applies to you too! How can you possibly recommend skin care treatments and give good home care advice if your skin is suffering, because you do not follow you own advice?

Sleep and the skin

Research has shown that we sleep an average of 90 minutes less per night now than we did in the 1920s. Even so, doctors still recommend 8 hours of good quality sleep, to recharge and replenish the body's systems.

While we sleep, growth hormone is released, and this, in turn, influences skin growth, even if the body has stopped growing in height. (Sleep is therefore very important in the very young – babies need nearly twice as much sleep as an adult for growth and development.) Collagen and keratin production within the dermis is increased, and the skin cells of the germinative layer (and therefore the rest of the epidermis) replicate faster than during the day.

Lack of sleep can affect other hormone production and is thought to be linked to adult acne and very dry skin conditions. As the body tries to cope with this lack of replenishment, and the general fatigue that goes with sleep deprivation, the blood is diverted towards the major organs, draining away from the face. This causes the skin pallor and the dark under-eye shadows associated with poor sleeping habits.

Long-term sleep deprivation is bad for the body: the hormone cortisol is released by the adrenal cortex, which is important both for normal carbohydrate metabolism and for the response to any stress. When stress levels and glucose levels are not functioning normally, the changes in the body are similar to those which occur with age. It can lead to high blood pressure, obesity and the onset of diabetes. The good news is that the levels will return to normal once the individual has a regular pattern of 8 hours' sleep.

Brain functioning and coordination are also affected by sleep deprivation, and account for a percentage of accidents at work, as well as poor performance generally in the workplace.

To encourage the client (and the therapist) to get good quality sleep, try the following.

- Avoid eating just before going to bed.
- Avoid stimulants such as tea, coffee and alcohol – alcohol may send you to sleep initially, but you will wake up in the night through dehydration.
- Try a gentle walk for half and hour in the evening to use the muscles.
- Stick to the same time for going to bed, where possible.
- Relax and unwind in a warm bath with a pre-blended bath oil containing essential oils, e.g. jasmine or chamomile.
- Avoid over-stimulating the mind just before going to bed.
- If a particular worry is going around in your head, write it down and then list what you will do to tackle it in the morning. Prioritise what you can deal with: allow yourself time in the morning to get help with what you cannot deal with, and avoid wasting time worrying about the rest!
- Try relaxation tapes or soft music to help relax the mind and body.
- Visualisation can be a great help – imagine relaxing on a warm beach, with the sun shining, and drift off to sleep.

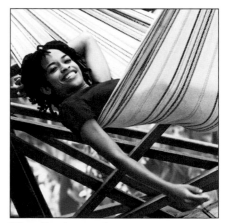

Visualisation, such as imagining you are swinging gently on a hammock, is an effective way of relaxing

Nutrition and the skin

Good nutritional habits are not just about keeping the skin functioning well and looking good, they are also about maximising health potential for the whole body. A sensible mixture of all the food groups is essential for good health, and will provide the essential vitamins and minerals needed.

Below is a suggested healthy eating plan recommended by the World Health and Coronary Prevention Group. It is not a diet for weight loss, which clients often view as something to be done for a set period of time and then forgotten. This is a sensible guide to eating for health and should last for life. Yo-yo dieting is very bad for the body, and is liable to encourage the body to store extra fat, as eating patterns are so erratic. (For information on metabolic functioning, see **Body treatments**, page 321.)

The benefits of eating healthily are a longer life span, better functioning of the body, a glowing skin, and the client may lose weight as a side-effect of cutting down on high-fat foods.

To follow the pyramid plan, a person's daily menu, or average daily menu over the course of a week, should consist of:

- 6 – 11 servings of grain products, e.g. breads, cereals, rice and pasta, with the emphasis on eating a variety of whole grains or organic products
- 5 servings (never fewer than 3) of vegetables from the three categories – dark green leafy and deep yellow; beans and peas; and starches such as potatoes
- 4 servings (never fewer than 2) of various fruits or juices
- 3 servings of fish, lean meats and chicken
- 2 servings of milk or milk products – skimmed or low-fat yoghurts and cheeses are good.

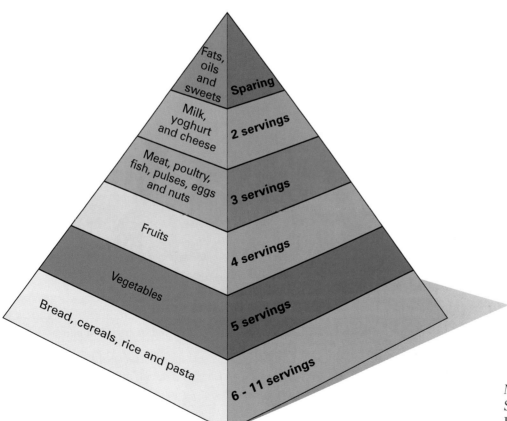

Make a meal of health
Source: World Health and Coronary Prevention Group

These guidelines are flexible over several days. There are no bad (or banned) foods, although high-fat food groups should be eaten in moderation.

You can also advise clients on how to cook their food.

- Avoid frying. Fried foods have a high fat content, which will cause weight gain and are not healthy for the heart. Frying also destroys much of the vitamin content of the food.
- Cook vegetables in a small amount of water for a short time, or preferably steam them, to retain their vitamin content. Some vitamins are fat soluble, others such as vitamin C are water soluble, so vegetables cooked in a large amount of water for a long time lose their goodness.
- Grilling and steaming are an effective way of sealing in the nutritional content of the food.
- Eat some fruit and vegetables raw – the fibre content stays intact and is very good for the skin and the rest of the body.

Nutrient	Sources	Why it is needed
Protein	Red and white meat; dairy products; pulses and lentils; seeds and nuts	Maintains and supports body growth
Iron	Red meat; liver; egg yolk; dried fruits, e.g. apricots, raisins; dried pulses	With protein, it forms haemoglobin to carry oxygen through the body. Vitamin C taken simultaneously helps absorption; tannin and antacid medication limit absorption. Deficiency causes anaemia resulting in fatigue
Calcium	Dairy products; whole fish (sardines); sunflower and sesame seeds	With other minerals and vitamin D, helps strengthen teeth and bones
Vitamin A (retinol)	Animal fats; fish liver oils; egg yolk; carrots; margarine; fortified dairy products; liver; green vegetables	An anti-infective vitamin necessary for growth, reproduction, the maintenance of a healthy skin and mucous membranes. Needed for the formation of rhodopsin, which is the visual purple contained in the retinal rods of the eyes
Vitamin B1 (thiamine)	Wheatgerm; liver; whole grains; nuts; offal; unrefined cereals and pulses; yeast and yeast extracts; fruit; milk; egg yolks; pork meat; legumes; leafy vegetables	Aids digestion and utilisation of energy. Essential for the carbohydrate metabolism and fats and nutrition on nerve cells
Vitamin B2 (riboflavin)	Milk; eggs; yoghurt; cottage cheese; liver; kidney; whole grains; green vegetables; whole grain and enriched flour	Essential for growth and good vision. Aids in digestion and carbohydrate metabolism
Vitamin B3 (niacin)	Oily fish; whole grains; liver; fortified breakfast cereals; peanuts	Aids digestion and normal appetite needs
Vitamin B6 (pyridoxine)	Meat; bananas; dried vegetables; molasses; brewer's yeast; whole grains; offal; fish liver	Helps to regulate body's use of fatty acids to fight infection
Vitamin B12 (cyanocobalamin)	Milk; eggs; meat; dairy food; liver and kidney; fish	Essential for the maintenance of red blood cells and nervous system, the metabolism of fats, proteins and carbohydrates. No vegetable source sufficient for daily needs. Vegans should see their doctor about synthetic forms

(continued on next page)

Nutrient	Sources	Why it is needed
Folic acid (folacin)	Green leafy vegetables; nuts; dried vegetables; whole grains; liver and kidney	Essential for blood formation, within the bone marrow
Vitamin C (ascorbic acid)	Broccoli; oranges and most citrus fruits; red, green and yellow vegetables; sweet potato; tomatoes	Helps build strong teeth and bones, for strengthening small blood vessels, muscles and connective tissue – for formation of the intercellular cement. Important in combating infections and prevention of scurvy. Increases resistance to infection, enables blood coagulation and iron absorption. More required during illness
Vitamin D	Fortified milk; oily fish; liver; eggs; butter. Also sunshine on the skin	Helps in absorption of calcium and builds calcium and phosphorus into bones and strengthens them
Vitamin E	Vegetable oil; green leafy vegetables; wheatgerm; egg yolk; whole grains	Protects fatty acids from destruction
Vitamin K	Fish liver; animal liver; alfalfa; cabbage; spinach; tomatoes; all leafy vegetables; green vegetables; soybean oil; fats; pork; cheese; egg yolk	Essential for the formation of prothrombin and the clotting of blood. Absorbed only in the presence of bile
Phosphorus	Milk products; meat; fish; whole grains; beans	Combines with calcium to strengthen bones and teeth
Iodine	Seafood; fortified salt	Regulates energy use in the body
Zinc	Lean meat; seafood; whole grains; dried beans	Makes up some enzymes and releases vitamin A from liver

Sources of nutrients and their importance to the body

Vitamin	Problems caused by deficiency	Special properties
A	Stunted growth; over keratinisation of the skin and mucous membranes; skin infections; likelihood of bladder and bronchial infections because of altered epithelial membranes; lowered resistance to infection; disorders of the conjunctiva and retina (night blindness)	Fat-soluble. Can be manufactured by the body and from carotene
B1 (aneurine hydrochloride/thiamine)	Loss of appetite; fatigue; mental apathy; impaired functioning of the nervous, digestive, muscular, circulatory and endocrine systems; and if long term, beri-beri. (The symptoms of beri-beri are neuritis, paralysis, muscular wasting, chronic constipation, progressive oedema, mental deterioration, and finally heart failure)	
B2 (riboflavin)	Inadequate functioning of cell enzymes; lowered resistance and vitality; cracks at the corner of the mouth and lesions on the lips; glossitis (inflammation of the tongue); anaemia; retarded growth; photophobia; cataracts	

(continued on next page)

Vitamin	Problems caused by deficiency	Special properties
B3 (niacin)	Affects carbohydrate metabolism; pellagra – leading to glossitis; dermatitis; spinal cord changes	
B6 (pyridoxine)	Symptoms of nervousness; can cause convulsions in infants; dermatitis; nausea; vomiting; affects protein metabolism	
BI2 (cyanocobalamin)	Pernicious anaemia and other types of anaemia	Absorbed by villi of small intestine and stored in liver
Folic acid	Has anti-anaemic properties, so is useful to prevent all types. Vital during pregnancy as lack leads to higher incidence of neural tube defects in babies	
C (ascorbic acid)	Sore and bleeding gums; dental caries; sore joints; tendency to bruise easily; fragility of capillary wall; lowered resistance to infection; retards tissue repair and wound healing; scurvy	Water soluble; readily destroyed by heat
D	Inadequate development of bones and teeth; rickets; osteoporosis. Overdose is possible which causes vomiting, diarrhoea, headaches and drowsiness, high blood calcium and calcium deposits in walls of blood vessels, heart and kidney tissues	Can be made in the skin by action of sunlight (UV rays) on ergo sterols present; fat-soluble
E	Rarely deficient in humans	Fat soluble
K	Tendency to haemorrhage	Fat soluble

Problems caused by vitamin deficiency

Water and the skin

Water is essential to good health and makes up a large percentage of the body. It is lost from the body through the sweat glands at the rate of approximately 100–150 ml every 24 hours, during respiration and through the digestive processes.

Ideally, the body's water balance should be maintained – the intake of water should equal the output. Drinking six to eight glasses of water daily is recommended and it is very beneficial to the skin and the digestive process, along with cell metabolism.

Body dehydration usually results in the sensation of thirst, and drinking to relieve it. However, clients often make the mistake of drinking stimulants, such as alcohol, tea and coffee, which may moisten the dry mouth, but are not as beneficial as water. Clients also misinterpret the sensation of thirst as hunger, or develop a headache, so take a pain killer instead of a glass of water. Drinking a glass of water prior to and during a meal provides the body with adequate fluid to function properly, and prevents over-eating.

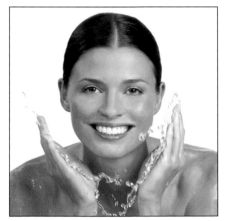

Keep the skin hydrated – internally and externally!

Skin dehydration is associated with clients who:

- do not drink enough water to replenish natural loss
- do not use the correct products to maintain the skin's hydro lipid (acid) mantle, so water is evaporated through the skin
- follow a completely fat-free diet, so are deficient in essential fatty acids, essential to the keratinocyte cell membrane, which results in low epidermal lipids, as well as reducing active and passive transfer of nutrients and oxygen within the cells

- work in a dry atmosphere, which also encourages water loss
- have a high alcohol intake, which is a factor in dehydration.

It is important to encourage clients (and yourself, as the therapist!) to maintain a good intake of water, daily. It can be in the form of water with added flavourings, or a low-sugar squash. The client should see the difference in a matter of days. Also check that clients are using the correct products for their skin type, so that water is not being lost unnecessarily through the skin's surface.

External environment

The external environment is a major factor in the ageing process. It is widely recognised by leading dermatologists that up to 90 per cent of skin damage is caused by external environmental factors, leading to ageing of the skin. The thickness of the skin can begin to decrease by the age of twenty, so in biological terms if the cells are losing energy, they will also lose their ability to protect themselves against the environment.

Free radicals

Besides smoking, wind, pollution, and so on, free radicals, or oxidants, are factors in the ageing of the skin. Free radicals are generated in the body as a reaction to the damage caused by environmental factors on the body, including UVA and UVB rays, petrol and cigarette smoke, and internal factors such as stress and tiredness. A consequence of this attack on the skin is an acceleration of the skin's ageing process, with the loss of radiance, elasticity and tone. Free radicals are controlled by enzymes, but should the production of the enzymes become poor, due to an unhealthy lifestyle, lack of sufficient nutrition, and so on, then there will be a build up of chemicals and toxins within the tissues.

Research is continuing into which chemicals within our environment stimulate free radical production. Crop sprays, pesticides and household cleaning items are some of the products under investigation.

This explains why so many clients are coming to the salon for advanced facial and body skin care techniques – some bodies are just not coping.

Skin colouring

The skin owes its colouring to:

- the carotene pigments within subcutaneous fat
- the concentration and state of oxygenation of the red haemoglobin found within the blood vessels
- the existence of other pigments such as blood bile pigments, reflected in the colour of the skin
- the amount of melanin present in the skin
- the general health and circulation of the client.

Various degrees of pigmentation are present in the different ethnic groups, but the differences are in the amount of melanin produced and are not dependent upon the number of melanocytes present.

Certain areas of skin are very rich in pigment, such as the genital area and the nipples, while practically no pigment is present in the palms of the hands and the soles of the feet.

Remember

Free radicals are harmful, unstable molecules within the body which attach themselves to the skin's surface.

Remember

People living in northern countries, with less UV exposure, have less skin damage. Although much UV damage is done in the early years, often the results are not seen until clients are in their forties and fifties. This is more of a problem now that international travel is so common, and clients often travel in search of sunshine!

The pigment is stored as fine granules within the cells of the germinative layer, although some granules may also be deposited between the cells. In pale skin types the granules occur only in the deepest cell layers and mainly in the cylinder-shaped cells of the basal row. In brown/black skin types pigment is found throughout the entire layer and even in the stratum granulosum.

All melanin is synthesised in cells called melanocytes from an amino acid (tyrosine) by a complex chemical reaction, which makes pigment granules called melanosomes. When the melanosomes are full of pigment they are then distributed to the epithelial cells, spreading the pigment throughout the skin. The melanocytes are scattered in the basal layers of the epidermis and mature as the embryo is developing in the womb – influenced by the units of inheritance in the gene code, so determining skin colour.

Melanin is the skin's main defence against acute effects of exposure to UV light, both occurring naturally through sunlight and through artificial tanning, using any form of sunbed. It acts as a density filter, reducing the harmful effects of UV radiation. The protective property of melanin is its ability to absorb and disperse radiation.

Some people are born without the ability to produce melanin within their skins and no hair pigment, a condition known as albinoism. They have white hair, pale skin and pink eyes.

Black skin

Black skin has more evenly distributed melanocytes, which are larger and more active than in a white skin. Black skin is also more robust: it has greater elasticity and strength of collagen fibres, giving support to the skin, so there is less possibility of dropped contours of the face. Sebaceous glands are larger and denser, giving good lubrication and moisture to prevent the formation of wrinkles and making it less prone to premature wrinkles. This also means the ageing process is slower in black skin, with less cell deterioration, and because black skin flakes and is shed more quickly than white skin, cell renewal is faster.

Skin cancer is not as common in black skin, due to its protection from the harmful UVC rays of the sun. Also, the epidermis is considerably thicker than in its white counterpart, and it is therefore less reactive, and not prone to allergies or infection. For example, warts are rarely found on black skin.

Due to the epidermis being thicker, black skin easily forms scars, which can turn into keloid tissue – seen as an over-thickening of the skin, in a pink/beige colour, which is more noticeable against a darker background.

Obviously each black skin should be considered individually, as skin reactions are a very personal thing. During the consultation, ask questions about product use and sensitivity, and the client will guide you by his or her own experiences about what works for his or her skin.

Remember

The palms of the hands and the soles of the feet are often referred to as 'glabrous' skin, which lacks hair follicles and sebaceous glands and has a thicker epidermis.

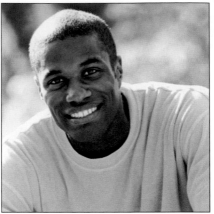

Each client's skin should be considered individually

Remember

Some black skins are quite sensitive to skin care products, and care should be taken to avoid harsh, abrasive products, or strong alcohol-based toners. These types of product are often used to treat an oily skin. Do not always judge black skin as oily, as there is often a sheen or glow on black skin which is actually a reflection of the light, especially under a spotlight or facial examination lamp.

The pH of skin

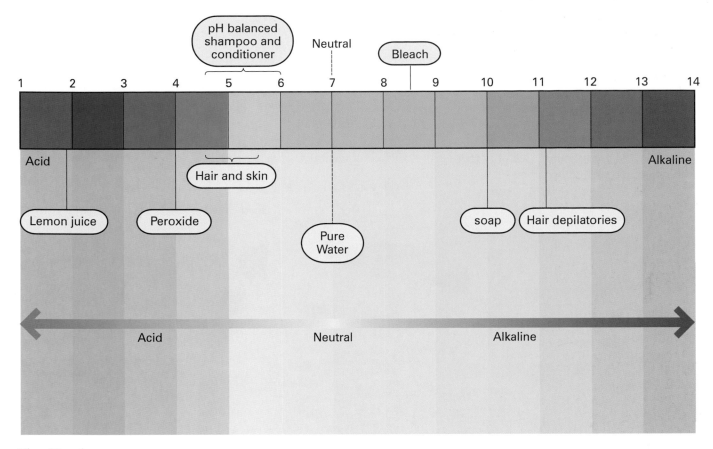

The pH scale

The skin acts as a defence against infection and has a protective barrier over the surface of the epidermis, which is often referred to as the acid mantle, or the hydro-lipidic mantle (see **Related anatomy and physiology**, page 147). The term comes from *hydro*, referring to the water from the sweat glands, and *lipid* as in fat or sebum from the sebaceous glands – the acid mantle is a mixture of both gland secretions. This is a kind of water-in-oil emulsion on the skin's surface, which also contains minerals, urea, lactic acid and amino acids, and it is this combination which gives the skin its acid pH of between 4.5 and 5.5 in a normal, healthy skin.

The average skin pH is about 5.4, and this inhibits the growth of bacteria. Fungi are controlled by sebum, which inhibits their growth, so it makes sense to maintain a steady pH balance in the skin, to help fight infection. Using products which are too harsh and strip the skin of its protective pH acid mantle will allow infections in and cause damage.

Desquamation

The process of desquamation, or exfoliation, enables the skin to rid itself of old cells and allow new ones to come up to the surface, keeping the skin healthy and able to fight infection. (For more information on desquamation and keratinisation, see **Related anatomy and physiology**, page 149).

Exfoliant products and brush cleansing are excellent methods of desquamating the skin prior to other treatments, especially if the client does not have the time for a steam treatment, or the full microdermabrasion process. Exfoliation both cleanses the skin and creates an erythema within the dermis, so the blood vessels are receptive to carrying absorbed substances further into the body. Avoid creating too much of an erythema, however, as another stimulating treatment may cause a skin reaction, and become a contra-action to treatment.

Desquamation is painless. Even controlled microdermabrasion (MDA), which is a skin peeling process for the treatment of skin problems such as scar tissue, pigmentation abnormalities and acne, is not felt, as the intensity of the peeling depth is firmly controlled by the therapist, and only restores the balance of healthy, well-functioning epidermal cells.

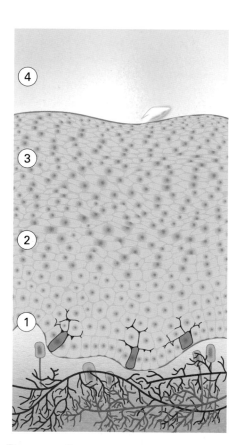
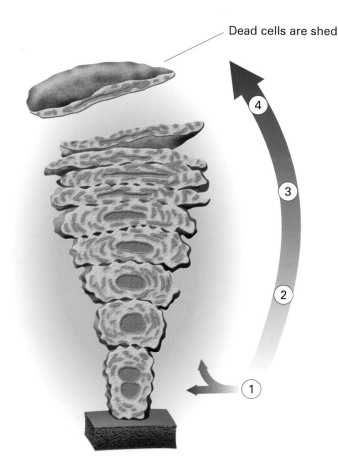

Dead cells are shed

Desquamation

Abnormal shedding

The shedding of skin can be affected by skin diseases such as psoriasis, where itchy, red, scaly patches form, most commonly on the elbows, knees, legs and scalp. Here the life cycle of skin cells drops to only five days (instead of 28) from the stratum germinativum to the stratum corneum. As this happens so fast, the nuclei in the cells are retained. The cause is not known, but it is a very common skin disease and is thought to be stress-related. Sunlight or UV exposure from a sunbed often helps the condition and there are creams available to help, too.

Allergic reactions

A method of defence used by the skin is the production of histamine, a compound derived from the amino acid histidine, found in nearly all tissues of the body. Histamine causes dilation of blood vessels and contraction of smooth muscle. It is an important moderator of inflammation and is released in large amounts after skin damage, producing flushing of the skin, irritation, itching within the area and often a wheal. Pain may be experienced and also there may be swelling.

This is not a common reaction, but can occur if clients are allergic to any active ingredients within a product, especially when using electrical currents to help penetrate the product into the skin. Galvanic creams/gels can produce an allergic reaction in clients with a sensitive skin, or those who have a low tolerance of other substances such as pollens, certain foods, animal hairs and so on.

Clients with a quick-trigger response of histamine to substances can be prescribed anti-histamine drugs, which suppress the response, and keep irritation from either products or allergic conditions such as hayfever at bay. Anti-histamine is used to suppress most allergic reactions, so the subject should arise within the consultation when you ask the client if he or she is taking any form of medication. This will indicate the level of allergic reaction the client has, and you can adapt accordingly.

Contra-indications to treatment

Specific contra-indications to each treatment are covered within the relevant section of this book. These should be discussed during the consultation for whichever treatment you are considering for your client.

Skin conditions

The following conditions are contra-indications that will not necessarily stop the treatment from taking place, but treatment may need to be adapted to avoid the contra-indicated area.

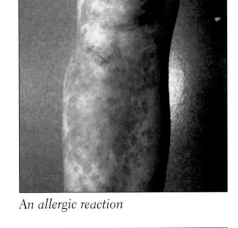

An allergic reaction

Remember

The client may have an allergy to nuts, and it is vital to find this out at consultation stage, as nut derivatives are included within many cosmetic preparations. If the reaction is severe, it can be life threatening – the client may go into anaphylactic shock which requires immediate medical attention. Symptoms include breathlessness, pallor, weakness, fever, convulsions and unconsciousness. In extreme cases, the client may carry an epi-pen – a form of injection which delivers a dose of adrenaline via the muscles to counteract the reaction.

Cuts, abrasions, broken skin

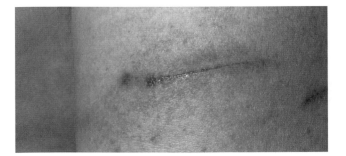

Cut

If recent, a scab will be forming, the skin may be tender and swollen in the area, and bruising may be seen. If cuts and abrasions are recent, avoid the area altogether. If the area has healed over, and is not too recent, get the client's agreement that gentle application can take place, with careful consideration of hygiene.

Bruises or swelling

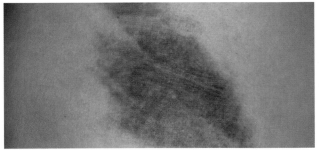

Bruise

Easily recognised as a swelling, with discoloration in varying shades. Avoid altogether if recent or painful to the touch. If healing has taken place, a gentle application of make-up will help to blend in the colour differences to the client's normal shade. Always ask for the client's agreement.

Recent scar tissue

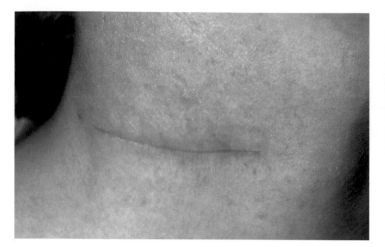

Scar tissue

Usually a different colour from the rest of the skin, following the line of injury. If the scar is recent, raised or angry looking, then avoid the area altogether. If the area is healing and not very large, gentle application is possible with the client's permission. Scar tissue less than six months old, or over a large area, should not be touched with make-up.

Eczema

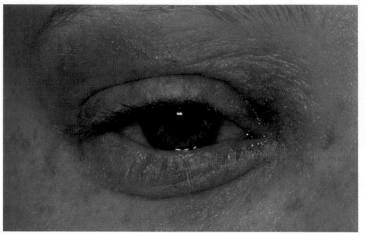

Eczema

Very dry skin, often scaly and flaky, can be red and often very itchy. If the eczema covers a large area, and is inflamed with broken skin, then leave alone, and suggest a visit to the GP. You may make it worse. If the eczema has irritated the eye area, it is unlikely the client would want make-up application. If it is only a small patch of eczema, and not angry, just exclude the area from treatment. The use of hypo-allergenic products is recommended and patch test if the client is very sensitive.

Dermatitis

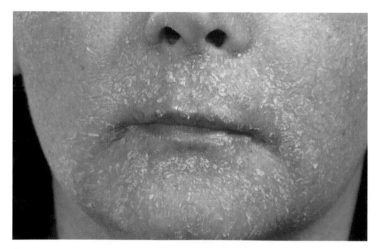

Dermatitis

This is similar to eczema in appearance, but the cause is not the same. A reaction or allergy to something in contact with the skin usually causes dermatitis.

Skin allergies may result in a contra-action so if the client's skin tends to react, do a skin patch test 24 hours prior to the make-up application. It may be wise to use hypo-allergenic make-up, and ask the client to bring in her own make-up if she knows she is safe using it.

Psoriasis

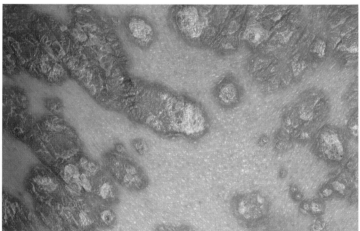

Psoriasis

Seen as scaly patches of red and/or silvery skin. This can break open and become sore. The cause is unknown but is thought to relate to the nervous system. A contra-indication would be if the psoriasis is open or bleeding. One of the common sites for psoriasis is the scalp, so the client may have a little patch visible along the hairline. If the client agrees to make-up application, and it is not directly over the area, then continue. A patch test 24 hours prior to the application of make–up is advisable to ensure that the condition is not aggravated.

Acne vulgaris

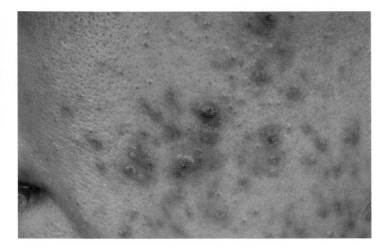

Acne vulgaris

Inflamed whiteheads, blackheads and pustules in various degrees of congestion. Mostly associated with hormones – and the presence of bacteria can make the condition infected.

Infected inflamed acne is a contra-indication. However, a client with mild acne can be treated in the salon, and a light water-based foundation applied. There may be a tendency to greasy skin, and therefore a light application of powder keeps the skin looking matt.

Acne rosacea

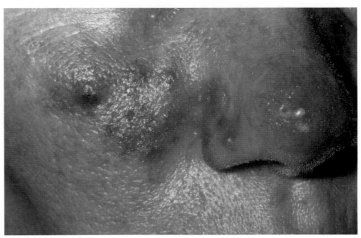

Acne rosacea

Seen as a flush of red over the nose and cheeks with a raised feel to the skin. Often those who have suffered acne vulgaris in youth are prone to rosacea in later life. If the skin is not tender and the client agrees, application of make-up can tone down the redness and therefore lessen the angry look of the skin.

Skin tags

These are usually found on the eye area or lids and/or on the side of the neck. They resemble little 'mushrooms' of skin on a stalk, which move when touched.

As these are not painful or dangerous, make-up application can take place. If they become enlarged and irritating to the client they can be removed under local anaesthetic, usually at the GP's surgery.

Milia

These are small white pearls under the skin, often around the eyes or on the side of the cheek, caused by a build-up of sebum. Make-up application can take place over milia, as they are not infectious.

(See also **Professional basics**, page 42, to refresh your knowledge of types of skin conditions which are caused by bacterial, fungal or viral infections, and which may contra-indicate treatment.)

Pigmentation disorders

These disorders are caused by irregularities in the skin's melanin production. They are not infectious and are not a contra-indication to facial or make-up treatments. Pigmentation disorders do affect the client's appearance, however, and may make the client feel embarrassed and self-conscious; as a therapist, you therefore need to treat them sensitively. The use of camouflage cosmetics may help more effectively with the matching of the pigmentation than ordinary foundations and concealers.

Melanoderma

This is a general term used to describe patchy pigmentation. This is usually an increase in melanin caused by applying cosmetics or perfume which contain light-sensitive ingredients (e.g. bergamot oil used in the perfume industry) – the skin becomes extra-sensitive to UV light. Some drugs have a similar effect. This can also follow inflammation and is sometimes the cause of brown patches following sunburn.

Vitiligo

This is also called hypopigmentation. It is a condition in which small patches of skin have lost their pigmentation, and appear a lighter colour than the rest of the skin. These lighter areas burn easily in the sun and need to be protected. It is not raised or painful to the touch. If the discoloration is in large patches a specialist camouflage make-up should be applied to conceal and match the skin tone. This may mean referral to a specialist. If the patch is small, clever choice of foundation and careful application is acceptable. Any pigmentation disorder may require the use of specialised make-up products to ensure even coverage, and the correct colour match of the skin.

Chloasma

This is also called hyperpigmentation. It consists of irregular patches of brown pigment caused by the over-production of melanocytes. This often appears on the face during pregnancy and is sometimes linked to the contraceptive pill. The discoloration usually disappears when the hormone balance is restored.

Freckles

These are tiny, flat irregular patches of pigment on fair-skinned people, particularly blonds and redheads. They are due to the uneven distribution of melanin, and this becomes more noticeable on exposure to strong sunlight. The freckles often increase in size and join together. The skin between the freckles contains little or no melanin so burns easily. As a therapist you should recommend a good sunscreen to the client.

Lentigo

Larger and more distinctive than a freckle, and may be slightly raised. This pigmentation does not increase in number or darken on exposure to UV light.

Haemangioma

This consists of various conditions caused by the permanent dilation of superficial blood vessels. Stimulating treatments will therefore be contra-indicated, but camouflage cosmetics can be used.

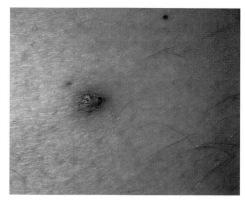

Haemangioma

Dilated capillaries

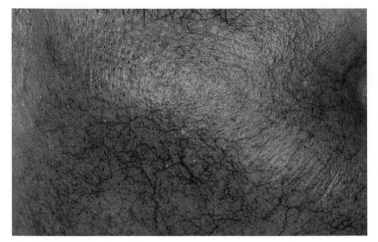

Dilated capillaries

This is the result of loss of elasticity in the walls of the blood capillaries – the cheeks and the nose are often most affected. Exposure to weather, harsh handling and lack of protection, along with spicy hot foods and alcohol, can also be contributing factors. Clients with dry/sensitive skin types are most likely to be affected.

Split capillaries

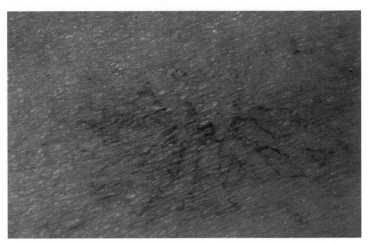

Split capillaries

Weakening and rupturing of capillary walls – clients should avoid stimulating treatments. This condition can be treated by diathermy.

Strawberry naevus

This is a raised and distorted area, often on the face, bright pink or red. It appears a few days or weeks after birth and usually clears up completely by the age of eight.

Spider naevus

A central dilated vessel with leg-like projections of capillaries. The face and cheeks tend to be most affected and this often occurs during pregnancy due to the increase in oestrogen levels.

Port wine stain

This is a bright purple, irregular shaped flat birthmark that can vary in size. These birthmarks are thought to be due to damage by pressure during foetal development. These birthmarks grow with the body and can be quite disfiguring to the client. As a therapist you should always treat such marks sensitively with good cosmetic camouflage make-up.

Sensitivity testing

Failure of thermal and sensitivity tests will indicate a malfunction of the skin, and would be classed as a contra-indication (see **Professional basics**, page 38).

Recognising skin types

You will be expected to treat all of the skin types within your treatment ranges, and you may need to refresh your previous training on how to recognise them (see **Facial treatments**, pages 230–2, for a full example of a facial record card and questions to ask the client).

The skin types are:

- normal
- oily
- dry
- combination
- sensitive
- mature
- dehydrated
- blemished/congested
- male skin.

The true skin type may not be easy to diagnose at first, as all skins react to the environment, products used and the lifestyle of the client. Some investigation is required and a patient approach within the consultation will help you identify the correct skin type.

Normal skin

This supposedly does not exist, as a 'perfect' skin is only found in teenagers unaffected by hormonal influences, when the oil and sweat glands are working in harmony. However, many clients who look after their skins, or who were born with a good skin, would class their skin as normal, in its behaviour and properties.

This type of skin has a good balance of moisture content and oil to keep the skin soft, supple and flexible, so this is the ideal skin type to aspire to, even if rarely found. The skin is finely textured with no visible pores and smooth to the touch; it is plump, clear and has a healthy glow. It should feel warm to the touch, and heals well if damaged. This type of skin has a good hydro-lipidic (acid) mantle, so control of bacteria and protection against germs is good, as is the moisture content, which is well contained within the skin. This skin type would be considered to be the most balanced.

Questions to ask the client

- Is your skin generally in this condition?
- Do you feel you have any problem areas?
- Have you had problems in the past?
- What skin care routine and products are you currently using?
- What electrical and mechanical treatments, if any, have you had, and which most suited your skin?

Dry skin

A dry skin is deficient in both oil and moisture, leaving the skin dry to the touch, and there may be some loss of elasticity depending upon the client's age, and a tendency to flakiness. All skins tend to dry out as they get older, because of reduced functioning of the sebaceous and sweat glands. However, a dry skin can be looked after and responds well to treatments.

Dry skin problems

The texture of the skin is usually fine and dry skin can often be thin, with small red veins (dilated capillaries) present on the cheek areas. Pores and follicles are often closed and inactive. Skin chaps easily and is inclined to be sensitive. Lines and wrinkles may form early with dry skin, especially around the eyes. This can be inherited, and this skin type has a predisposition towards eczema and dermatitis.

This skin type is hard to judge, as it is possible the client is drying out the top layers of the epidermis by using the wrong products, and the skin is actually not a dry skin at all. Environmental factors could be influencing the hydro-lipidic (acid) mantle and the skin could be dehydrated.

If a dry flaky skin has pustules and comedones present, then the oil production is very much in evidence, and the client may have used a harsh retail preparation to dry out the comedones, but has dried out the epidermis too much. To be certain of this skin type, a very gentle exfoliant should be used on the skin, to remove the dry flaky skin cells which have accumulated on the epidermis and look at the underlying skin.

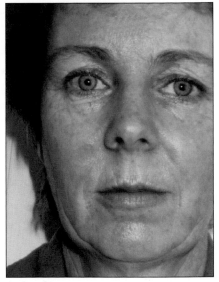

A *dry skin*

Questions to ask the client

- Does your skin feel tight and drawn?
- Does your skin sometimes flake?
- Does exposure to cold and wind make your skin sore?
- Do you burn easily?
- Is your skin prone to outbreaks of dermatitis or eczema?
- Would you consider your skin to be sensitive as well as dry?
- What is your product/skin care routine?
- Do you have comedones or pimple out breaks and if so, how do you treat them?
- What electrical and mechanical treatments, if any, have you had, and which most suited your skin?

Oily skin

This type of skin is the easiest to recognise if there are problems, but be careful with this skin category. It also suffers from poor product use, along with over-stimulation of the sebaceous glands, leading to misdiagnosis of the true skin condition.

True oily, or greasy, skin is caused by an over-production of sebum from the sebaceous glands. It looks shiny; it can be slightly thicker in consistency than normal skin, sallow, coarse and have problems associated with it. This skin is often referred to as seborrhoeic.

Oily skin problems

Enlarged pores, congested pores, comedones and infection may occur on greasy skins, so care must be taken. A greasy skin often develops during puberty, when there is a surge of hormonal activity under the influence of the sex hormones, as the teenager reaches sexual maturity. It often corrects itself when the hormone levels settle, and the use of the correct skin preparations can certainly help. Clients with an oily skin often use harsh, drying products as they feel they need to keep the skin 'clean' and oil-free. What they are doing is:

- stripping the hydro-lipidic (acid) mantle from the skin, risking infection and water loss, through lack of protection in the epidermis

- over-stimulating the sebaceous glands to produce more sebum, to replace the lost sebum contributing to the hydro-lipidic (acid) mantle. With vigorous pressure on the skin, the glandular activity becomes even more erratic.

Oil-based products will be inappropiate for this skin, as they interfere with the delicate hydro-lipidic (acid) mantle, so you will need to advise the client how to break the vicious circle of drying out the top of the epidermis, and trying to compensate by putting oil-based moisturisers on after a rigorous cleanse.

Unfortunately, acne can scar the skin quite badly and although the infection may be cleared up by the use of prescribed medication, the scarring left can be quite noticeable, and make the client self-conscious. Microdermabrasion is very successful in minimising the effect of scarring, through normalising the stratum corneum, increasing the number of living cells and helping to restore good function to the cells, so salon treatments can make a difference to this skin type.

The advantage to having an oily skin in youth is that although there may be skin problems caused by too much sebum production, as the skin ages, the sebum production slows down but still keeps the skin soft. An oily skin does not dry out as much as a dry skin, and wrinkles are less noticeable.

Questions to ask the client
- Is your skin prone to pimples and blackheads?
- Does your skin shine?
- Is it difficult to keep on make-up?
- What type of products are you using?
- Does your skin feel tight and dry to the touch?
- What type of exfoliating products do you use?
- What electrical and mechanical treatments, if any, have you had, and which most suited your skin?

Combination skin

Some skins are a combination of two or more skin types. The most common one is a greasy T-zone along the forehead and nose, with normal or dry skin on the cheek area. This is because there are more sebaceous glands along the T-zone which may therefore show all the characteristics of a greasy skin. This skin is very easy to recognise in youth – the nose may have comedones and the cheeks are noticeably drier than the rest of the face. As the skin gets older, and the sebum production slows down, the T-zone will become less oily. The cheek areas, if looked after well, should be stable and the skin looks more even and is not quite as easy to identify.

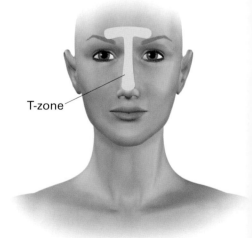

T-zone

The greasy T-zone

Questions to ask the client
- Is your nose shiny?
- Are you prone to blackheads in the T-zone area?
- Does the skin on your cheeks ever feel tight or dry?
- What products are you using?
- What electrical and mechanical treatments, if any, have you had, and which most suited your skin?

Sensitive skin

All skin needs to be sensitive for good health, but in beauty therapy a sensitive skin is one that is actually super-sensitive, that is, it reacts to even mild stimulus. Sensitive skins are often associated with pale skins or a dry skin that lacks the protection of enough sebum. They have a highly flushed look, with a tendency to colour easily, and may react to beauty products or chemicals used within the salon (see the information allergic reactions on page 199). A sensitive skin will certainly react with some of the active ingredients within galvanic gels, so a range for sensitive skins should be suggested.

Questions to ask the client

- Is your skin prone to allergic reactions?
- Are you taking any medication for allergies?
- Do you often have a high cheek colour?
- Does your skin show signs of being dry but slightly red?
- How does the sensitivity of your face compare with your body?
- Have you recently changed a household product brand for a new one, e.g. washing powder, fabric conditioner?
- Are you allergic to metal? (Important for epilation and the choice of needle used)
- What electrical and mechanical treatments, if any, have you had and which most suited your skin?

Mature skin

In a fine-textured, older skin the slower rate of the sebaceous secretions accompanied by loss of elasticity are contributory factors to the skin's appearance through the ageing process (see page 210). Wrinkles begin to form; the epidermis may become thinner, with a lack of springiness and loss of support from underlying muscles. Collagen becomes degraded and thinned out and the skin sags. Lack of oestrogen production in menopausal clients is a problem, as oestrogen helps maintain good levels of fat in the lower dermis, so fine lines and dryness are a result. Collagen and elastin fibre production is not as prolific as in youth, and this can produce a loss of firmness and slack contours to the face. Smoking, environmental influences and poor diet will be reflected in a mature skin, which is sallow and dry.

However, a mature skin, when looked after, and when a good lifestyle promotes good health, can look very radiant. Although some maintenance is required, a mature skin is rewarding to treat within the salon as it responds so well to electrical, rehydrating treatments. Many salons find that the mature skin is the most frequent skin type treated: the client wants to minimise the signs of a mature skin, and older clients often have more time to spend in the salon and more disposable income to pay for treatment courses. While a programme of facials will mean the client sees a dramatic improvement in this skin type, a mature skin still needs a high degree of care at home to sustain the effects of salon treatments, especially night care products. Mature skin also suffers from dryness, so the questions to ask will be the same.

Questions to ask the client

These would be the same as for a dry skin (see page 205).

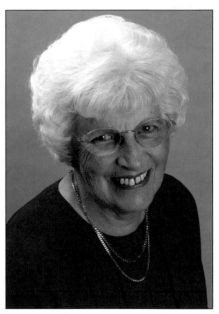

A mature skin

Dehydrated skin

Skin may have the normal sebaceous secretions and still suffer from flaking and tightness due to loss of surface moisture – a condition of dehydration. Any skin can suffer temporary dehydration, which may be caused through using harsh products on the skin or exposure to extreme temperatures, central heating or excessive dieting. Encourage the client to drink 6 to 8 glasses of water per day (see page 194).

Questions to ask the client:

* What skin care products are you using?
* Have you altered your diet recently?
* What is your product/skin care routine?
* What are you using as an exfoliant?
* What electrical and mechanical treatments, if any, have you had and which most suited your skin?

Congested skin

Congestion occurs because the pores become blocked and sweat and sebum cannot escape onto the skin's surface. It can be seen and felt as lumpy and coarse. Whiteheads and blackheads can build up and the epidermis may harden. Poor removal of make-up, using the wrong products and excess sweat building up all contribute to this skin condition. Congested skin will need a course of treatments to help with the deep cleansing and balancing of the glands' production. Often, several sessions of exfoliation and galvanic desincrustation can return a congested skin to normal, as long as the salon treatments are supported by good home product use combined with a healthy diet and an exercise programme. Bad habits of not cleansing, or not cleansing sufficiently, and poor diet, along with a sluggish lifestyle, need to be rectified, so that all factors contribute to the healing of the skin.

Infected skin

Any bacteria, fungi or viruses can penetrate the skin and cause infection. This is easily recognised as swelling and irritation, with pain and tenderness. The presence of pus is also a sign of infection (see **Professional basics**, page 40, for hygiene and safety information on all infectious conditions).

Acne vulgaris

Acne vulgaris is often called polymorphous adolescent acne, as it typically occurs in adolescence, and is more common in males than females. This is because it is linked to or triggered by the influence of testosterone, the male sex hormone. This hormone stimulates the epithelial cells, particularly in the upper layers, causing them to increase in bulk, resulting in an overgrowth of tissue, leading to obstruction of the follicle. The hormone also acts upon the sebaceous glands, making them increase in size as well as output. So, just as the sebaceous glands are working overtime, and have grown larger, the follicle is blocked and the sebum cannot escape onto the skin's surface. This results in:

* sealed comedones
* open comedones and whiteheads, often with a white/yellow column appearing during extraction, which is the column of horny cells embedded in the sebum
* papules, seen as hard, small, reddish lumps on the skin's surface
* pustules, often forming on top of a papule
* nodules of inflammation, seen as angry red lesions.

When bacteria enter the follicle, an infection is triggered and the skin forms deep abscesses of a violet colour, which can be very painful, and the result is often deep scarring, especially if cysts stay after the infection has cleared. The skin has a very unbalanced hydro-lipidic (acid) mantle, so the skin is more at risk from outside infection and dehydration.

Infected acne can really only be treated by internal medication, and some are very good at reducing the infection quickly. However, research is still going on with drugs to treat acne, as some of them are known to trigger depression and can have serious side-effects. With a GP's approval, and after the infection is completely cleared, a course of skin care treatments can make a remarkable difference to both the skin's appearance and the self-confidence of the acne sufferer.

Male skin

When looking at skin types and colours, it is important to include the male skin, as men are becoming big spenders in the skin care market. One of the fastest growing areas within the beauty industry is the demand for specific men's salon treatments and related care products.

Products designed for men have been developed to reflect the fact that the skin is more resistant, but conversely may also be more fragile, through neglect, misuse or total lack of protective products such as moisturisers and sun blocks.

Male skin is approximately 25 per cent thicker than female skin, due to the influence of the male hormones testosterone and androgens, so is it therefore more resistant but becomes thinner more quickly when ageing. Because of testosterone influences, male skin tends to be oilier than female skin, so men prefer lighter moisturising products and products which solve their particular problems – healing and soothing products, creams that reduce razor bumps, products which reduce the possibility of ingrown hairs and anti-ageing creams are popular.

Men who shave daily are automatically exfoliating the upper epidermal cells, so the skin stays healthy looking and clear. There are many products available for sensitive skins, both for dry and wet shaving, to avoid shaving rash, which can be very sore and unsightly.

Anti-ageing creams (a misleading term as nothing can stop the ageing process) are a fast-selling line because, although the signs of ageing appear later on a male face, when they do arrive the wrinkles are more intense and visible – men have fewer small lines, but more deep wrinkles.

Most men's basic product needs are for the daily routine of washing, shaving and moisturising, unless calming products are needed for the specific treatment of blocked pores, irritation from shaving and razor burn or folliculitis (inflammation of the hair follicle in the skin, commonly caused by an infection). Some men use salon treatments to enhance their natural good points – eyelash tinting and the application of tinted moisturiser are very common, and manicures and pedicures are also a favourite with male clients.

Remember

Acne can occur on the face, back and chest, so may become a body treatment as well as a facial treatment.

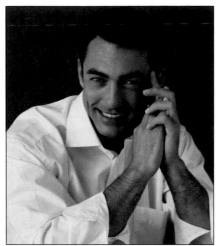

Male skin is approximately 25 per cent thicker than female skin

Ageing of the skin

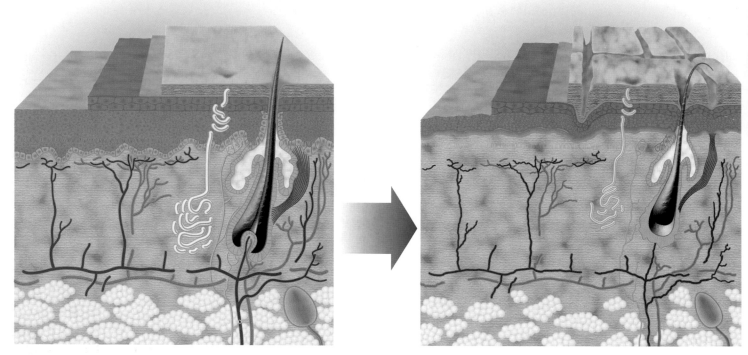

Differences in the epidermis and dermis of young and ageing skin

Along with the skin type clients inherit, the care they take of it and their general health, age is the other largest influence on the skin, not only because of the hormonal impact. Ageing is a natural part of the life cycle of a human being – it cannot be stopped or reversed, and skin cells begin to age from the age of 20 onwards.

Unfortunately, western culture is geared up to the young and growing older is not seen as a desirable trait – unlike eastern cultures where age is equated with wisdom and knowledge. Western society tries to push back the ageing process – there has been a marked rise in the demand for face lifts and extreme beauty treatments, such as Botox injections, to delay the ageing process.

Ageing happens to us all – and at generally the same rate, unless we are unfortunate enough to have a disease that interrupts these natural processes. The inherited factor comes into play again, with the ageing process – if your parents age well, enjoy good health and have good skin, the chances are that you will too.

The ageing process affects the skin for the following reasons.

- Cell renewal is always faster in youth; the older we get, the slower the renewal process becomes, until it stops altogether.
- The genetic information in each cell gets a little diluted every time the cell reproduces, so the cells of an 80-year-old do not have the same information as a young baby's.
- Hormone production in both sexes varies with age and contributes to the skin's development, health and deterioration.
- Fewer skin cells are being reproduced.
- The underlying structures supporting the skin begin to offer less support – the collagen and elastin fibres in the skin degenerate, muscular tension diminishes and wrinkles appear.

Remember
There is an old saying – 'You get the face you deserve', and this is partly true because if you lead a healthy lifestyle, follow a good skin care routine and protect against ultraviolet exposure, this will minimise the risk of skin damage and premature ageing.

- The adipose tissue supporting the skin diminishes and the skin starts to sag – the skin can no longer fight the gravitational pull.
- Sun damage and pigmentation disorders become more noticeable as the melanin production within the skin lessens, along with age or liver spots on the surface of the epidermis.

Age grouping of the skin

The teenage years: 14–20 years

Just as the body is changing with puberty, ready for the reproductive part of the human life cycle, so emotional development also begins, making teenagers acutely aware of themselves and their relationships with their peers. In females, the onset of puberty usually starts around the age of 10 or 12. Hormonal activity dictates the development of the body, changing both the sexual physical development and the emotional highs and lows that accompany this dramatic change.

At this age, the skin should be firm and compact, with a good supporting structure of collagen and elastin to give a firm, smooth feeling to the touch. Unfortunately, the hormone levels can be unbalanced and the sebaceous glands produce too much sebum, leading to blackheads and congested skin. Acne is common in this age group and may be directly related to high testosterone levels, so is more common in boys than girls.

Teenage boys may also cause skin problems by neglect – regular skin cleaning with the correct products can diminish skin problems but may be perceived as not a masculine pastime. However, with males taking a larger proportion of retail skin care sales than ever before, there is no reason for a male not to use a foaming facial cleanser designed for the male skin to help keep the skin clear.

A proportion of late-teen skins are not as clear as they could be, for self-inflicted reasons. Poor diet and an excessive alcohol intake, combined with the introduction of smoking, do little to enhance the skin. The only advantage is that this age group has youth on its side to recover more easily!

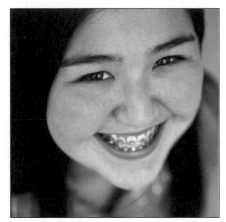

Teenage skin is firm and compact

Early adulthood: 20–30 years

This is when the chubbiness of the teenage years disappears and hormonal activity settles down, so the skin is at its peak. It looks fresh, radiant and glowing. The underlying structure is good; there are no fine lines developing yet, and providing good health is enjoyed, and a healthy diet gives the body the correct nutrients, the skin is good.

In pregnancy, hormonal changes may affect the pigmentation of the skin and darker patches, called chloasma, may appear – commonly found along the hairline and on the neck or hands. Also, tiredness in young parents, poor lifestyle choices and simply 'burning the candle at both ends' will take its toll on this generation, if care is not taken. Good choices in the appropriate skin care range and protection with a moisturiser, along with correct use of sunscreens, will be an investment for the future.

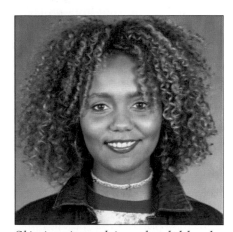

Skin is at its peak in early adulthood

Adulthood: 30–40 years

The skin begins to dry out and its reproduction slows down, with fine lines appearing, usually initially in the neck area. The jaw line is firmly defined at the beginning of the decade but can shows signs of change, either losing its definition or if the client puts on weight it will fill out and a double chin may form. Puffiness may be found in the cheeks – any weight gain in the face or body is instantly ageing.

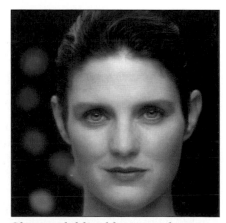

Skin in adulthood begins to show signs of ageing

The facial tissues begin to lose their fatty layer and tiredness can creep into the eye area. Creases and wrinkles remain after the depressions that form them have disappeared. Correct use of skin care products and protection against UV damage is essential in this generation, as prevention is better than cure! A neck and hand cream will prevent dehydration. Many clients forget this – they concentrate on their faces, forgetting that hands and neck areas are the true age reflector.

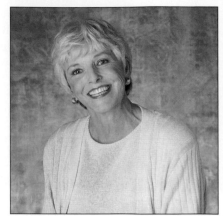

Elasticity diminishes during middle adulthood

Middle adulthood: 40–50 years

There is still a good clear definition of features, but 'temporary' double chins and wrinkles developed in the late thirties become a permanent fixture. Elasticity and the supporting structures of collagen and elastin fibres are diminishing, especially if the client is undergoing the menopause, which may start towards the fifties. Oestrogen levels start to fall and this affects bone density, elasticity in the tissues and skin thickness. The skin has begun to become thinner and more prone to damage from UV radiation and the environment. Blemishes, broken capillaries and pigmentation changes begin to occur.

Later adulthood: 50–60 years

All women will have begun, or completed, the menopause in this generation, and the skin will be loose and thin. It may feel coarse to the touch, and the eyes are lined and puffy. The muscle tissues around the eye and mouth develop depressions, seen as wrinkles around them, and the lip line loses definition. The sebaceous glands have slowed down the production of sebum and care must be taken to keep the skin lubricated and free from infection. With ageing, the skin loses some of its ability to fight infection and heal itself quickly. Facial hair growth may start to be obvious around the mouth and chin, and the hair is coarse and thick because of the influence of the male hormone testosterone, which is not being balanced by oestrogen.

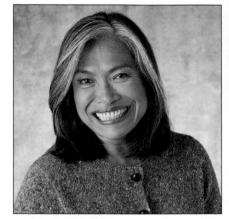

Skin will often be loose and thin in later adulthood

Late adulthood: 60–70 years

At this stage, the skin has the appearance of being soft, paper thin and pappy. There is very little underlying fat to support the facial structure, and deeper furrows appear from the corner of the nose towards the lips and from the outer mouth down to the chin. Darkened patches may appear, or loss of pigment can be seen, especially on the hands and arms. The throat, neck and chest are very lined and like tissue paper, with very little sebum to lubricate the skin.

Can we slow the rate of ageing?

Evidence suggests that the chances of living a long life are affected by your genes – long life seems to run in families. It is also known that cells have a programmed maximum number of divisions before they die off, so your life span is, to some degree, predetermined. However, there are some sensible precautions that clients should take.

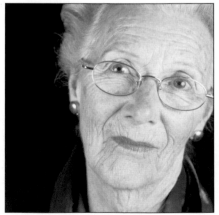

Skin can look soft and paper thin in late adulthood

- Eat healthily – people on lower-calorie diets tend to live longer, and meeting the body's additional demands as you age is important. A female who has heavy periods throughout her life will need more iron, but a menopausal client will need more calcium to help keep bones healthy.
- Keep physically active – three half-hour aerobic sessions a week helps keep circulation and metabolism going and stimulates the body to repair itself (this means a brisk walk or swim to get the cardiovascular system working).

- Get enough sleep or rest – rest allows the body to repair and heal itself and for the brain activity to slow and sift through all the stimulation it has received through the day. Sleep deprivation is very harmful to the body in the long term.
- Remain mentally active – the more you use your brain, the better it works, and the longer you remain alert. Doing a crossword, mental arithmetic, music and learning poetry are ideal brain activities as you get older.
- Remember good health maintenance – smoking ages the skin; a high alcohol intake is also damaging.

Anti-ageing treatments

The key here is 'prevention is better than cure'. In other words, encourage clients to look after their skin as early as possible, rather than waiting until the signs of ageing have begun to show. Anti-ageing treatments cannot turn back years of poor skin care and neglect, nor can it stop the ageing process. Some can significantly enhance the skin's appearance, but not on a long-term basis or without continuous treatments.

Scientific research into the different types of ageing is enabling cosmetic houses and beauty product manufacturers to develop anti-ageing treatments which target the symptoms of ageing more accurately than ever before.

Moisturisers

Contrary to popular belief, moisturisers do not add moisture to the skin, but rather they prevent moisture from being lost. This is achieved with the use of non-irritating oils and emollients such as lanolin and vegetable- or petroleum-based oils, which form a thin layer on top of the epidermis and stop water from literally evaporating out of the body. The result is that the outer most layers of skin absorb the water being released by the deeper layers, and so small wrinkles are filled out, and the skin looks and feels a lot softer. Moisturising the skin also helps protect it from air pollution, harsh weather conditions and the drying effect of heating and air conditioners. Most importantly, the majority of moisturisers contain ingredients that provide UV protection, which can affect the skin throughout the year, not just in the summer months.

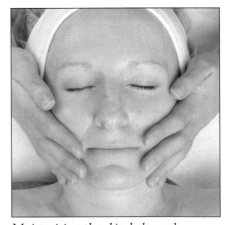

Moisturising the skin helps reduce water loss

Salon treatments

Any treatment which helps the desquamation process is going to help the skin look clean and fresh looking. Combine a treatment that deep cleanses and then rehydrates the skin using an electrical current, such as in a galvanic facial, and the result is instant – the skin looks plump and refreshed, and very clean. However, salon treatments will only last as long as the treatments are carried out regularly.

Scrubs, face masks and electrical treatments work on the outer layers of the epidermis, and will improve the look and feel of the skin, but under the Trade Descriptions Act a salon would be liable to prosecution if advertising these treatments as anti-ageing.

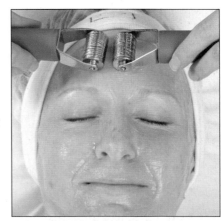

A facial electrical treatment can help reduce the affects of ageing

Alpha-hydroxy acids/skin peels

These treatments work by applying to the skin a chemical agent/acid (for example alpha-hydroxy acids (AHAs) or retionic acid/vitamin A) which dissolves the outer layers, thus temporarily reducing fine lines and other superficial signs of ageing. However, the long-term effects of such skin peels are not yet known, and adverse reactions are quite common, particularly if the concentration of the active ingredient is quite high, or if the product is left on the skin for too long. Peels also leave the skin far more susceptible to damage from UV rays and so sun protection is essential following treatment.

Laser skin resurfacing

Laser therapy for the skin is becoming a very popular salon treatment. Laser treatment can be used for skin ageing and wrinkles, as the light stimulates the capillary level, so improving the circulation. Acne and cellulite also respond well to laser treatment, as do pigmented lesions and the removal of tattoos. The pigment is broken down into minute particles and removed through the lymphatic system. Laser or intense pulsed light (IPL) treatments cross over from the beauty therapy field into medicine – lasers are used in eyesight correction, removing birthmarks and tattoos, treating and cutting through cancers and wound healing.

Within beauty therapy, lasers can be used for treating active acne, improving acne scarring and hair removal. Full training and a certificate of competence are required for insurance, as laser work is very specialised and has many contra-indications.

Collagen treatments

The protein collagen is the principal ingredient of white fibrous connective tissue found within tendons, skin, bone, cartilage and ligaments. Despite any claims made for collagen-containing products, the skin cannot absorb artificial collagen.

However, one collagen treatment that is temporarily effective and growing in popularity is collagen replacement therapy (CRT). This involves collagen being injected directly into the dermis to improve the appearance of fine lines and pockmarks. Collagen injections to the lips to create a 'bee sting' pout to the lip shape are common, but can go wrong if the client has an allergic reaction to the injection, leaving the lips very swollen and sore.

There are also treatments available where the patient's own collagen-producing cells – called fibroblasts – are collected using a biopsy from an unnoticeable area, say from behind the ear. These cells are then cultivated within the laboratory and mixed with nutrients to help them grow. They are then injected back into the patient, along the facial expression lines. The theory is that as they are the patient's own cells, there is likely to be no rejection reaction, as there is with some bulk-filling injections. The new cells stimulate growth in the existing collagen cells and within 4–6 months lines appear softer and acne scars are said to be practically invisible. This is not a salon practice, as it has to be carried out under local anaesthetic to harvest the biopsy, and can be expensive.

Botox treatments

Botox works by paralysing muscles located at the site where it is injected, thus reducing lines and wrinkles in that area. It is often used to treat frown lines and crow's feet around the eyes. Once again, the effects are temporary, and the treatments are required on a regular basis. The long-term effects of this botulinum-based treatment are not yet known. A recent report in the *Journal of Cosmetic Dermatology* suggested that people using Botox to defeat the signs of ageing may simply be developing more wrinkles in nearby areas, as neighbouring muscles try to compensate for those that are paralysed.

Cosmetic surgery

Surgery is a more invasive treatment and carries all the risks of any other medical operation. It is, however, considered an affordable treatment by many, and it can be very successful. Correcting sagging contours and removing wrinkles, by tightening the eye area, chin or a complete face-lift, will reduce the signs of ageing. However, there

Check it out

A protocol treatment plan is set out by most awarding bodies. Check what yours says regarding laser treatments.

is a danger of the skin looking too tight and not in keeping with the rest of the body – many film stars may look good facially, but their necks and hands reflect their true age. There is also a risk of the facial contours looking pulled and taut, which will look odd.

Cosmetic surgery should only be considered after a great deal of research and through a recognised medical referral. In some cases, corrective surgery can be very successful and most beneficial, especially if the physical problem causes psychological distress, too. The correction of a hare lip, reshaping of a broken nose or pinning back ears which protrude can give back confidence to clients and improve their perception of themselves.

Ageing and the sun

The effects of ultraviolet rays on the skin are well documented. Clients like a tanned, toned skin, which is usually associated with holidays and relaxation. An artificial tanning unit, in the form of sunbeds and showers, and fake tan application are very lucrative for salons. The government has now introduced a law banning under-16s from having sunbed treatments as many tanning shops are completely unsupervised and very few, if any, checks are performed to see if the skin is suited to the treatment.

Apart from helping to relieve certain conditions like asthma, aching joints and psoriasis, along with aiding vitamin D production, the sun's health benefits are primarily psychological. The truth is: too much sun can be positively harmful.

The immediate result of too much sun is sunburn, and many of us have experienced the painful blisters, fever and swelling that come from too much sun, too fast. Another result of sun exposure is prematurely aged skin. The sun causes the skin to thicken and gives a leathery, coarse appearance. With enough time, the sun weakens the skin's elasticity by cross-linking the collagen fibres in the dermis. This results in sagging and wrinkles on all sun-exposed areas.

The sun also causes dark pigmentation patches and scaly grey growths known as keratoses, which are often pre-cancerous. Sunburn and prematurely aged skin are not the worst results of constant exposure to the sun – skin cancer is. Almost all of the 300,000 cases of this disease developed annually are considered to be sun-related. Some people are more at risk than others of skin damage. Britain is fast catching up with Australia for numbers of skin cancer patients. In fact, the promotion of skin cancer awareness in hotter countries is bringing down their skin cancer patient numbers, as ours are growing.

Black skins are relatively safe because the darker skin provides good protection from ultraviolet light. Fair skins, notably in redheads and blonds, are at the greatest risk due to less melanin in the skin.

Certain drugs such as antibiotics, medicated soaps and creams, and even barbiturates and birth control pills can make the skin more susceptible to damage. The best cover-up of all is a chemical one, in the form of sunscreens and sun blocks. All clients concerned about premature ageing should be advised of the dangers of sun exposure, and recommended a sunscreen or sun block. Those clients who are sun worshippers should be educated to understand the relationship between the sun and skin cancer.

Once the ultraviolet light has caused cross-linking and thickening in the dermis and has predisposed the skin to premature ageing, no reversal of the damage is possible. Plastic surgery techniques can help disguise the sagging by re-draping the skin, but this does not compensate for the damage that has occurred. It is, therefore, the first topic that must be discussed with the client who expresses concern about ageing, and

> ### Remember
>
> As a beauty therapist, it is not within your job role to give medical advice or pass any judgment about medical matters, including cosmetic surgery. You may only recommend that the client seek medical advice, and nothing else.

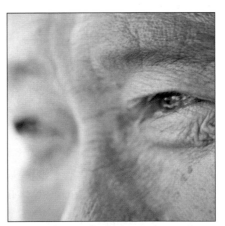

Too much sun damage results in the skin having a leathery, coarse appearance

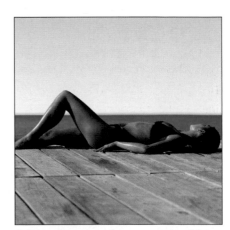

Advise clients to always use suitable sun protection

advice on sun protection should be given verbally and in a written fact sheet. Indeed, the only cosmetic product that can legally be labelled 'anti-ageing' is a sunscreen or sun block preparation.

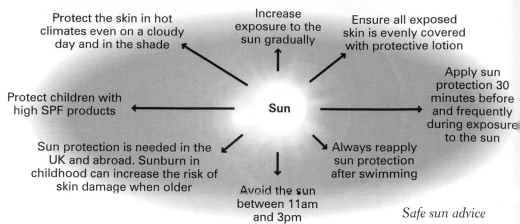

Protect the skin in hot climates even on a cloudy day and in the shade

Increase exposure to the sun gradually

Ensure all exposed skin is evenly covered with protective lotion

Apply sun protection 30 minutes before and frequently during exposure to the sun

Protect children with high SPF products

Sun

Sun protection is needed in the UK and abroad. Sunburn in childhood can increase the risk of skin damage when older

Always reapply sun protection after swimming

Avoid the sun between 11am and 3pm

Safe sun advice

Products and skin

Mechanical and electrical treatments for the skin are excellent at penetrating products into the skin, for various beneficial purposes. Most professional suppliers have their range of supporting products to be used with their own machine, and it is very important that you follow the manufacturer's instructions. What works with one machine might not be suitable or give the same benefits to the client as another. The active ingredients react with the various polarities and frequencies used (see Unit BT19, Improve face and skin condition using electro-therapy, for a full explanation of how the machines work).

During most professional training for new equipment and products there will be a practical test of competency and then a written paper on the benefits and effects of each product. Don't think that as you have left college, gaining knowledge and then testing that knowledge stops!

Remember

The active ingredients in the salon-size bottles for treatment use are also contained within the retail sizes, which you will be recommending for home use. It is important, therefore, that you learn your product ingredients and talk through with the client the added benefit of using the same ingredients on a daily basis.

Keys to good practice

Massage or mask – which comes first?

Product knowledge and research are advancing all the time, and professional suppliers will have their own procedures for performing the treatment. This may contradict the application knowledge you gained within Level 2 treatments. Some cosmetic houses would argue that you always apply a mask first, to cleanse and exfoliate the skin, in preparation for the massage and electrical treatments to follow. After all, why dry out the skin after all the benefits of a massage cream have been absorbed by the skin? Another product house would state that their mask content has the same active ingredients as the massage cream, and reinforces the treatment performed, and needs to be applied after the skin has been warmed and softened by massage. Who is right? They both are! As long as you use the procedure recommended for the product, then the benefits are not going to be diluted. It is only when you ignore the manufacturer's recommendations that problems occur.

Remember

When you qualify and start work at a salon, it may sponsor your training with a particular make of machine and product. In return, the salon will expect a period of loyal employment from you. What you learn in product knowledge may not be the same as the products you used at college, so be flexible – there are several procedures available for different machines. Be open to new training, which is the way to learn new skills and techniques.

Keys to good practice

Always use the correct product with its correct machine – the client deserves to have the treatment she is paying for, and the effects on the skin may not be as good if you cut corners. It may also invalidate your insurance if you have not followed the manufacturer's procedures.

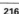

Knowledge check

1   What is glabrous skin, and what does it not have?

2   What gives the skin its colour?

3   Give four examples of good habits that the client will need to adopt to improve his or her skin.

4   Why does skin produce histamine?

5   What is the pH of skin?

6   What is desquamation?

7   What is keratin?

8   What happens in the horny layer of the skin?

9   Name two ways in which male skin differs from female skin.

10   What does collagen do?

facial
TREATMENTS

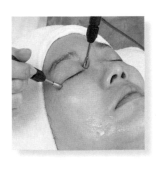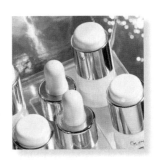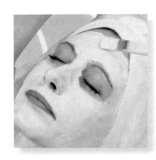

Facial treatments – theory and consultation

Electrical treatments are a large source of revenue for salons, and are very popular with clients. While therapists may argue that nothing is more relaxing than manual massage, electrical treatments are more effective for treating skin problems, figure problems and for deeper penetration of products into the skin.

> ### You will learn about
>
> - the benefits and effects of electrical treatments
> - choice of equipment
> - electrical therapies
> - properties of electricity
> - types of electrical facial treatments
> - the facial consultation.

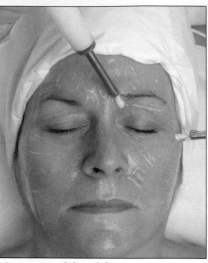

Non-surgical face lifting

The benefits and effects of electrical treatments

> ### Remember
>
> Any treatment using an electrical current, adapted to any of the machinery used with beauty therapy, will be more effective than manual treatments alone.

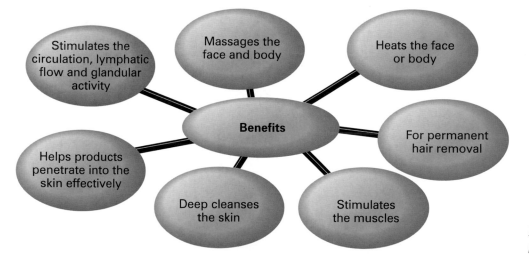

Benefits

- Stimulates the circulation, lymphatic flow and glandular activity
- Massages the face and body
- Heats the face or body
- For permanent hair removal
- Stimulates the muscles
- Deep cleanses the skin
- Helps products penetrate into the skin effectively

Benefits of electrical current for beauty therapy treatments

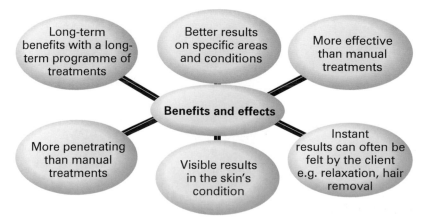

Benefits and effects

- Long-term benefits with a long-term programme of treatments
- Better results on specific areas and conditions
- More effective than manual treatments
- Instant results can often be felt by the client e.g. relaxation, hair removal
- Visible results in the skin's condition
- More penetrating than manual treatments

Benefits and effects of using electrical treatments

However, not all treatments are suitable for all clients.

Choice of equipment

This will depend on:

- the client's needs and any contra-indications present
- the client's likes and dislikes
- the area of the body to be treated – some equipment is suitable for the face, but would be impractical for use on the body
- the cost of a treatment or course of treatments
- the time constraints for a course to be fitted into a client's lifestyle
- the skin type and body condition/shape and fat type
- the type of business the salon caters for, and the clientele's requirements.

Keys to good practice

Make sure you are well-informed regarding all the options so that you can offer the client several alternatives. Always ask the client if he or she has any particular likes or dislikes. For example, it could be that the client's wishes are for relaxation, so the noise of a facial percussion machine might not appeal. Instead, offer the slow rhythm of a pulsation vacuum suction treatment to the face, which would be suitable.

Be informed about all the latest reports in the media about new electrical treatments within the beauty industry. You could be missing an opportunity to expand your business and offer clients something new and innovative. Talk to the clients about the benefits of the new treatments, and be specific about the benefits for the client's skin. Take extra training to learn new equipment usage and increase your client base by having the latest treatments available.

Electrical therapies

Electrical therapies use a range of different currents and frequencies. To understand the differences in equipment, you will need to know:

- the type of current used and how it behaves
- how each piece of equipment works
- its benefits to the client
- its risk assessment and hazard potential
- how to use it most effectively for the client's needs.

To appreciate these topics, you first need to understand the properties of electricity.

Properties of electricity

The atom

All matter, whether a solid, gas or liquid, is composed of units called atoms. Every atom has a nucleus and an external or outer layer.

- The nucleus contains positively charged particles, or **protons**.
- The nucleus also contains **neutrons**, which have no charge.
- The outer layer contains negatively charged particles called **electrons**.

Each electron rotates continuously around the nucleus, always in the same orbit.

An atom has one of the following three characteristics:

1   Atom without electrical charge – when the number of electrons and protons is equal and therefore the atom has no charge.
2   Negative ions or anions – if the atom gains an electron, the number of electrons will be greater than the protons, so the atom takes on a negative charge. The atom becomes a negative ion or anion.
3   Positive ion or cation – if the atom loses an electron, the number of protons is higher, and the atom becomes a positive ion or cation.

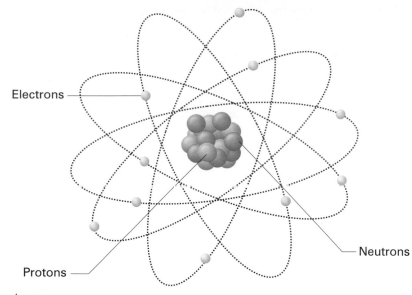

An atom

All ions relate to each other according to the physical laws of electricity: the same charged ions repel each other, while opposite charged ions are attracted to each other. Therefore, two negatives repel one another, so do two positives. A positive is only attracted to a negative, and vice versa.

This theory of opposites attracting is very important in galvanic work, when the active ingredients in the gels and solutions used have active ions, and they are used to aid skin penetration.

Electricity and electrical circuits

An electric current is a flow of electrons passing through a fixed point in an electrical circuit per second, measured in **amps**. Electrons flow from negative to positive as they are negatively charged. The pressure required to drive the electric current around a circuit in measured in **volts**.

The amount of electricity an appliance uses depends upon how much work it is designed to do – called the power rating. This is measured in **watts** or **kilowatts**.

Resistance is anything in the circuit which slows down the flow of electricity. There is a balance – the voltage is trying to push the current around the circuit and the resistance is opposing it. The relative sizes of voltage and resistance decide how big the current will be:

•   If you increase the voltage, more current will flow.
•   If you increase the resistance, less current will flow.

Resistance is measured in units called **Ohms**, but they cannot be measured directly. They need to be calculated from the volts and amps. The relationship between volts, amps and Ohms is called Ohms Law:

Ohms = volts/amps

For example, if the voltage of a lamp is 12 volts and the current flowing is 2 amps, the number of Ohms would be calculated as:

12 volts/2 amps = 6 Ω or Ohms

Electrical circuits can be seen as:

- a voltage pushing the current round with resistance opposing the flow
- energy transfer.

Anything which supplies electricity is also supplying energy. Electricity comes from different sources:

- cells
- batteries
- generators
- solar cells.

The most practical source of electricity is from the generators at power station via the National Grid. Cells and battery-operated equipment will need recharging and are not suitable for small portable pieces of equipment such as blood pressure machines. Solar energy is unreliable in countries that do not have a regular supply of strong sunlight.

An electrical circuit transfers the energy to components such as lamps, resistors, bells, motors, and so on. These components perform their own energy transfer and convert the electrical energy into other forms of energy, such as:

- heat, e.g. hairdryers, kettles
- light, e.g. light bulbs
- sound, e.g. speakers
- movement, e.g. motors.

Series or parallel circuits

Circuits are classified as either: series or parallel.

A series circuit is all or nothing – the components are connected in a line, end to end, and they all share the electrical current going through them, so once one part is broken the whole series breaks down. Think about the lights on a Christmas tree. If one bulb blows, the whole line of bulbs goes out, and it is a process of elimination to find out which one has gone. This is not very practical and, generally, few things are connected in series.

In a parallel circuit each component is separately connected to the supply. This type of circuit is sensible to work with, as removing or disconnecting one component of the circuit will not disrupt the whole circuit. Household electrics are run this way, so you can switch everything on or off separately.

Where does electricity come from?

Electricity is generated in power stations throughout the country and is distributed through the National Grid to local electricity substations, where the electricity is converted to a lower voltage for use in factories, businesses and homes. Factories require very high voltages (33,000 volts), whereas small businesses such as your salon will receive a 240-volt supply. In urban areas, the 240-volt supply comes into individual premises through underground cables beneath the street. The supply cable enters the building underground and arrives at the meter, fuse board, or circuit breaker, where usage is measured, and once the meter is read, electricity bills can be calculated.

Most electrical equipment in a beauty salon runs from the 240 volts coming through the wall sockets (mains electricity), and the machine will convert it into the type of current it is built to provide, e.g. faradic, high frequency or galvanic. The exceptions to this are the bigger electrical units, which require a higher voltage, such as saunas and steam cabinets. They require a greater supply than 240 volts and have to be connected

Remember

A complete circuit is needed for the current to flow. If the circuit is broken, there will be no current flow and no transfer of energy. This is important during electrical treatments when you think your machine is not working properly. Often you have not completed the circuit by giving the client the saturator, or passive electrode, to hold, so completing a circuit.

Remember

Conductors are materials which are good transmitters of electricity, that is they are substances that allow electricity to flow through them quite easily. Metal, the human body, water, saline solution (salts in water), silver and gold are all good conductors of electricity.

Insulators are materials which are not good transmitters of electricity, that is they do not allow electricity to flow through them easily. They are used as protection from an electrical current. Examples include glass, oil, plastic, rubber and wood, and they either inhibit or prevent the flow.

using a special consumer unit, by the installation company. The local electricity supplier will have to be informed and special rates of payment will be required – a sauna, shower unit and spa may need more than double the amps/volts normally available.

Topic	Measured in	Symbol used	Information
Electric current – a flow of electrical charges called electrons	Amps, using an ampmeter	A	Named after the French electrical pioneer, André-Marie Ampère
Pressure needed to drive current (driving force)	Volts, using a voltmeter	V	Named after Alessandro Volta, the Italian inventor of the battery
Power used to run equipment	Watts and kilowatts	W and kW	Named after James Watt, who invented the steam engine (1000 watts = 1 kilowatt)
Resistance which slows the current down	Ohms	Ω	Named after Georg Ohm, another electrical pioneer. Often referred to as potential difference
Alternating current (AC) flows in one direction, then in the reverse direction in the circuit. One complete back and forth is called a cycle	Hertz (one Hertz = one alternation per second)	Hz	Named after a pioneer in sending and receiving radio waves, Heinrich Hertz. Mains electricity has a frequency of 50 Hz

Summary of electricity terms

Effects of an electrical current

An electrical current is able to produce:

- chemical change
- heat
- sound waves
- magnetic fields
- light rays
- mechanical movements (kinetic effects)
- changes of matter from one state to another, e.g. water to steam through heating.

All of this is put to good use within the beauty salon equipment for the benefit of the client. An electrical current adapted for use on or through the body is able to:

- help improve skin function and appearance
- stimulate glandular and cellular activity in the region being worked upon
- improve the tone, functioning and appearance of the muscles
- provide relaxation to the tissues through heating them
- stimulate the systems of the body to encourage better functioning, that is the lymphatic system, circulation, cell reproduction and growth and repair.

Effects of electricity	Type of equipment	Effect on the body
Heating	Sauna, steam units, infrared heat lamps, spa pool, foam baths, showers, paraffin wax heaters	Relaxes the muscle fibres and raises body temperature; induces perspiration and therefore cleanses the skin; rehydrates the skin
Chemical	Galvanic treatments to the face, galvanic body treatments, galvanic hair removal	Deep cleanses the skin; forces substances into the skin; treats cellulite; removes hair
Magnetic	Mechanical massage units such as G5 vibro mat and Pifco units for facial massage. (The coil within the motor makes the head cause a circuit break and so the head taps the skin)	Stimulating massage movements encourage the skin's functions, glandular activity and desquamation of the dead epidermal cells; also helps soften and relax the muscle fibres
Light waves	Electro-magnetic waves used in infrared lamps and ultraviolet lamps	Warms the tissues, preparing them for other treatments such as massage or used as a counter-irritant – soothes the nerve endings; encourages production of melanin within the skin to produce a tanned skin, healing and helps with vitamin D production
Kinetic effects	Kinetic = movement, so muscular contractions caused by a faradic machine are classed as kinetic	Helps build tone and strength within the muscle fibres. May also have other benefits such as improvement in posture and confidence
Sound	Audio-sonic machine	Sound waves penetrate deep into the tissue for relaxation of the muscle fibres

Effects of electricity

Within beauty therapy, these electrical currents can be further broken down into categories of pattern, and the equipment can be adapted to alter the pattern to suit the client's needs, especially if it is a course of treatments and the body is getting used to the pattern and needs a little extra stimulation.

Types of electrical current

- A current which flows in one direction only is a **direct current** (DC).
- A current which alternates its directional flow is an **alternating current** (AC).

Type of current	Description	Wave form
Galvanic Used for: • iontophoresis • desincrustation • epilation	Constant and direct (DC) – has no break in the flow of electrons	

(continued on next page)

Type of current	Description	Wave form
Faradic Used for: • muscle toning • passive exercise	Surged and interrupted – alternating and low frequency. The current and wave formations can be adjusted on the machine to suit the client's needs	
High frequency Used for: • direct application • indirect application	Oscillating, high in frequency, higher in voltage with lower amps. Alternates rapidly at more than 50 times per second. Can be applied directly or indirectly to the body	
Microcurrent Used for: • uplifting facial contours • uplifting body contours	Modified direct currents (DC) – a galvanic current which can be altered on the machine for the client's needs and differing stages of treatment	

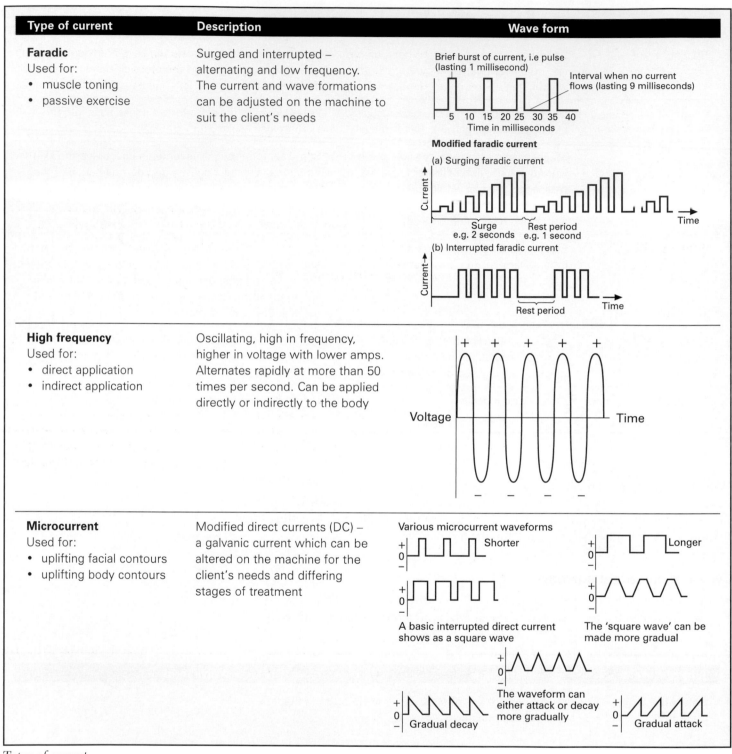

Types of current

Types of electrical facial treatments

The next pages show a general breakdown of facial treatments, and their role in client care.

Remember

Refer to Unit BT19, Improve face and skin condition using electro-therapy, for a full explanation and procedure of use for all equipment.

Prewarming:

Equipment	Uses and client needs	Suitable skin type/body type
Steaming (facial unit) 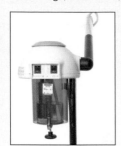	A heating element is used to boil the water, creating moist heat, i.e. a jet of steam from a nozzle. • Used to warm the tissues of the face, upper chest or back. • Helps open the pores, and cleanses the skin. • Warms the facial muscle fibres and relaxes them, making other treatments after steaming very effective. Very good prior to comedone extraction, but be careful to time the treatment, as if an erythema occurs too strongly, it may contra-indicate other treatments.	Most skin types, except where contra-indications present. Timing of treatment can be adjusted to suit skin type
Infrared lamp 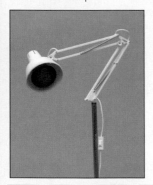	An infrared light bulb is fixed into a fitting with a swivel arm on a stand, making it easy to place the lamp into a suitable position. • Used to create extra blood flow, which generates heat for the skin and underlying tissue. Muscle fibres will soften and it can be used effectively on any part of the body. But can only treat small areas at a time, due to the limited arc of light from the lamp. Can be used on the face, chest or upper back – time the treatment, as if an erythema occurs too strongly, it may contra-indicate other treatments. • Can also be used on the face with a hot oil mask.	As above. Where used with hot oil mask, dry skin only
Brush cleansing 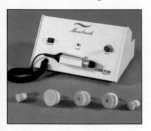	A brush-cleansing machine has a motor, which rotates a hand-held head that can have a variety of brushes inserted into it. The speed of the rotations is adjustable to suit the client's needs and preference, as is the direction of the revolution – clockwise or anticlockwise. Brushes of various thickness and stiffness will alter the treatment effect, as will the accompanying products used with the machine. Most water-based products are suitable, from basic foaming facial wash used to cleanse the face, back or congested chest area, to cleansing grains and specialist creams for particular skin problems. The effect of the treatment is one of exfoliation and stimulation to the skin and circulation. Can also be a useful tool in the removal of peels or masks from the face	Most skin types, except where contra-indications present. Product use will be determined by skin type or problem
Facial scrub 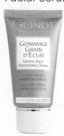	An exfoliant can be applied prior to most facial electrical treatments and is most convenient if the client does not have the time to have a steam treatment. The product is applied using the hands, in small circular motions, and then removed with sponges and warm water, once the entire face and neck have been covered. Some manufacturers provide mitts or facial sponges with a rough surface to enhance the exfoliation, so always follow manufacturers' instructions.	As above

(continued on next page)

Massaging treatments:

Equipment	Uses and client needs	Suitable skin type/body type
Manual massage 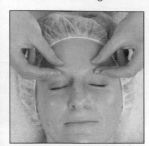	Using the hands, the tissue is manipulated in a series of movements for the neck, upper back, head and face. Can be stimulating or relaxing depending upon the movements used, but the most sought-after treatment outcome is for removal of tension nodules within the muscle fibres and total relaxation of the mind and body.	Most skin types, except where contra-indications are present. Timing and use of product/massage medium during treatment can be adjusted to suit skin type
Audio-sonic 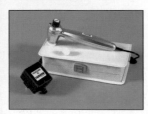	Deep penetrating sound-wave emissions used on any condition where deep massage helps, e.g. fibrocystic nodules, or tense muscle fibres, of the upper back. This is a small hand-held device and therefore only suitable to treat small areas in one treatment: not suitable for a whole body massage, as it would be too time consuming and not cost-effective. When using on the face, it is most comfortably applied over the therapist's fingers, so they absorb some of the sound waves. The facial structure does not have the depth of muscle tissue to absorb the sound waves that the body has, and it is not as relaxing directly on the skin.	Most skin types, except where contra-indications are present. Not suitable on fine-featured clients with very delicate facial contours – it may be uncomfortable
Percussion vibrators 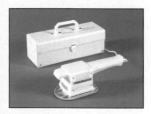	A hand-held smaller version of a G5 machine (see **Body treatments – theory and consultation**, page 320) with a smaller motor and therefore not as deep in its effect on the tissues. Has small detachable heads to provide a variety to the massage movements, but generally, the unit tends to produce a tapotement effect. Only suitable on smaller areas, such as the shoulders and neck area. Some clients find it uncomfortable on the face, while others enjoy it.	Most skin types, except where contra-indications are present
Vacuum suction 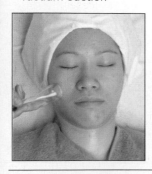	This machine uses a pump to create a vacuum within an attached cup, which picks up the tissue. Can be used either: • to glide to the lymphatic nodes, in a single movement, or • to create a pulse within the vacuum, for extra stimulation. Vacuum suction promotes the face's lymphatic and circulatory systems, thus helping the removal of toxins from the area. It is desquamating; it stimulates glandular activity and improves the general skin texture. Very relaxing facial treatment, and can replace manual massage as part of a routine: many clients find it very soothing and drop off to sleep!	Check for contra-indications, as treatment will not be suitable for all skin types, especially thin or fine skin with a tendency to bruise easily. Also, will not be comfortable on thin, bony clients or clients with older, crêpey skin.
Indirect high frequency 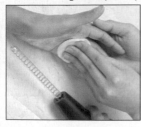	Often called a 'Viennese massage', indirect high frequency involves creating a circuit of current, flowing through the client via a hand-held glass rod, called a saturator, connected to the machine. The therapist's hands make contact with the client and the current is discharged through her fingertips, as she is massaging, creating warmth in the area. This deep massage will improve a dry skin, relax the tissues and help increase a poor or sluggish	Most commonly used on dry or fine skins, as the medium used is oil which will help the glide of the treatment and lubricate the skin

(continued on next page)

circulation to the area. Can be used in place of the facial massage routine, although if clients become too relaxed, they will lose contact with the saturator which they should be holding. Avoid losing contact with the skin, as this breaks the circuit. Most frequently used on a dry face or for back massage.

Other treatments for cleansing, healing, moisturising and exercising

Equipment	Uses and client needs	Suitable skin type/body type
Direct high frequency	Using a high-frequency machine, the current is transmitted into a glass electrode, which is in direct contact with the skin. Light circular motions then disperse the current. This is a drying germicidal treatment, ideal for a seborrhoeic skin, one that is congested or has blemishes. 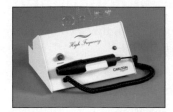	Most commonly used on oily, congested or acne skin types, to the face, back of chest area
Galvanic	A galvanic machine uses a direct constant current for both face and body work, and the results depend upon the method of use and the gels and products used. The current has to create a circuit flowing through the client, either by using rollers with a connection in the client's hand or a pad under the shoulder, or by the use of body pads, to complete the circuit. Can be used in two ways: • Desincrustation – removes the incrustation, i.e. the excess sebum, and gives a deep cleansing to the skin. • Iontophoresis – introduces beneficial substances into the skin, to rebalance and rehydrate the skin, or to get active substances to stimulate the body's systems, which aids lymphatic drainage. 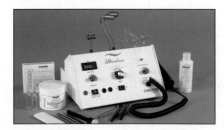	Most skin types, except where contra-indications present. Desincrustation – for oily skins or skins in need of a deep cleanse; iontophoresis – for a dry skin or to rebalance the skin or just to improve the skin texture
Microcurrent	A modified direct, low-frequency current which is used on its own for lifting of the facial contours and in conjunction with a galvanic current for skin improvement. Can help with fine line reduction, stretch mark minimising and scar reduction, and deep cleansing. 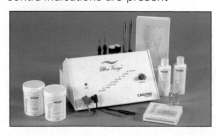	Most skin types, except where contra-indications are present
Faradic	Using a surged and interrupted current, a faradic machine can stimulate muscular contractions on both the face and body. It is often referred to as passive exercise, and you can actually see the muscles contracting under the pads, with no effort on behalf of the client – the client is lying still on the couch. The pads for the face are smaller than those used in body work, so it is possible to target specific muscle groups for improvement in tone and suppleness. Treatment is ideal for double chins, dropped jaw line and cheekbone definition. 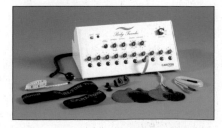	Most skin types, except where contra-indications are present

Types of equipment

Keys to good practice

Whichever pieces of equipment you choose as the most suitable for the client's treatment plan, always follow the five golden rules:

1 Complete a full consultation.
2 Complete a contra-indication checklist.
3 Carry out thermal and sensitivity tests.
4 Follow the manufacturer's instructions.
5 Test the equipment on yourself before using it on the client.

The facial consultation

As you work through this section, refer closely to all the information you learned in **Professional basics**.

Facial record card

The facial consultation begins with you and the client talking through the record card. Below is a typical completed card.

Personal details	Medical details
Name of client: Mrs Jane Jones	**Name of doctor:** Michael Springfield
Address: 2 The Farthings, Faith Hill, Canley, Oxford OX19 7PQ	**Practice address:** The Surgery, 1 Sale Avenue, Canley, Oxford OX19 3XY
Daytime tel. no: 012345 67890	**Tel. no:** 091834 923456
Home tel. no: 091834 567834	**Present medication:** Anti-inflammatory for IBS Anti-histamines for allergies
Date of birth: 13/10/50	
No. of pregnancies: 3	**Past medication:** Contraceptive pill for 20 yrs
No. of children: 2 aged 16 and 18 years	**Allergies:** Dogs, cats, most animal fur; eggs
Occupation: Nursery teacher	

Remember

Although most equipment used would be classed as electrical because it works from mains electricity, in beauty therapy equipment is also grouped according to the effect it has on the body. Electrical treatments are those which send an adapted electrical current through the body such as galvanic current, microcurrent, high-frequency and faradic treatments. Equipment that has an external effect only on the body is called a mechanical treatment and includes G5, vacuum suction and small massage equipment such as audio-sonic.

Lifestyle: Quite busy with work and family, and husband in a demanding job	**Client's general health:**
Sleeping pattern: Not always good	Client is trying to lose weight; with the Weightwatchers programme and so her eating habits are healthy, and the weight loss is slow, but good. The client does like to unwind with a glass of wine with her meal in the evening, and is going to the gym twice a week. Her job is quite stressful – not the children, but the paperwork is heavy and they are going through an OFSTED inspection, which is more stress. The client feels it is affecting her sleep pattern, which is disturbed at the moment. More relaxation would be a good thing, the client feels.
Smoker (yes/no)/no. per day: No	
Alcohol units per week: 0–10	
Diet: Client is trying to lose weight and is on the Weightwatchers programme, so she is recording all food and drink intake, which is very healthy. A good ration of fruit and vegetables and the client is drinking 2 litres of water per day, which is very good for the skin	

Facial condition — please ✓ if present and use comments box	✓	Comments box
Muscle tone scale 1—3 (1 being poor; 3 being good)		Client's muscle tone is good for her age (54). Chest, neck and jaw would benefit from some facial faradic stimulation and home exercises, but the facial contours are good, and the eye and cheek area is lovely – great cheekbones! Elasticity good – skin springs back quickly.
For: Chest area	2	
Neck	2	
Jaw line	2	
Cheek area	3	
Eye area	3	
Forehead	3	
Skin colour and tone		Warm, pink and healthy looking, no yellow present and in good condition. Client's colouring: pale blonde with pale, fair skin.
Skin texture (lines present)		Fine – soft and smooth, with no obvious problems, and only fine lines visible around eyes.
Skin damage (broken capillaries, etc.)		Small dilated capillary on left nostril – caused in childbirth, client would like to have it cauterised – refer to our electrologist
Pigmentation areas (any sun damage or loss of pigmentation)		Small pigmentation around the hairline – very faint, as a result of pregnancy and hormonal changes. Hardly noticeable, and client has hair in a fringe
Pores (fine, large, comedones, blocked, pustules, etc.)		Fine and clear. No shine, matt and dry to the touch.

Skin type (oily, dry patches, etc.)		Client's skin is fairly dry, but in good condition, with correct products used, so no sign of dry patches, although client is prone to dry, chapped lips in the winter.
Other (skin tags, scarring, superfluous hair, etc.)		Client has soft downy hair on the cheek and upper lip areas, not noticed as they are so fair in colour, but client is quite conscious of it.

Overall comments

Client has taken care of her skin: she is not a smoker, and drinks plenty of water throughout the day. Her general health is reflected in her healthy skin, with no obvious signs of any problems. Not keen on sunbathing as she is fair, and has always worn a hat when abroad.

Client's previous treatments/results

Mrs Jones has had no electrical facials with this salon, but did enjoy the paraffin mask and would like to have some form of moisturising mask again.

Recommendations:

A course of facial faradic treatments and galvanic facials to keep skin exfoliated and rehydrated.

Warm oil mask would be enjoyed, and a galvanic facial would rehydrate the skin.

Speak to Elaine regarding removal of capillary damage around the nostrils.

Upper lip wax as client is aware of hair on the upper lip.

Facial record card

Once you have filled out the client's record card, place it on the trolley for additions during the treatment, and you will be ready to begin the facial observation. You should note any adaptation of treatment necessary should the client have a small contra-indication which is not a barrier to treatment.

The client may also have questions for you, for example 'What can I do about my open pores?' or 'Why does my face itch when I put on moisturiser?'. This will open up the consultation and you will have created a trusting atmosphere where the client feels able to say exactly what his or her concerns are and what he or she is most conscious about, allowing you to give professional advice.

The facial observation

When you are confident that no contra-indications prevent the client from having the treatment, you should invite the client on to the couch in readiness for the skin analysis. The positioning of the client is the same as for manual facial treatments. The client should be cocooned within the bedding, with only the face showing, turban on, and jewellery on the trolley in a bowl. The client should feel warm and secure.

An electrical facial consultation is very similar to a Level 2 consultation/observation, except that your treatment recommendations will involve electrical equipment, so try to be meticulous and thorough. You will need to see the skin in its natural state, that is without make-up – if a client is adept at make up application, then the true condition of the skin could be hidden.

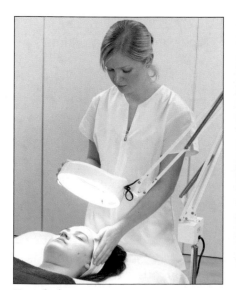

Facial observation

Keys to good practice

Ask your client if he or she is wearing contact lenses. The client may be happy to keep them in, or might prefer to remove them. For steaming and electrical treatments, the client may prefer to take out the lenses.

Client modesty

For the female client
- Tights and half-slip may be kept on, but shoes should be removed.
- Bra straps may get oily and should be dropped off the shoulder, or the bra may be taken off altogether, especially if the bra has a metallic strap adjuster. Metal is a good conductor of electricity, and the client may find there is an accumulation of current, and a stronger sensation under the metal, if she keeps her bra on.
- If the client chooses to push her straps down on to the top of the arm, there is still a danger they will get massage medium on them, as you will be going halfway down the upper arm with your movements. Encourage the client to remain topless, but with a small modesty towel around the bust area, which she may wish to keep with her at all times.

For the male client
- Since facial massage includes the upper back and shoulders, the shirt or T-shirt should be removed, and the client's chest covered with towels and/or blankets to prevent his upper body getting cold.
- Most male clients are not as sensitive to current as a female, as their skin is slightly thicker, but the current is attracted to the moisture in hairs, so if the client is hairy, he may transmit the current quite well!
- Metal facial piercings should be removed, and if the body is pierced, cover with a plaster, where appropriate.

Skin analysis

Once the client is comfortably positioned on the couch, and you have washed your hands, you will be ready to begin skin analysis (for information about the skin, see **You and the skin**, page 187).

Ask the client if he or she would prefer to have his or her eyes covered with cotton wool rounds, or if the client would just like to close them.

Look closely when doing a skin analysis. Use a magnifying lamp to illuminate the face, and study the facial contours, jaw line, chin, nose, cheeks and forehead. You are looking for:

- the skin's general condition
- pore size
- any area of shininess
- dry flaky patches
- comedones or blocked pores or papules
- skin problems, e.g. acne rosacea or acne vulgaris
- the contours of the face – any loss of elasticity or dropped contours
- dilated capillaries
- the colour and texture of the skin
- areas of pigmentation.

What you see is very important, and you need to use your consultation skills to confirm verbally with the client exactly what you have seen and how this may affect the client and the treatment plan. Questions such as 'How long have you had a broken capillary on your nose?' will lead into a discussion as to whether the client regards it as a problem, if she is conscious of it, and would like to have it treated, or if she is happy because it is covered with make-up and does not bother her.

When looking at the skin, you can also talk about the client's current skin care range, and how happy the client she is with the results. For example:

- Is she using a regular exfoliant to help slough off the dead skin cells?
- Does the colour look a little flat and dull?
- Would the skin benefit from having the circulation stimulated, bringing oxygen and nutrients to the cells?
- Are the current products drying out the top layers of the skin?
- Does the skin look plump and full of moisture, or dehydrated and dry, with lines?
- How firm is the jaw line? Is the client developing a double chin?
- How much water is the client drinking every day to keep the skin clear and healthy?

Manual examination of the face

Most of the information gathered on the record card is from questioning the client and observation of the facial skin condition, but you will also need to feel the skin's texture, warmth and contours. This will be done when carrying out the superficial and deep cleansing routine – your fingertips will alert you to rough patches of skin, moles and raised areas of skin, which may not be visible but can be felt.

A cold face will often indicate poor circulation, or a hot face may be a sign of the client's age, and the onset of the menopause, which often affects body temperature regulation. In fact, hormones are one of the key factors in the skin's behaviour, along with diet, water intake and environmental aspects and product use. (To refresh your knowledge of factors that influence the skin, see **You and the skin** and **Related anatomy and physiology**.)

Be aware that the client may be very adept at applying make-up, so the skin might look flawless and there may be no visible problems. However, with make-up removed, your light massage technique during cleansing, may tell a different story. Feel for cysts, raised moles and indentations. You are also feeling the firmness of the tissue, whether there is good muscular support, if the skin feels firm to the touch and springs back easily when manipulated. Older skins are less springy because the supporting collagen fibres begin to weaken, resulting in the skin and underlying tissue feeling a little slack. (For a full breakdown of skin types and questions to ask the client, see **You and the skin.**)

Another factor affecting the contours of the face is if the client has had extensive dental work done, or has recently had dentures fitted – this affects the gums, cheek muscles and jaw line, especially if the client is not yet comfortable with new teeth. If this is the case, avoid any heavy pressure along the lower face, as it will be uncomfortable for the client.

Once you have completed the facial examination, you are ready to discuss and then carry out facial treatments with the client's permission.

Check it out

Contact several companies that supply facial electrical equipment and ask for a sample of their record cards. Compare the cards. How are they different? Do they all ask for the same information? Are the contra-indications all the same? Which one do you find most helpful, and why?

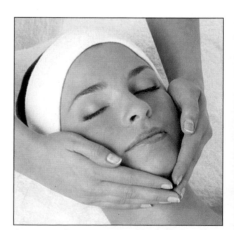

A manual examination can be relaxing too

Improve face and skin condition using electro-therapy

Unit BT19

Choosing the right pieces of equipment for the client and then using them in a safe and appropriate manner will ensure the client receives a first-class treatment, with instant results. All of the electrical treatments used on the face perform several functions and offer a combination of the following benefits.

- They improve the skin condition.
- They improve muscle condition and the contours of the face.
- They improve lymphatic drainage to the face.
- They aid in relaxation, both physically and mentally.

In this unit you will learn how to achieve all of this using:

- a high-frequency unit
- vacuum suction
- a galvanic unit
- a faradic unit
- a microcurrent unit.

Using equipment safely and with confidence is essential, and it is very important that you follow the manufacturer's instructions for the machine you are using, since these will vary. Products used, treatment times and the dials showing strength of current will differ from one make of machine to another. The only way to be totally safe and competent for your assessments is to understand each machine thoroughly and know its capabilities. This will provide you with the confidence to treat clients in a professional manner, which in turn will instil the client with confidence in your abilities.

Within this unit you will cover the following outcomes:

BT19.1 Prepare for the facial treatment
BT19.2 Consult and plan the treatment with the client
BT19.3 Perform electro-therapy treatments
BT19.4 Complete the treatment

Before beginning a facial electrical treatment, you will need to refer closely to all the information you have learned so far – see **Professional basics** and **Facial treatments – theory and consultation**.

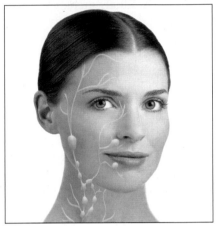

Electro-therapy improves skin condition and lymphatic drainage

Keys to good practice

When learning a new piece of equipment gain dexterity skills by using it without current for a few sessions. This will help you gain confidence in using the rollers, prongs or pads, without the fear of breaking contact with the skin, or worrying about hurting the client. Once you feel comfortable and able to control the application of the equipment on to the skin, then use current.

In this unit you will learn about	
• preparing the skin for treatment	• galvanism
• high frequency	• faradism
• vacuum suction	• microcurrent.

Preparing the skin for treatment

Let's assume that the facial consultation has gone smoothly – the client has no contra-indications, the client is in a suitable position for treatment and you are ready to use your chosen electrical equipment. The skin has been cleansed and is grease free. It is still essential to further prepare the skin to be receptive to the electrical treatment you are about to perform.

Cleansing/exfoliants

Most commercial companies have a complementary pre-treatment cleanser, which varies from a make-up removal cleanser. Usually, it is an exfoliant containing micro beads to slough off any remaining dead skin cells from the surface of the epidermis, which may hinder the benefits of the treatment. Plant extracts and essential oils within the products such as lavender, coconut, apricot kernels and aloe extracts ensure that the skin is gently exfoliated – too harsh an abrasion and the skin would be too red and irritated to have further treatments. These are massaged into the skin and then removed with warm sponges and water, or flannel mitts, which leave the skin softened and receptive. This form of pre-treatment is especially ideal for those clients who do not have the time for a full facial steam or brush cleanse treatment.

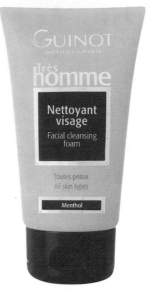

A *pre-treatment cleanser*

Keys to good practice

Whichever pieces of equipment you choose as the most suitable for the client's treatment plan, remember the five golden rules – see **Facial treatments – theory and consultation**, page 230.

Step-by-step

Facial cleanse and exfoliation

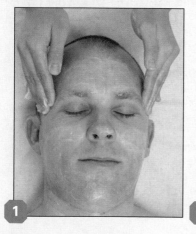
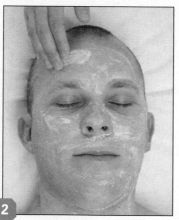
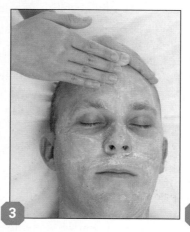
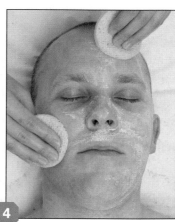

1. Emulsify the product between the hands and begin application
2. Apply product to face and neck (the client may wish to have eye pads on)
3. When product has dried use light rubbing motions to exfoliate dead skin cells
4. Remove remaining product with clean sponges and warm water

Remember

The different types of electrical currents have various effects on the body. Most of them will warm the skin and muscles through the increase in circulation to the area, lymphatic drainage will be stimulated by using the equipment in the direction of the nodes, and the nerve endings will be soothed by the heat generated. Only the faradic current is used to cause muscular contractions, and no electrical current has any effect on the skeleton.

High frequency

High frequency is a very useful multi-purpose machine: it can be used both directly and indirectly on most skin types and gives excellent results. However, the nature of the frequency means the machine is quite noisy to use, and some therapists are put off by this. However, use the machine often and with practice, you will hardly notice the noise!

The high-frequency current

This is a dampened alternating, oscillating, high-voltage, low-amperage current. A high-frequency machine produces a frequency of 100,000–250,000 Hertz (cycles per second).

Most beauty therapy equipment has a transformer within it, to alter the AC current but not the frequency (see **Facial treatments – theory and consultation**, page 225). This 'special transformer' in the high-frequency machine is an **induction coil** called an Oudin coil. The high-voltage, high-frequency current is not easy to confine with the insulation of a wire, so the Oudin coil is inside the hand piece which holds the **electrode**. This is why the electrode holder is round and fat. (Some manufacturers' instructions refer to the hand piece as the Oudin resonator.)

The cabinet of the machine contains the **capacitor** and the 'make-and-break' vibrator to recharge it repeatedly. In most modern machines an electronic 'make-and-break' is used and this contributes to the buzzing noise when the machine is working.

As it alternates so rapidly, at more than 50 times per second, the current does not stimulate motor or sensory nerve endings. It is also the alternation that produces the high-pitched sound that is the characteristic of high frequency. High frequency is one of the few machines that does not require two connections to make a full circuit – the current is carried through the client's body, creating warmth by increasing the circulation.

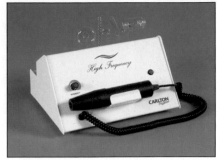

A *high frequency unit*

Key terms

Induction coil – a device for producing a very high electrical force from a very small electrical force.

Electrode – a conductor through which electricity enters or leaves a vacuum tube.

Capacitor – a device for storing an electric charge.

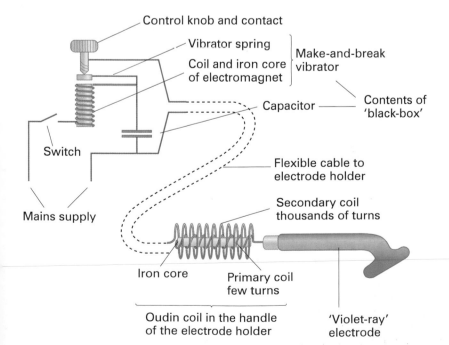

How a high-frequency unit works

It is very important that you are confident in the use of the machine, as the noise level can be disturbing to the nervous client, especially if applied on the face. A thorough explanation should be given during consultation.

Application

High frequency can be used in two ways:

- **Indirect** – the current flows through the client's body using the therapist's hands to perform massage which conducts the current. The client holds the intensified saturator electrode (called saturation).
- **Direct** – application is directly on to the skin using an Oudin resonator (glass electrode).

High-frequency equipment may vary in general appearance between manufacturers, but the basic operations of the equipment will be similar. There are generally two main control switches – the on/off switch and the intensity control. A mains lead connects the unit to the power supply. A flex leads from the unit to the handle, which is used to house the glass electrodes. There are a variety of electrodes that the therapist can select to use, depending upon the method of application and the area to be treated and the desired effects. You will need to refer to individual manufacturer's instructions.

Contra-indications to high-frequency treatments

- Cuts or abrasions to the skin in the area to be treated.
- Skin diseases or disorders.
- Highly vascular conditions.
- Sensitive skin.
- Highly nervous clients.
- Excessive metal in the area.
- Swellings in the area.
- Very hairy areas.
- Sinus blockages.
- Heart conditions.
- Epilepsy or diabetes.*
- Circulatory problems.*
- Pregnancy.*
- Asthmatics.*

* Only to be carried out with medical approval.

Indirect high frequency

This method of applying the high-frequency current involves creating a circuit of current which flows from the saturator to charge the client. The therapist massages the client, which allows the current to discharge from the client's face or body to the therapist's massaging fingers or hand. This provides heat in the fingertips and creates a really deep, warming massage.

> **Remember**
>
> - Clean the heads with either warm soapy water and dry thoroughly, or wipe with surgical spirit or a hibitane. The heads are made of glass, so be careful when handling them and store them correctly.
> - Within each electrode a small quantity of inert gas is sealed, usually argon. As the current flows through the gas, a coloured glow is produced. The electrodes glow either blue/violet if they contain argon, or red/orange if they contain neon.

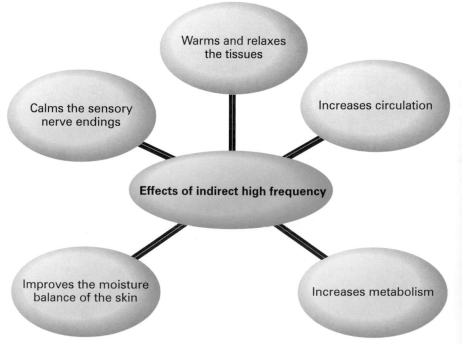

Effects of indirect high frequency

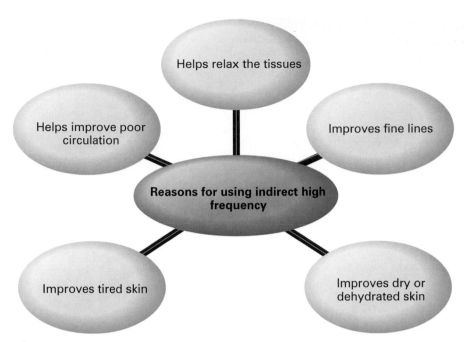

Reasons for using indirect high frequency

Precautions during indirect high-frequency treatment

- Care should be taken around the hairline as sensation will be increased because hair is a good conductor.
- Contact must not be broken.
- Rings must not be worn by the client on the hand that holds the saturator.
- The client and therapist must not touch any metal conducting material while giving the treatment.
- The intensity of the current in the tissues will be increased when lifting one hand off.
- In the past, talcum powder was used as a medium for good conductivity, but its drying effects are not beneficial for a dry or dehydrated skin. Contact your own professional association for recommendations. Large quantities of talc should not be used as it is believed to have carcinogenic effects on some people, and its use is not recommended near the nose or mouth in case of accidental inhalation, especially if the client has a history of asthma or respiratory problems.
- Care must also be taken with any belts that have metallic buckles that the therapist may be wearing as part of her uniform, or worn by the client if clothing is kept on.
- Try to avoid contact with the couch.

Remember

Your normal massage routine can be followed, but you must not break contact with the skin, so avoid all tapotement-type movements and concentrate on giving a relaxing, deep, penetrating, warm massage to those tense muscles.

Important note:

Indirect high-frequency application is the same for face and body. Follow the same steps, as shown on the next page, for a facial treament.

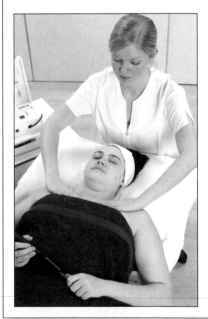

Step-by-step

Indirect high frequency – preparation and method

1. Observe general safety precautions for using electrical equipment.

2. Place the machine on a stable trolley.

3. Select the products required for treatment and place them on the trolley.

4. Check the machine and test to ensure it is working correctly.

5. Great the client at reception and escort him or her to the treatment area.

6. Ensure a full consultation is carried out, contra-indications are checked, and the treatment is explained.

7. Help the client onto the couch, and protect hair and clothing in the usual manner.

8. Ask the client to remove all jewellery. Clean and prepare the skin with suitable products.

9. Carry out skin sensitivity testing.

10. Select a suitable medium and apply it to the client's back – a massage oil or nourishing cream is ideal – to feed the skin.

11. Ensure the mains lead is plugged into the mains supply and that all switches are off and all dials are at zero.

12. Test the machine in front of the client and reassure him/her where necessary about the buzzing noise that can be heard.

13. Apply talcum powder to the client's hands to absorb any perspiration; wipe the saturator with disinfectant and place it firmly in the holder.

14. Place one hand to make contact with the client's skin, using small circular effleurage movements, while with the other hand turning the intensity dial slowly to suit the client's tolerance. Always ask the client if he or she is comfortable with the intensity.

15. Place the other hand on to the skin by sliding over the first hand and begin your usual massage movements, ensuring that contact is not broken, i.e. no tapotement-type movements are used. This will break contact and make the sensation of current uncomfortable.

16. The treatment time will vary between 8 and 12 minutes, depending upon the client's skin condition, skin reaction and the manufacturer's recommendations.

17. At the end of treatment, reverse the procedure of hands by taking one hand off, reducing and then turning off the current and then removing the other hand.

18. Remove the massage medium and continue with facial procedures most beneficial to the client, i.e. tone and moisturise.

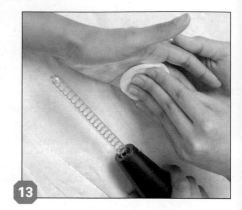

13

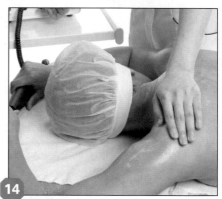

14

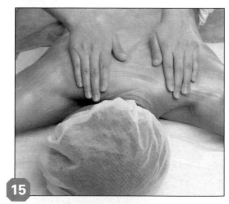

15

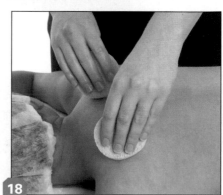

18

Remember

- Indirect high frequency should be used on a dry skin with a suitable massage medium.
- It should be used in place of the normal manual massage.
- The client should hold the saturator in a talced hand
- The therapist must make contact with the skin before turning on the machine.
- All dials on the high-frequency machine should be set at zero to begin with.
- Do not use tapotement movements – these break skin contact.
- After massage is completed, remove one hand from the client, and turn off machine before removing the other hand.

Keys to good practice

Remember the five golden rules – see **Facial treatments – theory and consultation**, page 230.

Indirect high frequency

- Used on dry skin with suitable massage medium.
- Used in place of normal manual massage.
- Indirect contact – client holds saturator in a talced hand.
- Make contact with the skin before turning on the machine.
- All dials at zero to start.
- No tapotement movements.
- After massage is completed, remove one hand and turn off machine before removing other hand.

Neck electrode – direct high frequency electrode specifically contoured for working on the neck area but equally versatile for use in any curved area, such as arms and legs

Roller electrode – this versatile roller can be used on any large area, especially a large back, and is ideal for a nervous client as it does not spark. Glides easily and does not necessitate any gauze or sliding agent should the client prefer not to have any.

Large facial bulb – used for direct high-frequency facial and body work. Particularly useful for larger areas such as the chest and back (can be used for sparking – check with your awarding body)

Saturator – electrode used for indirect high frequency only. The metal spiral inside the glass ensures that only a gentle current is required to give maximum effect

Small facial bulb – smaller facial direct high-frequency bulb for use on smaller areas such as the nose and around the ears

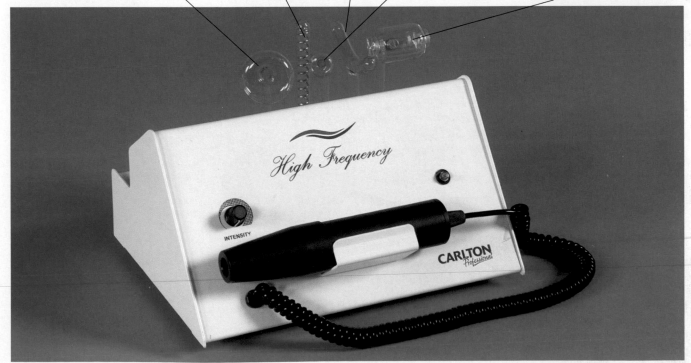

High-frequency electrodes

(continued on next page)

Saturator
Wide comb electrode – some machines have a comb-like electrode which hairdressers can use over the scalp to stimulate blood circulation to the hair follicles. All the same procedures should be followed during treatment

Types of saturators used within high frequency

Keys to good practice

After each treatment, wipe the electrode with an antiseptic solution, dry it and then store it safely.

Direct high frequency

This method of application uses glass electrodes which are placed in direct contact with the client's skin. The current is dispersed at the point of contact with the client and as the effects are concentrated around the electrode, they are superficial but very beneficial to the skin.

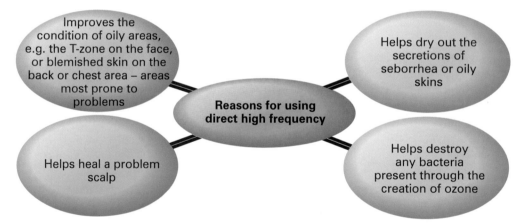

Reasons for using direct high frequency

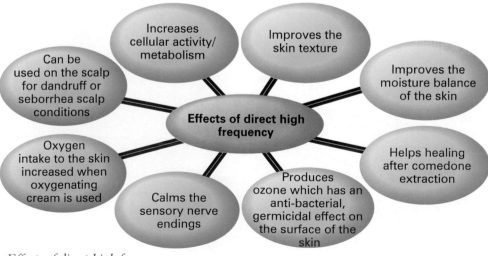

Effects of direct high frequency

Step-by-step

Direct high frequency – preparation and method

1 Observe general safety precautions for using electrical equipment.

2 Place the machine on a stable trolley.

3 Select the products required for treatment and place them on the trolley.

4 Check the machine and test to ensure it is working correctly.

5 Greet the client at reception and escort him or her to the treatment area.

6 Ensure a full consultation is carried out, contra-indications are checked, and the treatment is explained.

7 Help the client onto the couch, and protect hair and clothing in the usual manner.

8 Ask the client to remove all jewellery. Clean and prepare the skin with suitable products.

9 Carry out skin sensitivity testing.

10 Select a suitable medium and apply it to the client's face and neck – a massage oil or nourishing cream is ideal – to feed the skin.

11 Ensure the mains lead is plugged into the mains supply and that all switches are off and all dials are at zero.

12 Test the machine in front of the client and reassure the client where necessary about the buzzing noise that can be heard.

13 Apply the electrode in one of two ways. Either place the electrode in contact with the client's skin and move it around using small circular movements while turning up the intensity to suit the client's tolerance, or place the finger in contact with the electrode before turning the machine on, then turn the intensity dial up and place both finger and electrode in contact with the client's skin before removing the finger.

14 The treatment time will vary depending upon the client's skin condition, e.g. oily skin 8–15 minutes, but follow manufacturers' instructions and recommendations.

15 The facial can then continue in the normal way with appropriate products.

13

Keys to good practice

High-frequency currents should not be used on areas of skin that have been in contact with flammable liquids, such as alcohol toners, as there is a small risk that if sparking occurs, then they could ignite and cause burns.

Precautions during direct high-frequency treatment

- Some manufacturers recommend the use of an oxygenating cream with direct high frequency, and because of the loose consistency of some creams (like beaten egg white), a gauze mask may be put over the skin to hold the product in place.
- Always use eye pads. Cut a nose hole for the client, to prevent the client feeling claustrophobic, and follow manufacturers' instructions.
- Sparking may occur when the electrode is lifted away from the skin. The spark produces ultraviolet rays which destroy bacteria. The germicidal effect is created by the ionisation of the oxygen in the air, which creates ozone. Controlled qualities of ozone help to promote the healing process; however, there are risks involved. The distance between skin and electrode should be only a few millimetres, causing the current to jump across the gap in an attempt to maintain contact. Check with your individual awarding body regarding use of ozone and the practice of sparking.
- Always follow the procedure recommended for the machine you are using. Some companies recommend finishing with oxygenating cream and direct high frequency, especially after a galvanic facial, so the client's skin benefits from the oxygenating cream as the final product; others continue with a mask and massage. This is especially true of companies whose products all contain the same active ingredients and therefore the mask and massage are continuing to bring benefits to the skin. Both of these methods are acceptable, so ensure you follow the product specifications fully.

The following table gives a risk assessment for high-frequency treatments.

Remember

The application of the direct high-frequency electrode creates warmth on the skin and converts the stable oxygen molecules in the oxygenating cream to unstable ozone molecules which may have a germicidal effect.

Direct high frequency

- Drying, germicidal effect, often used with oxygenating cream or talc.
- Place saturator on to the skin before switching on.
- Use small, circular movements – avoid breaking contact.
- Switch off before removing the saturator from the skin.
- Often done after galvanic to finish treatment.

Identify the hazard	What is the risk?
Danger from electric shock	Low
Risk of sparking the client	High
Risk of small burn to the area	Low
Talc inhalation	Low
Postural problems for the therapist	Low

What should I do to prevent the hazard from becoming a risk?

Follow manufacturers' instructions
Make sure the saturator or mushroom is firmly inserted into the handle
Test on yourself before treatment
Ensure no jewellery is worn by the client or therapist, especially using the indirect method, as current can be attracted to the metal and the client may experience a burn in the area
Avoid inhalation of talc – especially if the client has respiratory problems
Make sure the machine is positioned close to you, so that you have full control over the intensity dials and the saturator/electrodes – do not lean over the client or make contact with the couch
Ensure correct posture and chair height to allow you to be in control of equipment
Do not make sparks by breaking contact with the skin, especially around the eyes and mouth
Not recommended for use with any flammable liquid, such as alcohol toner, as there is a small risk that if sparking occurs, they could ignite and cause burns
The electrode should always be in contact with the client's skin before turning on the current and machine should be turned off before removal of electrode

Risk assessment for high frequency

Aftercare and home care for high frequency

- Discuss the client's normal product use – this is often the cause of recurring skin problems, where clients are not using the correct product type for their skin's needs.
- Often the skin is so completely clean and has a germicidal finish (with direct high frequency) that no other care, such as cleansing or toner, and moisturiser are required for 24 hours after treatment.
- Advise the client to avoid picking or touching the skin, especially with unclean hands.
- See **You and the skin**, page 188, for other skin recommendations.

Vacuum suction

When used properly, vacuum suction is a gentle and effective treatment, and so relaxing that the client should fall asleep when this treatment is being carried out! The only rule of thumb with vacuum is that you should work towards the lymph nodes, to reinforce the natural draining ability of the lymphatic system. Vacuum suction is effective when used in conjunction with other treatments, or it can be offered on its own, and good results will be seen in the skin's appearance after a course of treatments. It is equally effective on the body: the principle being the same, just with bigger cups.

The vacuum suction current

A vacuum therapy treatment to either the face or body is classed as a mechanical treatment performed with the aid of a compressor, as there is no electrical current flowing through the body.

A vacuum suction machine works using a pump action which creates a vacuum in the various cups attached to the tubing. A cup is referred to as a ventouse, and they come in a variety of shapes, depending upon the client's needs.

Most vacuum suction machines are very straightforward and have an on/off switch, an intensity control to adjust the vacuum pressure within the cup and a pulsation switch to alter the vacuum, which creates a mini pressure within the cup.

> **Remember**
>
> In the United States this technique is referred to as non-invasive sub-dermal therapy (NIST).

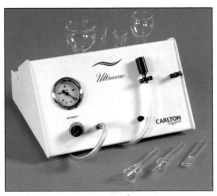

A vacuum suction machine

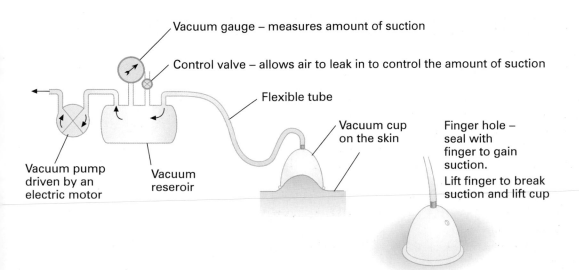

How a vacuum suction machine works

Vacuum gauge – measures amount of suction

Control valve – allows air to leak in to control the amount of suction

Flexible tube

Vacuum cup on the skin

Finger hole – seal with finger to gain suction.

Lift finger to break suction and lift cup

Vacuum pump driven by an electric motor

Vacuum reseroir

Application

By compressing the tissue into a cup and using a gliding and/or pulsation method of application, you will be aiding the body to move the lymph fluid nearer to the nodes to be filtered and improve the skin's condition.

Care must be taken not to have too great a vacuum within the cup as this compresses the tissue and capillaries may burst, causing bruising. However, facial cups are quite small, and testing on yourself prior to application should prevent this.

To ease application and removal, most cups have a small inlet hole, which needs to be covered with the finger so that the tube is sealed to create the vacuum. This means that when you want to break the vacuum and lift the cup away from the skin to go on to the next movement, you can do so easily, without having to flick the cup off the skin, so giving a smoother sensation and preventing possible damage.

Application is always carried out over a lubricating product, usually oil-based, to prevent dragging of the skin. Always glide the ventouse towards the nearest lymph nodes. Avoid pressure on the skin; instead try to create a little lift away from the skin, while keeping the vacuum inside steady, to avoid bruising and to make the gliding action pleasant for the client.

Keys to good practice

If you are unsure whether the client is suitable for a facial vacuum treatment, try to pick up on the facial tissue around the jaw line. If you cannot pick up any tissue, the client's skin is too thin for a vacuum treatment; offer an alternative treatment.

Contra-indications to vacuum treatments

- Delicate, sensitive skins
- Broken capillaries or thread veins
- Couperous conditions
- Loose, older skin with little underlying tissue
- Infected skin sites
- Acne with the presence of pustules
- Recent scar tissue
- Cuts, bruises and abrasions
- Sunburn
- Thin, bony areas
- Undiagnosed swelling
- Fine skin texture, e.g. found in diabetics
- Epilepsy
- Herpes simplex
- Any glandular swelling

Very hairy areas, while not strictly a contra-indication, may not be very comfortable for the client. This may apply to facial hair, as well as body treatments.

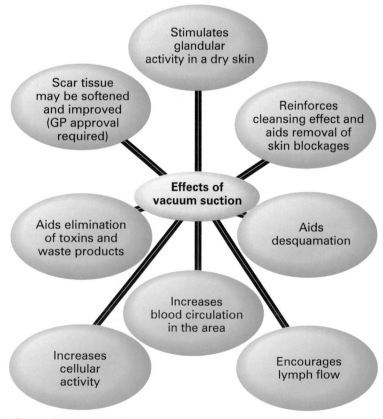

Effects of vacuum suction

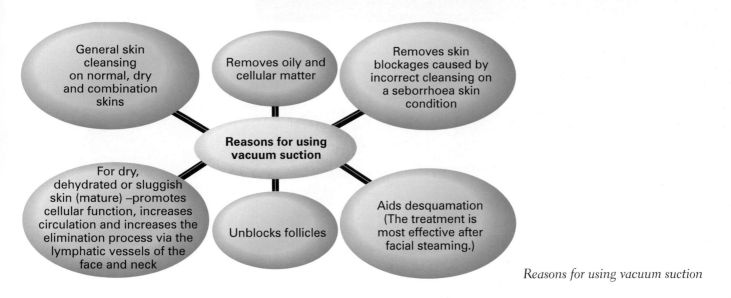

Reasons for using vacuum suction

The table below describes the use of glass vacuum applicators.

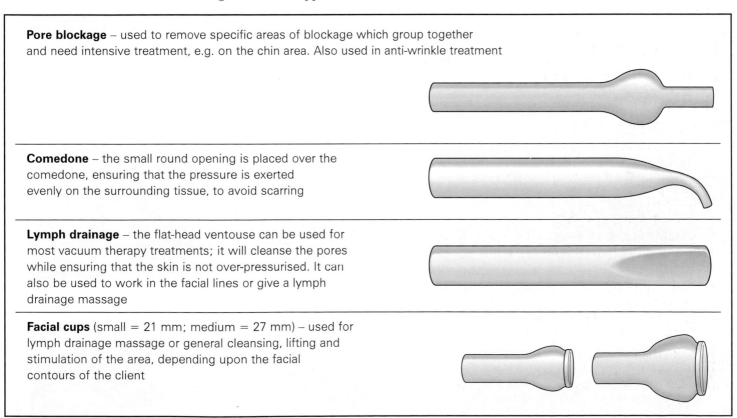

Pore blockage – used to remove specific areas of blockage which group together and need intensive treatment, e.g. on the chin area. Also used in anti-wrinkle treatment	
Comedone – the small round opening is placed over the comedone, ensuring that the pressure is exerted evenly on the surrounding tissue, to avoid scarring	
Lymph drainage – the flat-head ventouse can be used for most vacuum therapy treatments; it will cleanse the pores while ensuring that the skin is not over-pressurised. It can also be used to work in the facial lines or give a lymph drainage massage	
Facial cups (small = 21 mm; medium = 27 mm) – used for lymph drainage massage or general cleansing, lifting and stimulation of the area, depending upon the facial contours of the client	

Glass vacuum applicators

Each glass ventouse, except the comedone extractor, has an air hole on the side, which when covered creates the vacuum. This provides easy release and prevents skin drag or bruising.

Step-by-step

Preparation and method – vacuum suction treatment

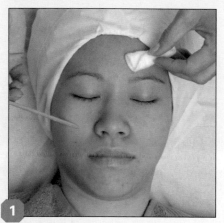

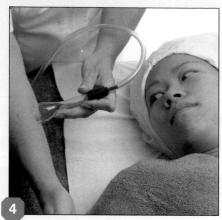

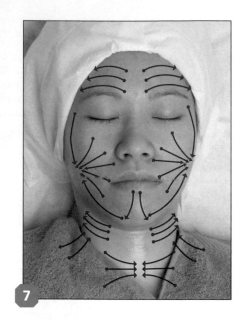

1. Ensure the skin is thoroughly cleansed. Carry out sensitivity testing on the face.

2. Carefully insert the selected ventouse into the black coupling connector at the end of the tubing. (Often referred to as a universal fitting, as it should house all sizes of ventouse.)

3. Set switch to 'on' and check that intensity dial is at zero.

4. Test machine on yourself in front of the client by turning up the intensity control clockwise until sufficient suction is obtained to glide on the skin, while maintaining a vacuum.

5. Turn off, then apply the massage medium to the face and neck with a mask brush or manual massage strokes.

6. Apply the applicator on the chest below the clavicle in an easy flowing stroke over the surface – adjust the intensity to the skin's reaction and resistance. The lift into the applicator should not exceed 20 per cent.

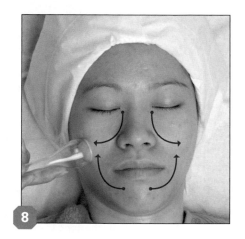

7. Follow the diagram for the pattern of strokes. The duration of the treatment may vary from 3 to 5 minutes for general cleansing to 10 to 12 minutes for massage and lymphatic drainage.

8. Always follow in the direction of the nodes.

9. Check client's skin for reaction. If a strong erythema occurs, this would be a contra-action to treatment – do not continue with the treatment.

10. The size and shape of the applicators used depends on the skin's sensitivity and the effect required, e.g. general cleansing, toning or removal of skin blockage.

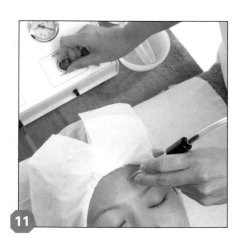

11. Turn off the machine with one hand, or break contact by releasing the air hole in the side of the ventouse.

12. The treatment concludes with the removal of the oil followed by a cleansing mask or further manual application, according to the routine chosen.

Keys to good practice

When using the pulsating programme of the machine, always start and finish with gliding only to help waste materials drain into the lymph nodes.

Keys to good practice

Remember the five golden rules – see **Facial treatments – theory and consultation**, page 230.

Vacuum suction

Always work towards the lymph nodes in the area.

Remove the ventouse by breaking the vacuum – release the finger from the hole.

Never flick or pull the ventouse from the skin.

Precautions during vacuum suction

- Choose the most appropriate-shaped ventouse and cup size.
- Cover the hole at the side of the ventouse to create the vacuum.
- Always test on yourself, even when changing the ventouse for a different-shaped one. When testing on yourself, only fill to 20 per cent of cup.
- Place ventouse on client before turning up intensity.
- The lift into the applicator should not exceed 20 per cent of the cup's volume.
- Put on plenty of product to lubricate the gliding movements.
- Always work towards the lymph nodes in the area.
- Always remove the ventouse by breaking the vacuum, by releasing the finger from the hole.
- Never flick or pull the ventouse from the skin.
- Keep a hand towel on the trolley and remove all oil from your hands before attempting to change the ventouse. With slippery hands, the ventouse can easily break and become a hazard. Always change the ventouse over the trolley, and not near the client.
- After each treatment, place glass applicators into warm soapy water with a little antiseptic solution, and clean thoroughly, then dry, to leave the glass clean and oil-free, or follow the manufacturer's recommendations. Be careful, the applicators are very delicate and can easily be broken.
- Place applicators in the back of the machine for safe storage, or wrap them up in cotton wool or similar, to prevent damage when not in use.

The following table gives a risk assessment for vacuum suction.

Identify the hazard	What is the risk?
Danger from electric shock	Low
Bruising to the area	High
Dragging on the skin resulting in pain for the client	High
Spreading of infection	High
Skin damage from broken ventouse	Low
Postural problems for the therapist	Low

(continued on next page)

What should I do to prevent the hazard from becoming a risk?
Follow manufacturers' instructions
Test on yourself before treatment to ensure less than 20 per cent tissue in the cup
The ventouse should always be in contact with the client's skin before turning on the vacuum and the machine should be turned off before removal of ventouse
Always start on zero intensity
Always have sufficient product on the skin to keep it well lubricated
Constantly monitor for any developing contra-actions
Choose the correct size of ventouse for the area
Always carry out a consultation and never treat a client who has an infection present
Never flick or pull the ventouse from the skin, always use the hole in the tube to release the pressure
Always change the ventouse over the trolley top and not near the client, and always remove oil from your fingers when attempting to pull the ventouse from the nozzle, to avoid slippery fingers dropping the glass ventouse
Always clean and sterilise the ventouse thoroughly after each treatment
Make sure the machine is positioned close to you, so that you have full control over the intensity dials and the saturator/electrodes – do not lean over the client or make contact with the couch
Ensure correct posture and chair height to allow you to be in control of equipment

Risk assessment for vacuum suction

Recommended course of treatment

This treatment should be appropriate for most skin types.

- **Dry, mature skin** – within the normal treatment course.
- **Oily, seborrhoeic skin** – used in conjunction with steam treatment, desincrustation or specialised cleansing masks. Course of six to ten treatments or until desired effects achieved; once a week.
- **Normal skin** – within the normal treatment course.

Salon treatment

Vacuum suction can be used with any appropriate treatment or electrical therapy suitable for the client's skin type. It is especially beneficial after facial faradic treatment to aid with the elimination of lactic acid build-up in the muscles.

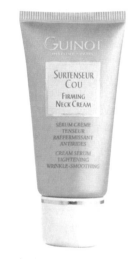

Aftercare and home care for vacuum suction

- Recommend suitable skin preparations and masks.
- Suggest a regular skin cleansing routine and regular salon treatments.
- Stress the need for regular use of a good moisturiser and night cream.
- If skin is congested and comedone extraction is required in the salon, recommend an exfoliant suitable for the skin type.
- Advise the client to avoid picking and touching the skin after treatment.
- See **You and the skin**, page 188, for other skin recommendations.

Galvanism

Most commercial companies offer treatments using a galvanic current, and although the products and names may be slightly different, the underlying principles are the same. Once you understand the theory of how a galvanic current is used, any other external training you receive should make sense.

Larger salons are offered training when they initially invest in a branded galvanic system such as Guinot, Perfector or Carlton, and they also purchase a stock of

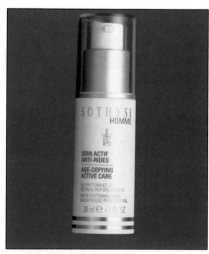

Suggest appropriate aftercare products

products for retail and salon use. The financial outlay may be quite high, but the training of staff is often included within the price and in return for training, the therapist is expected to be loyal to the salon for a period of time (anything from 1–3 years, depending upon the contract of employment).

Along with understanding how to use a particular machine, the therapist receives very thorough product knowledge, which supports the salon treatments, and also becomes certificated and insured for that machine. The therapist also receives a badge to state that she has trained with the company. So, although your NVQ Level 3 training will be sufficient to operate a machine, you will still be expected to undergo further commercial training for galvanic use when you join a salon.

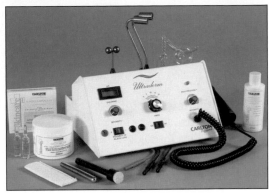
A galvanic unit

The galvanic current

The galvanic current is a direct, constant current, with low voltage, which can be used in two ways on the face and body. It is measured in milliamps. This is shown on the front on the machine in either a window with a metal arm moving along a series of numbers, or a digital reading, or crystal display unit. (Refer to Unit BT18, Improve body condition using electro-therapy, for galvanic body treatments.)

A galvanic machine

A galvanic machine contains:

- a rectifier, to change the alternating mains current into a direct one
- a capacitor, which smoothes any irregularities within the constant stream of electrons
- a transformer, to reduce the voltage from the mains supply.

Application

A galvanic current can be used in two ways:

- **desincrustation** – deep cleansing of the skin, usually to prepare the skin for iontophoresis, but it can also be used on its own
- **iontophoresis** – used to penetrate beneficial creams, ampoules or solutions into the skin for a specific treatment depending on the client's needs. It is also used in cellulite treatments on the body to penetrate diuretic-based gels into the skin to stimulate lymphatic drainage.

Both methods have two fundamental principles for correct use:

- the polarity of the product used on the skin
- the polarity setting of the machine.

> **Remember**
>
> A galvanic current is an electric current produced by a chemical action, and can be used for hair removal (electrolysis), and the penetration of substances into the skin for deep cleansing and hydration.

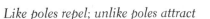

Like poles repel; unlike poles attract

Penetration of products into the skin is only successful because of the action of the ions, when forced into action by the current. According to the basic laws of polarity, the same poles repel each other but opposite poles are attracted to each other, because the atoms want to hook up and be complete in their formation. We can use this information to help the products penetrate into the skin.

The client forms a circuit by holding a covered electrode in the hand, which is linked to the machine. The rollers are also linked to the machine and when placed on the face, a circuit is formed for the current to flow through. If the polarity of the rollers is the same as the cream, then they will not attract one another – and the ions in the cream will be attracted to the electrode in the hand, therefore going through the skin to get there. (If the polarity is set wrongly, and the cream is negative and the rollers are positive, or vice versa, then the cream is attracted to the rollers, and the client's skin receives no benefit at all!)

Manufacturers produce many differing creams, ampoules and gels with electrolytes (or ions) in them, so you will always have to check which polarity to use, but as long as the rollers and the gels are the same polarity, they will not be attracted and as the client has an opposite electrode in the hand, the cream/gel will penetrate.

That is the basis of any galvanic treatment, regardless of which system you are using.

This table below shows some common terms used when dealing with the principles of galvanism.

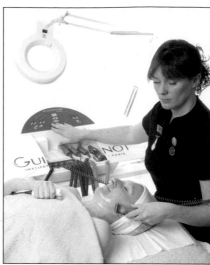

The client holds the passive electrode while the rollers are applied to the face

Ions	Atoms, or group of atoms, which have a positive or negative charge
Anion	A negatively charged ion
Cation	A positively charged ion
Electrolytes	Atoms dissolved in a liquid or gel
Electrodes	The conductors of the electrolytes in contact with the skin
Active electrode	The 'working' electrode at the skin site where the electrolytes are penetrating into the skin – this can be rollers, a single ball probe, a double-pronged probe or covered pads for the body
Passive electrode (sometimes called neutral, inactive, indifferent)	The electrode held in the hand to complete the circuit. On new machines, it can be a covered pad which sits under the shoulder or strapped to the upper arm
Cathode	The negative electrode – if the ions are positive, they will be drawn to this
Anode	The positive electrode – if the ions are negative, they will be drawn to this
Saline solution	A solution of water and salt – one teaspoon of salt in one pint of water – often used in desincrustation because it is a good conductor and contains sodium chloride. Most of the liquid in our body tissue is saline, so humans are good conductors of electricity
Saponification	Conversion into soap or a soap substance so sebum becomes emulsified and is easy to remove
Electrolysis	Chemical decomposition of a substance by passage of an electric current through it. Also used in the destruction and permanent removal of hairs, moles, spider naevi, etc.
Moving coil meter	The window at the front of the machine with a metal arm moving along the milliamp readings
LED	Light emitting diode – for reading milliamps on the front of the machine

(continued on next page)

LCD	Liquid crystal display – for milliamp registering
Polarity switch	Dial found on the machine. It can reverse the polarity of the electrodes, without having to remove them from the body – although on most machines you have to turn off the current before you reverse the polarity. If you were doing desincrustation only, you might want to reverse the polarity for just a minute to reduce the erythema on the skin. For anti-cellulite treatments, you may find you do the same thing for the same reason – check with individual manufacturers' instructions
Red lead	Often referred to as a jack lead. Some machines are colour coded – the red lead is inserted into the red socket. Usually positive, and is mostly used for roller or prong insertion, but check with individual machines and manufacturers' instructions
Black lead	Inserted into the black socket on the machine, and is negative so tends to be the electrode that the client holds or is placed under the shoulder

On some machines, the current will not work if you insert the coloured leads into the other coloured socket, e.g. the black lead into the red socket. Also be careful that you do not put one of the rollers into the red socket and the other one in the black – this will not work either, as you are not completing a circuit. *The rollers must be of the same polarity* – usually, they come out of the red socket, and the hand-held electrode is out of the black. Confusion occurs because the rollers are a pair, but often have a linking wire into the red lead, so check to make sure they are not plugged into the different sockets.

Contra-indications to galvanic treatments

- Failure to respond to thermal and sensitivity testing, which would indicate a loss of skin sensation.
- Very sensitive skin.
- Recent sunburn/windburn.
- The presence of skin infection or diseases.
- Broken skin, such as cuts, abrasions or acne with open pustules.
- Pregnancy.
- Epilepsy.
- Metal plates in the head.
- Metallic pins or bridge work or excessive amalgam fillings in the mouth.
- Heart conditions, pace makers fitted or any heart condition requiring medication.
- Headache or migraine sufferers.
- High or low blood pressure.
- Pregnancy.
- Highly nervous clients.
- Contact lenses should be removed.

If in doubt, always seek the client's doctor's approval before treatment.

Keys to good practice

- Some manufacturers state that pregnancy, extensive dental work and bridge work are not contra-indications as the current is low. Never assume this is the case, however – always follow specific instructions.
- Some manufacturers recommend the client waits at least 12 hours before and after any heat treatments, including facial waxing, electrolysis, sauna, sunbeds, hood hair dryers and swimming.
- After collagen injections, galvanic facials should be avoided until the consultant's approval is gained (approximately 2 weeks).

Contra-actions to galvanic treatment

- Clients may experience a metallic taste and a tingling sensation in the mouth, as the current is drawn towards the metal in amalgam fillings.

- Some clients will feel the current quite strongly; others may have quite a high tolerance to it, and not feel very much at all. It is important not to turn the intensity up higher than is recommended, as a galvanic burn can occur. Always reassure clients that even if they cannot feel it, the treatment is working.

- It is rare, but some clients have been known to develop a heat rash and irritation in response to galvanic preparations, so if this happens, turn off the machine, remove the rollers and then remove the product and place a cool water compress over the face. Allow the skin to calm down, and recommend the client uses a calamine-based lotion at home if the sensitivity continues, and avoids any other products which would cause further irritation. Remember to put this on the client record card for future reference.

Using the negative pole rollers, as the active electrode changes the gel which contains sodium carbonate

Sodium carbonate interacts by electrolysis with the moisture in the skin – the moisture is turned into sodium hydroxide, which is alkali

This saponifies – forms a soap

Results in a deep cleansing effect which softens the skin

Effects of galvanic desincrustation

Keys to good practice

Desincrustation is usually carried out using the negative polarity, but always check because some manufacturers have changed their desincrustation gel for use under positive polarity. It is a good idea to write the polarity required on the lid of the gel for future reference, both for yourself and for colleagues.

If the polarity is not stated on the box or in the instructions, look for the pH value of the product:

- if it states it is acidic and *below* a pH reading of 7, use the positive polarity
- if it states it is alkaline and *above* a pH reading of 7 – use the negative polarity.

(For more information on the pH scale, see **You and the skin**, page 197.)

Remember

When testing galvanic equipment on yourself, you have to form the circuit and should be holding the neutral (covered) electrode in one hand, and make contact with the roller on your arm. Gradually turn up the current until sensation is felt. If you have the roller on your arm and the client is holding the neutral electrode, you will not form the circuit and will feel nothing.

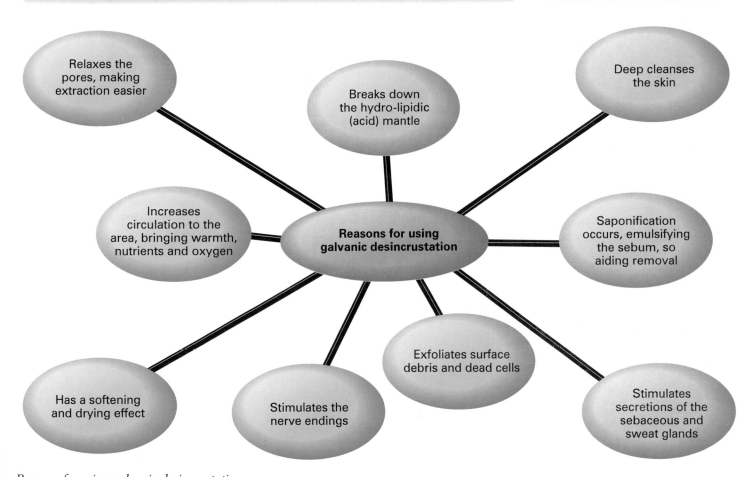

Reasons for using galvanic desincrustation

Keys to good practice

Recommend that a male client has a very close shave prior to galvanic treatment as the current is attracted to the moisture content in the hair and may cause a concentration of current in one area.

Step-by-step

Preparation and method – galvanic desincrustation treatment

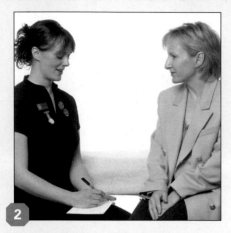 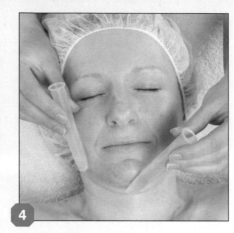 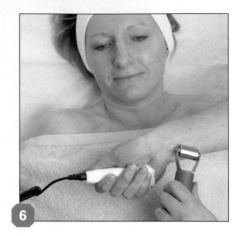

1 Set up machinery with all appropriate equipment required. Check polarity of the desincrustation gel and set machine accordingly.

2 Carry out a full consultation.

3 Prepare client on the couch, with turban in place to keep hair away from the current, and remove eye-make up, then cleanse the skin thoroughly – twice is ideal to remove both make-up and perform a deep cleanse. Remove cleanser and blot, so the skin is clean and grease-free.

4 Carry out thermal and sensitivity testing on the face.

5 If steaming or pre-warming of the skin is required, it should be carried out now, but remember not to over-stimulate the face and adjust timings accordingly – some manufacturers do not recommend steaming, but prefer a mild exfoliant to be used in place of the second cleanse.

6 Test the machine on yourself and in front of the client – if required, test it on the client, too – so the client feels the sensation and is comfortable with it.

7 Give the client the covered, neutral electrode (bar) to hold in a hand without jewellery on, and make sure the sponge glove is damp, but not wringing wet – some companies do not require the bar to be covered (always check).

8 Decant desincrustation gel into a bowl, and apply to the face with either massage movements or a mask brush.

9 Make contact with the roller on the skin, and turn up the current gradually, until the client feels a tingling sensation; turn down the intensity slightly and introduce the other roller to the face.

10 Use slow, even, rhythmic movements all over the face, but do not allow the rollers to come into contact with one another.

11 Follow the directions of the arrows (see the next page) and work all over the face and neck area – approximately 5–7 minutes depending upon skin type and reaction, etc.

12 When roller use is completed, remove one roller; keep the one in contact with the skin moving and turn current down and then off. Remove other roller.

13 Change to ball or double-pronged electrode and start machine again, with electrodes in contact with the skin, working around the crevice of the nose and chin area.

14 Turn off the current, remove the electrode and thoroughly remove all the product with damp sponges.

15 Comedone extraction with sterile probe or covered fingers can now be completed.

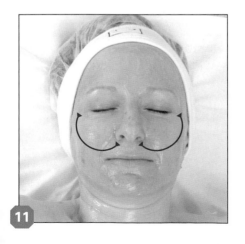

9

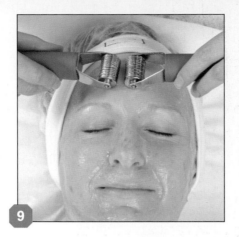

9

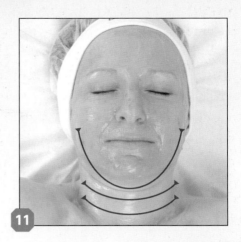

11

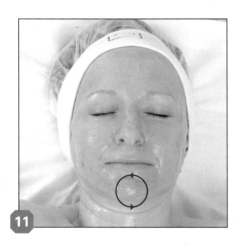

11

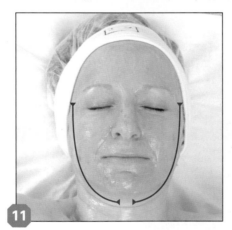

11

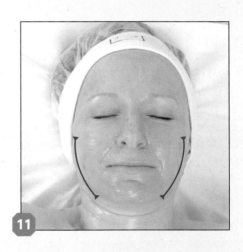

11

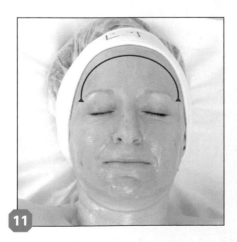

11

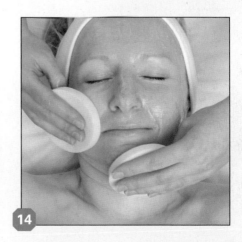

11

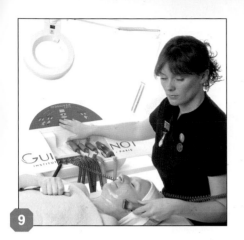

14

If you are not continuing with iontophoresis, then some companies recommend reversing polarity for the last minute of desincrustation to calm the skin down. If you are moving on to iontophoresis, then carry straight on to that procedure.

Keys to good practice

Before the treatment, rub the rollers in the palm of your hands (with no current on) for a few minutes to pre-warm them and discharge any ions sticking to them from a previous treatment. This also helps the flow of the ions once in contact with the face. Some manufacturers recommend soaking the rollers in surgical spirit after treatment, both to clean them and to discharge any residue of cream/gel.

Keys to good practice

Initially, the skin has a natural resistance to the current and the client may have little or no sensation. However, once the skin's resistance has been broken down, through the warming of the tissue, there may be a rise in the sensation felt – in which case the intensity will need to be turned down slightly.

Type of skin	Setting
Dry/sensitive	0.15 milliamps
Normal/combination	0.20 milliamps
Oily/problem	0.25 milliamps

Suggested galvanic settings for desincrustation
Always check individual manufacturers' instructions.

Ingredient	Description
Sodium chloride (10%)	Common table salt; astringent and antiseptic properties
Sodium carbonate (5%)	Soda ash found in sea water and lakes
Sodium bicarbonate (10%)	Baking soda; alkali

Reasons for use

Used under the negative (–) polarity for saponification of fatty acids and desincrustation; especially effective on an oilier skin

Common ingredients in desincrustation gels

Keys to good practice

Always adjust the intensity of the current and the duration of the treatment to suit the client's needs – some skins will need, and respond to, more current than others and the ratio of time spent on desincrustation and iontophoresis is proportional to the skin type and the client's needs.

Recommended treatment course

If the skin type is normal, the client would benefit from desincrustation at least once a week for three weeks. Oily or congested skins would require slightly more treatments. A rest of two weeks should be suggested, to avoid over-stimulation of the sebaceous glands, which may worsen the condition – this will depend upon individual reactions and the manufacturer's recommendation for the particular system used.

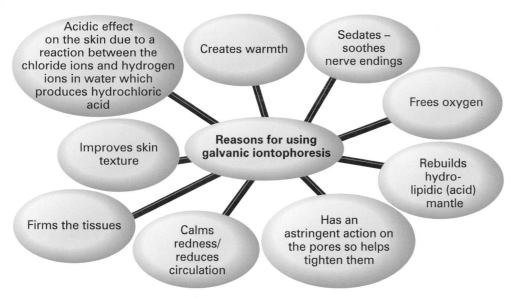

Reasons for using galvanic iontophoresis

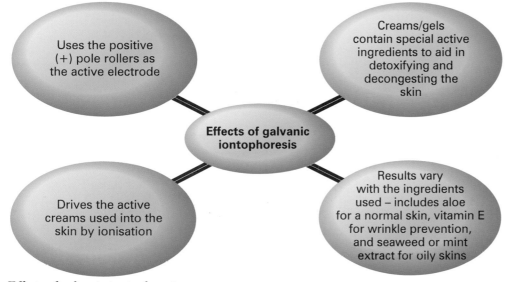

Effects of galvanic iontophoresis

Flowchart (right column):

- Test on self – form a circuit by holding the covered neutral electrode in one hand and a roller on the arm, while turning up the current.
- Rub rollers in the hand for a moment to warm them.
- Check product polarity needed for desincrustation.
- Place roller in contact with skin, and then turn on and increase current.
- Work all over face and neck with rollers.
- Remove one roller, then the other.
- Remove desincrustation cream and carry out extraction.
- Apply iontophoresis gel/ampoule/cream.
- Change polarity, if required.
- Work all over face and neck with rollers.
- Follow recommended steps from product supplier and finish with direct high frequency.

Keys to good practice

Remember the five golden rules – see **Facial treatments – theory and consultation**, page 230.

Precautions during galvanic treatment

- Make sure the client holds the bar in a hand that is wearing no jewellery.
- Check product polarity required for desincrustation (usually negative) – rollers and cream must be the same polarity.
- When carrying out desincrustation on the face, place the roller in contact with skin and only then turn on and increase the current.
- Remove one roller, turn current down and off, and then remove the other roller.
- Check polarity required for iontophoresis – usually positive.

The table on pages 260–1 shows possible product use for iontophoresis.

Step-by-step

Preparation and method – galvanic iontophoresis treatment

1 Carry out desincrustation procedure before beginning iontophoresis (shown on pages 256–7).

2 Check polarity of product most suitable for skin type and change polarity of active roller to positive. Always test machine on self in front of client.

3 Some products for iontophoresis come in ampoule form and care should be taken when breaking the glass – always use a tissue and break the ampoule over the trolley, not over the client.

4 Apply product all over face and neck with mask brush or fingertips.

5 Set the intensity to 0.15–0.25 milliamps, depending upon machine and recommendations.

6 Follow steps 9–14 from the desincrustation procedure (on page 256). Allow 7–10 minutes for the routine, ensuring that the roller movements cover all the face and neck area.

7 Use rollers or fork electrodes.

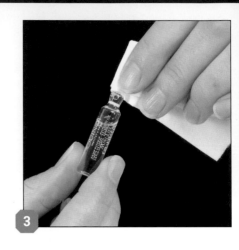

3

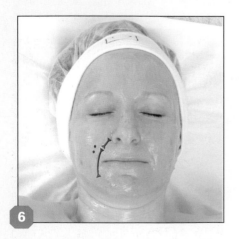
6

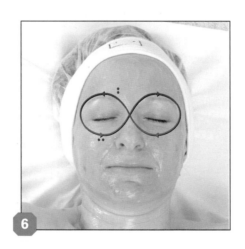
6

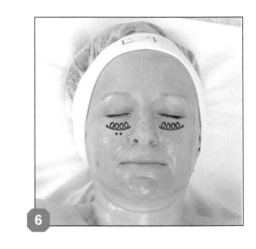
6

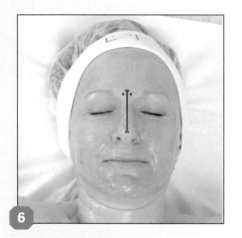
6

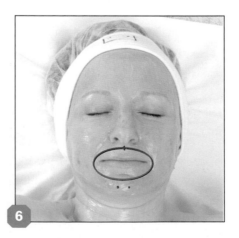
6

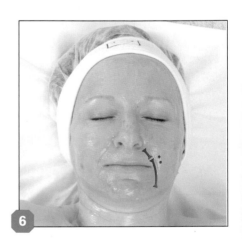
6

8 Manual massage. Follow the suggested routine given for the products you are using – some companies recommend leaving on the iontophoresis cream/gel, adding more and then carrying out a manual massage with no current involved. This ensures that the active ingredients work on, through the massage.

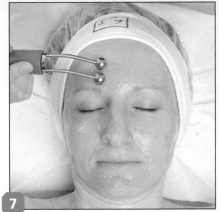

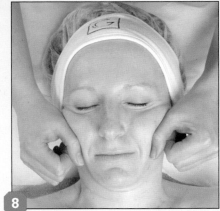

9 Remove the residue of the massage cream and apply a suitable mask. It is usually a good idea to use the one recommended by the same product suppliers as again the active ingredients will be in the face mask so that the good work of balancing and rehydrating the skin continues. Other routines may suggest that a mask at this point would be too drying, so you will need to be flexible in your learning, and appreciate that different companies follow slightly different routines, suitable for their own products and equipment.

10 Carry on with direct high frequency application with oxygenating cream to increase oxygen levels in the skin, and finish the treatment with a drying germicidal finish to the skin. Some companies recommend a toning gauze mask and a moisturiser to complete the treatment; others recommend that the skin should be left alone after high frequency, so that the benefits of the treatment are not disturbed – always follow the procedure of the system you are using. Moisturise using appropriate products.

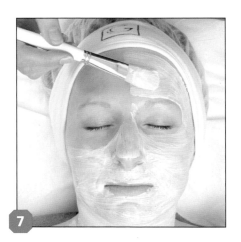

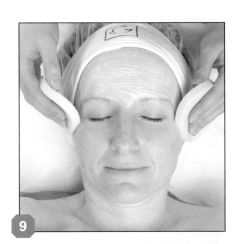

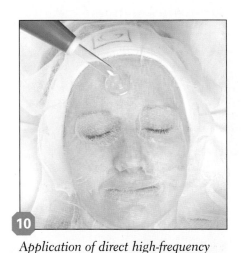

Application of direct high-frequency

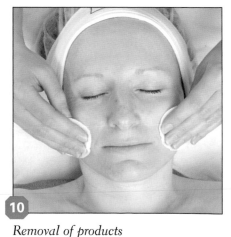

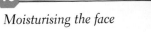

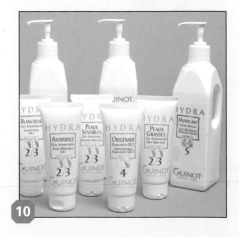

Removal of products

Moisturising the face

Active ingredient	Skin type	Result
Collagen Aloe Hylauric acid Wheat (vitamin E) Malt	Dry/mature skin	Highly active gels to improve skin tone and rehydrate and restore elasticity Wrinkle prevention on a maturing skin
Sulphur Seaweed Mint	Oily/problem skin	Gels/creams to calm and stabilise the skin
Active herbs	Normal/revitalising skin	A blended gel to revitalise a dry skin while maintaining the balance of more normal skin
Aloe vera Chamomile Centalla	Sensitive skin	Gels/creams to soothe and calm
Vitamin C Horse chestnut	Hyperpigmentation skin or generally dull	Lightens the skin and gives radiance Anti-inflammatory

Possible product use for iontophoresis

Aftercare and home care for galvanic treatment

- Avoid touching the face where possible.
- Avoid application of foundation and powder to the face for 24 hours after treatment – lipstick and eye make-up may be used. After treatment the skin is especially sensitive to the pigments contained in make-up.
- Try to use the most suitable skin care products for the skin's condition and stick to this regime daily.
- Drink plenty of water throughout the day and eat a diet rich in fruit and vegetables to help the skin heal and repair itself.

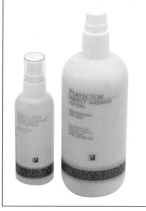

Use suitable skin-care products for client's skin type

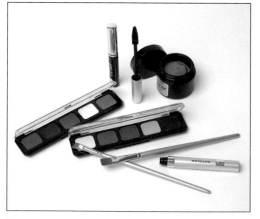

Advise client that skin may be sensitive to make-up

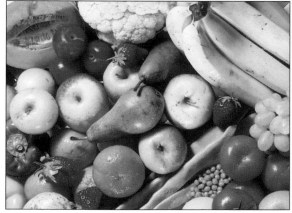

A diet rich in fruit and vegetables helps keep the skin healthy

For a full programme of steps the client should follow for skin improvement, see **You and the skin**, page 188.

Identify the hazard	What is the risk?
Danger from electric shock	Low
Galvanic burns	High
Postural problems for the therapist	High
Allergic/sensitive reaction	High

What should I do to prevent the hazard from becoming a risk?

Follow manufacturers' instructions
Carry out thermal and sensitivity tests
Test on yourself before treatment
Always have sufficient product on the skin to keep it well lubricated
Constantly monitor for any developing contra-actions
Remove all jewellery
Never exceed recommended current intensity
Always start on a zero current intensity and confirm that the client is comfortable
Always carry out a full consultation and never treat a client who has an infection present
Never use a broken spontex cover for the neutral electrode cover
Always break the ampoule over the trolley top, using a tissue, and not near the client, and dispose of the broken glass safely
Always clean and sterilise the rollers/equipment thoroughly after each treatment
Make sure the machine is positioned close to you, so that you have full control over the intensity dials and the rollers/electrodes – do not lean over the client or make contact with the couch
Ensure correct posture and chair to allow you to be in control of equipment

Risk assessment for galvanic unit

Faradism

The faradic current

Modern beauty therapy equipment combines various types of medium- to low-frequency currents. The type of current used is an alternating, low-frequency, surged and interrupted current. The source of electricity can be either the mains or a battery.

Application

The aim of facial faradic treatment is to intensively exercise the individual muscles, or groups of muscles, in the face to firm and tone them, which produces a firmer look to the contours of the face. Most modern faradic machines have both face and body outlets on them (see **Body treatments** for information on body procedures).

The faradic unit

The faradic unit is named after Michael Faraday, who studied the nature of electricity, but it is in fact an electrical muscular stimulation (EMS) unit, often referred to as neuro-muscular electrical stimulation

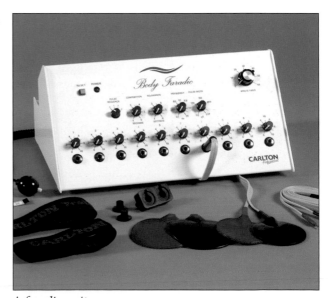

A faradic unit

(NMES). Some beauty therapists simply call the unit by its trade name such as Ultratone, Slendertone or Slim Master. (In the United States, faradic current is known as excitomotor current).

Whatever the name, a faradic unit is a machine which induces the muscles to contract and relax through stimulation of the motor nerves within the belly of the muscle. As the client has no control of this muscular contraction and there is no physical movement of the body from A to B, it is called passive exercise, and as there is no movement of the joints or limbs it is a form of isometric exercise. It is extremely effective on both the smaller facial muscles and on the larger muscle groups within the body. (For information about the muscles, see **Related anatomy and physiology**, page 160.)

At first, the machine may seem daunting to understand because of the range of settings available – the machine is designed to personalise treatment by altering the time, strength and pattern of the contractions. It may take some time for you to become familiar with it, but the more you use it, the more knowledgeable and confident you will become.

Dial settings

The machine has three dial settings that must be switched on and active for the equipment to work:

- a master on/off switch – some machines also have a timer that has to be set, and the machine will not light up ready for use unless the timer has been activated.
- a reset button at the back of the machine, which will not allow the machine to work unless the outlets where the pads go in are set to zero – this prevents the therapist from switching on the machine and giving the client a very strong initial contraction.
- a 'panic button', which is a switch on a lead plugged in at the back of the machine for the client to hold. Should the current be too strong or any discomfort be felt, the client can cut out the current and stop the treatment. This is very reassuring for the client, but as the therapist would never leave a client unattended, it should not be necessary to use it.

Some machines make a loud whining noise to alert the therapist to incorrectly set dials. The reset button needs to be pressed and the dials set at zero, and the noise alert will stop.

To help you understand the dials, it may help to study how a muscle contracts, its origins and insertions, in **Related anatomy and physiology**, page 160.

The other dials control the contraction patterns.

Pulse sequence

This is the wave form, or phasic control, and has four types.

- **Bi-phasic** regular pulse. The electrical impulses pass in both directions between the pads, giving a good firming, toning and strengthening treatment to the muscles. In normal body treatments, the pads should ideally be bi-phasic for comfort and to work the muscles to their full potential. The lights above this dial alternate to show that the current is alternating between the pads.
- **Mono-phasic** regular pulse. The electrical impulses pass in only one direction, helping to lift the muscles being treated. When a mono-phasic pulse sequence is selected, the black (negative) pad should always be placed on the insertion of the muscle and the red (positive) on to the origin (remember this as BIRO – black

> **Remember**
>
> Muscle contraction can be controlled by the strength, speed and variation of current, impulse duration, direction of the current (polarity) and frequency. All contribute to the duration and strength of contraction.

insertion red origin – so that the black pad is below the red). The muscle fibres are then lifted towards the origin. This is recommended for use on face and neck muscles, and also indicated for physiotherapy work. When the mono-phasic pulse sequence is in operation, only the positive (+) light will illuminate on the unit. Although not usually used on the body, this setting is sometimes used by body builders who require more muscular definition for shows and competition work. After several courses of treatment, the muscles get used to the contractions and may even begin to anticipate them – this does not work the muscle to its full capacity and the machine has the facility to change the pattern sequences to an irregular pattern to keep the muscle working. Always start on the regular phase settings, but introduce irregular pulses during the course of treatment.

- **Bi-phasic** irregular pulse. This adds variety and is useful for the nervous client who clenches the muscles in anticipation of the current – neither the client nor the therapist knows the pattern. This would only apply in body treatments.
- **Mono-phasic** irregular pulse. The irregular pulse sequence is designed to aid in the treatment of nervous or tense clients. The pulses come in groups of three and five, and due to the irregularity of the impulses, the client cannot anticipate the muscle contraction, thereby avoiding discomfort during treatment. This would apply in facial faradic work and can be used half-way through the course of treatment to keep the muscles working hard.

Contraction and relaxation settings

This setting may be altered to give a longer or shorter length of muscle contraction, and will vary according to the client's muscle tone. Weak muscle should be exercised on a lower setting, that is 1.5 seconds on and 1.5 seconds off, with the setting increased as muscle tone improves.

You will need to adjust the timings of the contraction and relaxation so that the relaxation time is never less than the contraction time.

Type of work	Setting
Normal body	80–100 Hz
Facial	**120 Hz**
Deep muscle	60 Hz

Suggested frequency settings

Type of work	Setting
Normal body	160 μs
Facial	**90 μs**
Deep muscle	240 μs

Suggested pulse width settings in microseconds

The frequency and pulse width settings can be altered to ensure the impulse penetrates to the correct depth of the muscle being contracted, ensuring the maximum comfort is achieved for the client.

Precautions during facial faradic work

- Just like normal exercising, the muscles work more efficiently after some form of warm-up – for a facial treatment, this could be a steam treatment, infrared application, hot towels or manual massage. This will prevent muscle damage.
- After treatment, lymphatic drainage should be carried out for a few minutes as lactic acid will have accumulated in the muscles as a by-product of oxygen and nutrient exchange.
- Ensure surge speed is not too slow as this would make the muscle contraction too long, which would be uncomfortable for the client.

Remember

For facial faradic work, the setting should be:

- Mono-phasic regular pulse, 120 Hz, 90 μs

- Never exercise a muscle to the point of no reaction, that is muscle fatigue. Always reduce the current around the eye area, bony areas, or where there are fillings or dentures.
- Never give treatment over areas where metal has been replaced as tissue, or around a mouth with extensive fillings.
- Always re-adjust the placement point if the client experiences discomfort or the required exercise is not being produced.
- Keep pads dampened with saline solution throughout the treatment.
- Ensure the amount of current flowing is minimal at the beginning.
- Always have the machine facing the therapist so that you can constantly check the dials.

Keys to good practice

Test the pads on yourself, in front of the client, and fully explain the treatment.

Contra-indications to facial faradic treatments

There are not many contra-indications to faradism because it is an action very similar to natural movement, but there are instances where it should not be applied or where medical guidance should be sought before treatment.

If clients are unaware of the state of their health, then it is advisable to ask them to check with their doctor before treatment, especially as a facial treatment plan will probably include other treatments and factors (e.g. vacuum suction, preheating treatments, microcurrent or galvanic treatments). Contra-indications include the following.

- Failure of the sensitivity or thermal tests.
- Muscle disease or spastic, paralysed muscles.
- A history of strokes, facial paralysis or bells palsy (which responds well to EMS but should only be carried out in a medical/ physiotherapy context).
- Skin cuts, grazes, inflammation, sunburn, etc. Small breaks in the skin may be protected by a small piece of plaster. With certain minor skin complaints, wet a sponge disc and position it between the pad and the body. Sponge discs should also be used for anyone found to be allergic to the rubber surface of the pad.
- Pregnancy (especially the early stages) and after birth until a doctor's clearance is given (usually six weeks).
- After operations.
- Old scars in the treatment area can cause discomfort if the skin has underlying adhesions or is taut or puckered.
- Epilepsy.
- Asthma – only with a doctor's approval.
- High blood pressure or heart conditions (particularly in the obese client) – only with a doctor's approval.
- Metal plates or pins in bones adjacent to treatment area.
- Implanted electronic devices, e.g. pacemaker.
- High temperature.

Effects of facial faradic treatment

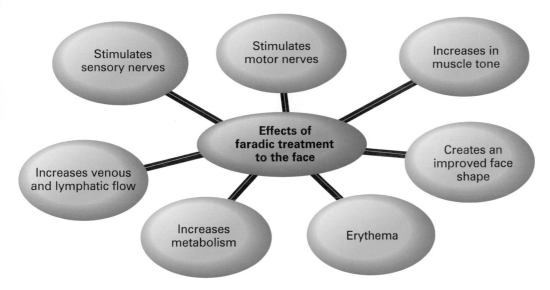

Effects of faradic treatment to the face

Stimulation of sensory nerves

The primary reaction is one of a mild prickling sensation underneath the pads. This is due to the stimulation of sensory nerves and ceases as soon as sufficient intensity of current is applied and muscle contraction is brought about. This sensory stimulation causes reflex vasodilation of the superficial blood vessels producing a slight erythema in the area.

Sensation may be increased once the skin's resistance has been broken down, and the current is able to penetrate further into the skin.

Stimulation of motor nerves

A faradic-type current stimulates the motor nerves, and provided the current is of sufficient intensity, causes contraction of the muscles which they supply. To avoid tetanic contractions, the current is surged. To avoid muscle fatigue developing, the current is also interrupted to allow the muscle to rest between contractions.

Increased venous and lymphatic flow

As the muscles contract and relax, they exert a pumping action on the veins and lymphatic vessels lying in and around them.

Increased metabolism

There is an increase in demands for oxygen and nutrients and an increase in waste products.

Erythema

A mild erythema is produced under the pads due to dilation of the superficial blood vessels.

> **Remember**
>
> Although muscle has a good blood and fluid supply, so conducts current well, adipose tissue does not, and a larger client will have less sensation and may require a higher intensity than a thinner one.

> **Remember**
>
> Tetanic contractions get their name from the medical condition tetanus, which causes muscles to go into spasm, as in lockjaw. Tetanic contractions are muscular spasms or stiffness. The current is surged gradually to increase stimulation in a smooth contraction, to avoid such spasms.

Increase in muscle tone

When a muscle is exercised it increases in 'tone', i.e. it responds more readily to a stimulus and becomes firmer. It becomes stronger and more able to hold the contours of the body more firmly and effectively without strain.

Increase in muscle bulk

In order to increase the bulk of a muscle, it is necessary for it to contract an adequate number of times against the resistance of a suitable load. When a muscle is very weak, the weight of the part of the body that it moves forms an adequate load and therefore electrical stimulation can be of assistance in restoring muscle bulk.

Preparation and method – facial faradic treatment

For facial faradic work, there are three types of electrode:

- facial block electrode
- mushroom electrode
- faradic mask electrode.

Facial block electrode

The facial block electrode is most widely used. It is easy to hold in the hand, has both the anode and cathode in its casing, which is made of rubber for insulation, and both wires red and black go into one outlet on the machine. Some of facial block electrodes have an intensity built into them, but most commonly, the block is held in one hand, placed on the face and the current turned up on the machine by the other hand.

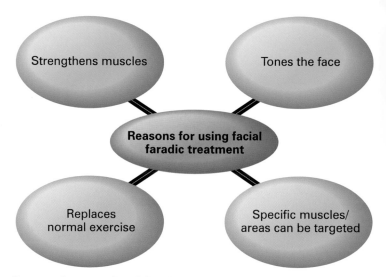

Reasons for using facial faradic treatment

Mushroom electrode

A mushroom, or disc, electrode is not widely used, but some companies still provide them. The mushroom needs another pad to complete the circuit. The electrode is the active pad, making contact with the muscle motor nerve, and the indifferent pad is either under the shoulder or strapped to the upper arm. The mushroom and the indifferent pad need to be covered with several layers of lint to prevent the client coming into contact with the metal, which could cause a burn. The advantage of the mushroom electrode is that as a single application, rather than the dual application of the block, the individual muscle can be easily isolated, and contracted.

Face mask electrode

The face mask electrode has the advantage of several points of contact and so multi-application of the current is easy. It consists of a facial mask as the active electrode and a covered arm pad to go either under the shoulder or strapped to the arm. Its drawback is that it would not be suitable for claustrophobic clients and the therapist cannot actually see the contractions taking place to monitor them and therefore control them for client comfort.

> **Remember**
>
> Faradic treatments are like any exercise – a regular course of treatments, say twice a week for six weeks, is far more effective than just one treatment. Results will be even better if the client also does the home care exercises and has a good skin care regime.

Keys to good practice

Only turn up the contraction intensity when the block is in contact with the skin, and the contraction light is on. This will ensure you do not exceed the client's tolerance. If turned up in a relaxation phase, the client may have too strong a sensation – it will be uncomfortable and may hurt.

Aftercare and home care for facial faradic treatment

See **You and the skin**, page 188, for suitable skin care recommendations.

The best form of home care for muscular development is some simple facial exercises which the client can carry out several times a day, to continue the work done in the salon.

Face and neck exercises

Face exercises

1 In a sitting position, tilt the head back, keeping teeth together. Contract neck and chin muscles for 30 seconds.
2 Repeat exercise 1 – with teeth slightly apart when head is tilted back, close the teeth. Repeat (30 seconds).
3 Say the word 'cue' pushing your lips forward.
4 Say the word 'ex' pulling the muscles back towards the ears. Repeat 20 times.
5 Open the eyes wide and drop the mouth open, stretching all the muscles as far as possible for 30 seconds.
6 Repeat exercise 5, but stick out your tongue as far as possible for 30 seconds.
7 Close your eyes and screw your face into a ball for 30 seconds.
8 Tilt head slightly, push lower jaw and teeth forward.
9 Try to reach your nose with your lower lip. Hold for 30 seconds.
10 Turn the lower lip down, stretching neck and jaw muscles.

Relaxation – neck rolling

Sit straight in a chair, drop the head onto your chest, then slowly swing your head up to the right shoulder, following through the back and down to the left shoulder, then back on to the chest. (Do not roll the head right around over the back – this is not recommended.)

Repeat six times clockwise and six anticlockwise.

Facial faradic

Remove all make-up and jewellery.

↓

Test on yourself in front of the client.

↓

Insert lead into facial applicator.

↓

Adjust pulse sequence, frequency and pulse width settings.

↓

Check all intensity dials are in the off position.

↓

Switch on minute timer and press reset button.

↓

Dampen facial electrodes and place on muscle.

↓

Turn up intensity control and contract ten times (this can increase with subsequent treatments). Pulse width settings may be increased if required until the most comfortable contraction is obtained.

↓

Turn down intensity control, move electrode to next muscle and repeat.

↓

Continue until all required facial muscles have been treated.

Step-by-step

Facial faradic treatment

1 Carry out a full consultation to check for contra-indications.

2 Prepare the client and ensure comfort.

3 Remove all make-up, jewellery and accessories.

4 Carry out thermal and sensitivity tests. Ensure the area is clean and grease-free and that the muscles are relaxed by some form of heat treatment or good massage.

5 Place the client in a semi-reclining position to enable you to see the contours of the face quite clearly (when the client is in a supine position, the contours of the face are distorted slightly by the forces of gravity). Check the machine, ensure all dials are at zero and set up ready for treatment.

6 Position the machine so that all dials are useable by the therapist without restricting movement and without wires causing discomfort. Prepare a warm saline solution – one teaspoon of salt to one pint of water. Wash hands.

7 Test the equipment on yourself in front of the client, by holding the pad in the palm of your hand. Switch on slowly until a current causes a mild contraction. Turn machine off. Briefly describe what the treatment will do, and the sensations felt as treatment begins and is built up. Warn the client of any noises and flashes which may cause alarm.

When the client is confident, position the surge and interval periods for one second each, dampen the electrodes with a warm saline solution and ensure the output dial is still at zero. Place electrodes on to the lower part of the sides of the neck, locating the motor point for the sternocleidomastoid and platysma muscles, turn on the output switch to release the current and slowly increase during surge periods only until exercise can be seen. Ensure that the client is not experiencing discomfort and never apply the current beyond tolerance level. As the muscle becomes more relaxed, an increase in surge and discomfort may become apparent. It is most important to watch the client's face throughout the treatment to make sure no pain is experienced. It may be necessary to reduce the current once the muscles increase their reaction to the current and this should be done during an interval period. Discomfort may also be experienced if the motor point has not been located accurately – a slight alteration in placement should solve the problem. Never remove the electrodes from the skin during a contraction period, and then reapply! Having stimulated this point for the required number of contractions (usually 10–15 for a general toning treatment) turn down the intensity control and move the electrode to the upper part of the neck (great oracular point of cervical nerve).

8 Work upwards exercising all of the main facial muscles.

9 When treatment is completed, carry out lymphatic drainage, either manually or with vacuum suction to the face, to help the lymphatic system drain the build-up of lactic acid within the muscles.

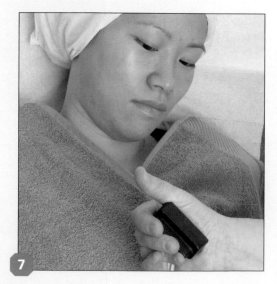
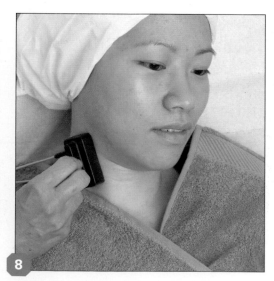

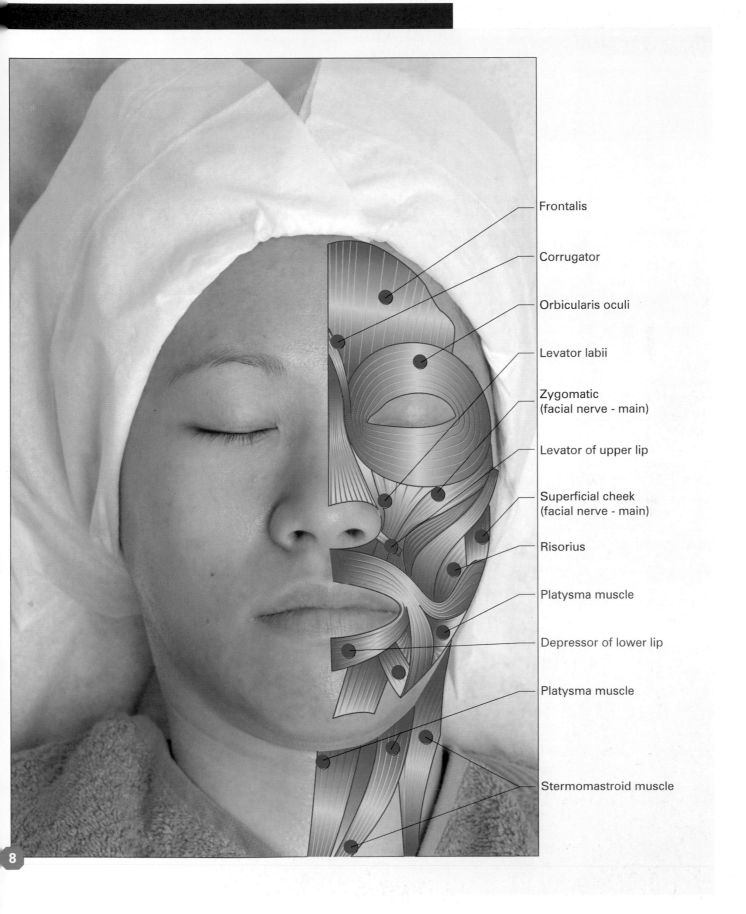

Frontalis

Corrugator

Orbicularis oculi

Levator labii

Zygomatic
(facial nerve - main)

Levator of upper lip

Superficial cheek
(facial nerve - main)

Risorius

Platysma muscle

Depressor of lower lip

Platysma muscle

Stermomastroid muscle

Identify the hazard	What is the risk?
Danger from electric shock	Low
Minor shock from current sensation	High
Muscle fatigue from over-exercising the muscles	High
Allergy to the pads	High
Postural problems for the therapist	Low
Allergic/sensitive reaction	High

What should I do to prevent the hazard from becoming a risk?

Follow manufacturers' instructions
Carry out thermal and sensitivity tests
Test on yourself before treatment
Always have sufficient product on the skin to keep it well lubricated
Constantly monitor for any developing contra-actions
Remove all jewellery
Never exceed the recommended current intensity
Always start on a zero current intensity and confirm that the client is comfortable
Never over-exercise the muscle – count the contractions and never exceed client tolerance
Make sure the machine is positioned close to you, so that you have full control over the intensity dials and electrodes
 – do not lean over the client or make contact with the couch
Only turn up the intensity in a contraction phase
Use damaged sponges as a barrier between the skin and the pad
Ensure correct posture and chair height to allow you to be in control of equipment

Risk assessment for faradic unit

Keys to good practice

Remember the five golden rules – see **Facial treatments – theory and consultation**, page 230.

Microcurrent

Microcurrent has been used for about 25 years in medicine. Good results have been achieved in the treatment of bells palsy, facial paralysis, stroke, wound healing and pain control. The 'Mens' and 'Tens' system for pain management utilise microcurrent.

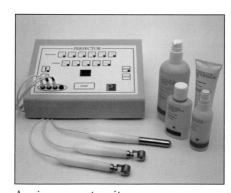

A microcurrent unit

Microcurrent mimics the body's own natural bio-electrical impulses. Our brain is continuously sending out impulses through the spinal column to muscles and soft tissues. As we get older, the body slows down, the muscles start to age and the skin begins to deteriorate (for the effects of ageing on the skin and the contributory factors for healthy skin, see **You and the skin**, page 188).

Microcurrent has the ability to speed up the whole metabolism of the tissue and cellular activity. It works in two ways – preventative and corrective. It heals the tissues so that a visible result will be seen after only one treatment. The skin will tighten, and lines and wrinkles will be softened because of the cellular activity being stimulated. In addition, because the muscle and tissue is then in a better state of repair to receive the body's own natural bio-electrical impulses, there is preventative care as well. The ageing process is being delayed and a healing effect is produced.

Most progressive salons offer microcurrent treatments for both face and body treatments and incorporate it into skin enhancement programmes as well as facial lifting.

Application

There are many microcurrent machines on the market, and they are so well developed that they use pre-set programmes and a variety of wave forms to penetrate different levels of skin tissue.

The more advanced machines are also self-calibrating to compensate for varying conductivity levels among individuals and this ensures constant results. The current is applied by dual-tipped probes, using cotton bud heads, rollers or pads, depending upon the manufacturer. Some microcurrent treatments also combine the galvanic current for iontophoresis treatments and the combination is very effective in treating the skin; a course is highly recommended, rather than just one treatment.

About the current

Microcurrent is a thousand times smaller than a milliamp and a million times smaller than an amp – that's how tiny it is!

We measure microcurrent in Hertz (Hz) – the frequency or speed of the current. Medical research has shown:

- 600 Hz touches the skin and bounces off
- 500 Hz penetrates just below the skin level
- 300 Hz stimulates lymphatic drainage
- 20 Hz stimulates circulation
- 10 Hz lifts superficial facial muscles
- 0.8 Hz gives a lift to deep facial muscles.

Microcurrent uses four wave forms:

- synergenic
- rectangular
- square
- ramp.

Synergetic wave form – used in face lifting programmes 1,5,6. Superficial effects

Ramp wave form – used in face lifting programme 2. Pumping effect

Square wave form – used in face lifting programme 3. Lifting effect

Rectangular wave form – used in face lifting programme 4. Lifting effect with a longer hold

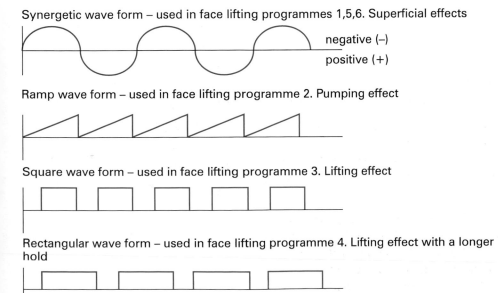

Microcurrent wave forms

These allow penetration through different levels of the tissue. So, for instance, if working on a muscle, the most suitable form is the square wave – this builds the current up quickly, holds it, then drops it off very quickly. If working on the skin, a very gentle wave form is required as no depth is required, so the synergenic, which is a wavy, very mild form, is used.

Microcurrent uses the different combinations of current, frequency and wave form to penetrate through different levels of the tissue.

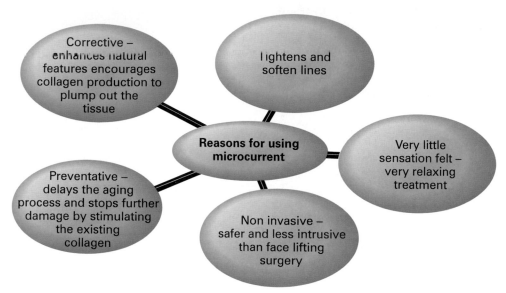

Reasons for using microcurrent

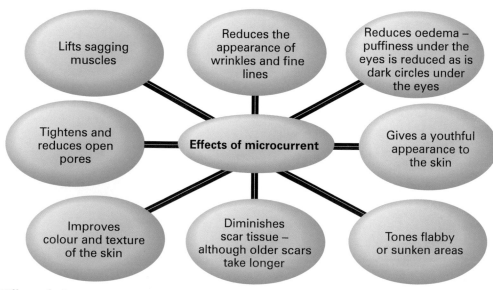

Effects of microcurrent

Contra-indications to microcurrent treatments

- Recent operations with general anaesthetic – within nine months add two more treatments to course, as it can act as a barrier to microcurrent.
- Anti-depressants – add two more treatments to course, as they can act as a barrier to microcurrent.
- Heart conditions – do not treat.
- Collagen injections – avoid area for 6–8 weeks.
- Botox injections – avoid area totally as microcurrent will stimulate the area.
- Pregnancy – do not treat.
- Epilepsy – do not treat.
- Metal implants – do not treat if the metal implants are in the head or neck area.
- Diabetes – be aware of any skin reaction during treatment.
- Smokers – due to the thickening of the skin and premature ageing, the advice is to add a further six treatments to the course.
- Chemotherapy/radiology – client must be totally clear of cancer for four years before starting.
- Retin A or Ro-Accuntaine – this medication used in the treatment of acne can cause thinning of the skin, so avoid treating for one year.

Effects of non-surgical face-lifting treatment

Circulation

This part of the treatment stimulates the epidermal and dermal blood circulation. It also has an activating effect on the lymph circulation.

Drainage/relaxation

This part of the treatment:

- increases circulation of the upper arm and lower layers of the connective tissue, providing increased nourishment of the epidermis
- detoxifies by activating the lymphatic system, ridding the tissue of waste, so reducing puffiness and fluid retention
- increases mitotic activity within the basal layer of the skin, so improving texture.

Lifting – short and long

This part of the program reprogrammes the muscles. Each muscle is stretched or relaxed, that is the muscle length is modified, which results in:

- reduction of deeper wrinkles – has a long-term lasting effect
- general firming up of loose tissue, e.g. jowls
- general toning of the dermis and reduction in the size of pores.

Firming

This program concentrates on the epidermis and dermis. The probes follow the weft of the skin. It results in:

- stimulating and speeding up the rate at which the skin produces its own corrective tissue fibres (collagen and elastin), so increasing the supportive framework of the dermis

- reducing large pores
- softening scar tissue
- refining the texture of the skin
- reducing fine lines and wrinkles
- increased local circulation causing increased nourishment, thereby increasing the regenerative process, and so firming up the tissue
- increased detoxification which improves the general colour of the skin and gives a more refined texture.

Ionisation

This part of the program allows ionised substances, in this case collagen and elastin, to pass into the epidermis of the skin with the aid of a galvanic current. Collagen and elastin promote the natural regenerative process of the skin and give added tone and elasticity to the tissue. Other ionisable products may be used.

Preparation and method – microcurrent treatment

Programme	Current (in micro amperes)	Wave form	Duration (in minutes)	Frequency (in Hz)	Polarity
1	300	Synergenic	2	20	Alternating
2	50	Ramp	10	300	Alternating
3	160	Square	16	10	Alternating
4	80	Rectangular	8	0.8	Alternating
5	500	Synergenic	10	500	Alternating
6	200	Synergenic	3	30	Direct

Treatment programmes for face lifting

Face lifting – setting up the machine

1 Plug machine into mains using the lead provided.
2 Switch on machine at rear.
3 All indicator lights will light up and a single audio signal will be heard. The lights stay on for a few seconds while the machine checks all circuits.
4 The LED will go to zero indicated by two lines (- -) and the on indicator (represented by a tick) will stay lit up.
5 Plug the probe leads into one channel – positive (+) and negative (–).
6 When ready, press the panel switch to start programme 1 (2 minutes). Then press start. The LED will begin counting down and the audio signal will sound every eight seconds.
7 At the end of the programme, the LED will return to zero (- -) and the light on the programme 1 button will go out. A single lower-toned beep will sound at the end of each programme.
8 Proceed through the remaining five programmes.

The programme you are working in can be paused or stopped at any time using the appropriate button on the right of the display panel.

If the (!) light comes on, you do not have conductivity. Check all leads and ensure you are using sufficient gel.

> **Remember**
>
> Not all microcurrent machines are the same – always follow the manufacturer's recommendations for timing and settings.

body
TREATMENTS

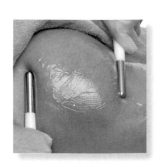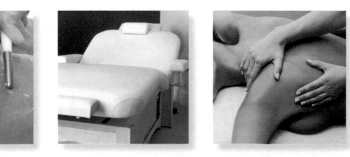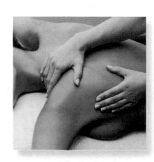

Body treatments – theory and consultation

A client's body image is linked to his or her self-confidence, so a body consultation requires tact and careful handling. To undergo a body consultation – opening up to a therapist and allowing your body to be scrutinised – takes a great deal of courage. Even clients with a 'model figure' have insecurities about their bodies. The average client comes to you because he or she believes you will be able to improve his or her body shape. It may take a couple of sessions before clients feel sufficiently comfortable with you to discuss their body image.

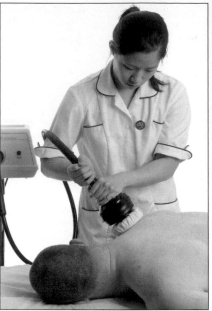

Using a G5 unit for a relaxing body treatment

You will learn about

- consultation techniques
- body consultation record card
- posture
- body types and conditions
- other factors to check in figure diagnosis
- manual examination
- fat and fat stores
- weight problems and obesity
- equipment used in body treatments.

Consultation techniques

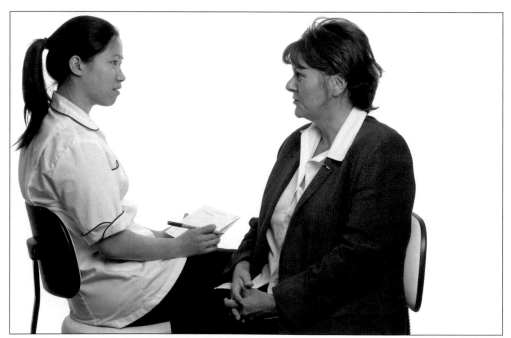

Consultation for a body massage

Remember

There are common threads running through the consultation for all body treatments. To refresh your knowledge of consultation techniques, refer to **Professional basics**.

Consultation techniques include a variety of methods to determine the best course of treatment to meet the client's needs. These include:

- observation
- questioning
- manual examination.

The initial assessment of the figure and posture of the client is a visual one. The next part involves the client removing clothing as far as underwear to allow a thorough physical and manual assessment.

Observation

Although you will be looking at the skin in the area to be treated for visible signs of damage, correction required and possible contra-indications, you will first observe the whole client for:

- posture/postural problems
- weight and height ratio
- mobility problems or a disability requiring treatment adaptation
- general body language reflecting confidence or self-esteem.

Your observation will need to begin before the client is aware of you, as this is when you will be able to see the client's unconscious body language and posture. How is the client carrying himself or herself? Does he or she look weighed down, or confident? Store your first impressions for when you complete the physical examination – you will only then see the true state of posture, with the client undressed, when you can observe the spine and balance of the shoulders and hips, and the distribution of body weight (see Posture on page 289).

Keys to good practice

A client who has poor self-esteem will not easily make eye contact. It might be that the client's visit to the salon is because of a facial or body problem which is causing negative feelings. This will be reflected in the individual's posture, demeanour and lack of enthusiasm. You will need to observe this and handle the client with care.

Questioning

Personal details and medical records will be recorded in the same way as for facial consultation (see **Facial treatments – theory and consultation**, page 230, to refresh your memory). These details will only need updating or revising if, for example, the client moves home or changes doctor.

However, on every visit you will need to check contra-indications and allergies, medication taken and any lifestyle changes. Any or all of these can change on a weekly basis, and a client can develop an allergy to a product he or she has been using for years.

Keys to good practice

At this stage, the client should be sitting with outdoor clothing removed to discuss his or her lifestyle and treatment requirements.

Body consultation record card

Use the body consultation card to guide you through your questioning. This is often printed on the reverse of the facial record card. On the next page is a typical body consultation card.

Body condition – please ✓ if present and use comments box		Comments box
Height: 1.65 m		Client is following the Weightwatchers eating programme to lose weight – she says her ideal weight would be about 63.5 kg, and she has already lost 6 kg over the past three months.
Weight: 79.5 kg Frame size (small, medium or large): Small Body mass index: 30		Her frame size is small, with tiny hands and a size 3 shoe. BMI needs to be 25 for a desirable weight – 30 is too high for good health.
Body type: Ectomorph Endomorph Mesomorph Combination	✓	The client is a classic endomorphic shape, small hands and feet, fat distribution around the hips and stomach. Heavy breasts and a tendency to fluid retention when her period is due.
Muscle tone: Medium (Good/medium/poor)	✓	Client has joined a gym and has been walking on the treadmill and cycling and swimming, so muscle tone is improving. Client was very athletic when younger and is keen to get back into shape.
General posture:	✓	Good – client stands upright with no visible signs of any postural problems. She does sometimes suffer with a frozen left shoulder as she does a lot of her work on the computer, and feels her posture could be better when sitting at her desk.
Postural faults: (Scoliosis, kyphosis, lordosis)	N/A	
Areas of fat deposits: Type of fat: (Hard/medium/soft/cellulite)	✓	Lots of soft fat deposited on the trunk area mainly. Tummy muscles quite weak but the leg muscles are improving due to work at the gym.
Circulation: Good (Good/poor/fluid retention)		Circulation is good and skin is pink and firm – although the client says she does get cold feet at night. No sign of fluid retention.
Circulation damage: (Varicose veins/broken or dilated capillaries)		One varicose vein from her pregnancies in her left leg, just behind the knee. Plays up if she has been on her feet all day, but not very visible and not swollen.
Lifestyle analysis:		Improving weekly – although the client would like to cut back on her wine intake; her diet and exercise routine is good since she joined Weightwatchers and she feels the exercise at the gym has reduced her stress levels. The exercise has also improved her sleeping pattern and the client feels positive and encouraged to continue with the new programme to lose weight for the summer. The client is happily married and enjoys an active social life, but does get stressed sometimes with two teenage girls in the house!
Diet and exercise:		Good – writing down all foods to count points, with a steady weight loss of 0.5–1 kg per week. At the gym once or twice a week, and swimming regularly.

Reasons for treatment:	The client has two reasons: 1 Tension in the shoulders, so relaxation through massage and heat. 2 Muscle tone improvement especially in the tummy area, to help the exercise along, and body wraps to give inch loss and encouragement.
Suggested treatment plan:	Infrared and massage for the back. G5 and manual massage. A six-week course of body faradic treatment on the hips and thighs, with a seaweed wrap every month.

Lifestyle and eating patterns should be discussed as well as sleeping patterns, stress levels and the client's perceptions, goals and wishes, as well as your professional advice. The client's physical well-being is only one part of the whole picture: discuss the client's relaxation choices, hobbies and family commitments and physical recreation – all play a part in how the body behaves and reacts. For example, repetitive muscle movements can cause tension and problems in the muscle fibres, such as fibrositis, and a simple chat about using a wrist support when typing, or changing the height of the chair in relation to the screen, may be enough to prevent the problem, along with heat and plenty of massage to release the muscular tension.

Posture

A good posture is one in which the body is in a relaxed and balanced, in an upright position, allowing the organs and systems of the body to work efficiently and effectively. This depends largely upon the tone of the muscles at the front and back of the trunk and legs working together, so that the body is balanced and not strained in any way – allowing muscles, ligaments and joints to move freely in their range of movement, without pain or injury. The muscles supporting posture are the antigravity muscles. They balance the front and the back of the body, using as little energy as possible.

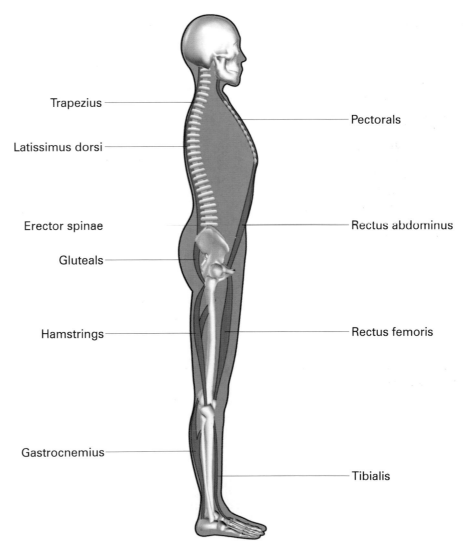

Trapezius

Latissimus dorsi

Erector spinae

Gluteals

Hamstrings

Gastrocnemius

Pectorals

Rectus abdominus

Rectus femoris

Tibialis

The antigravity muscles

Imagine there is an invisible thread or cord, holding the body upright (rather like a puppet on a string, but with one central string) from the centre of the top of the skull, through the middle of the body, shoulder and pelvic girdles, right to the ground. This is often referred to as a plumb line.

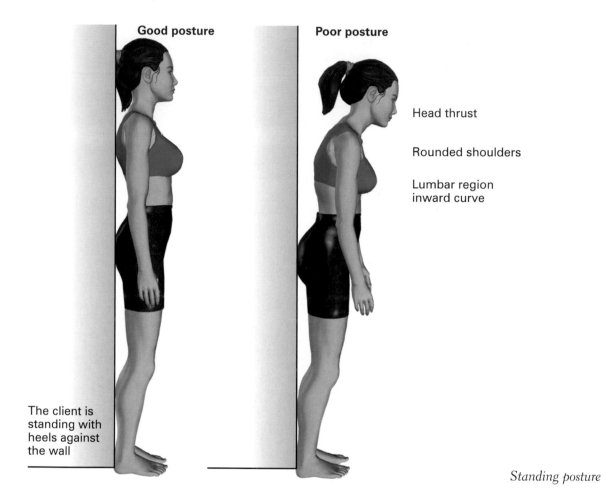

Good posture

Poor posture

Head thrust

Rounded shoulders

Lumbar region inward curve

The client is standing with heels against the wall

Standing posture

The benefits of good posture include the following:

- Breathing is easy as the lungs can be filled deeply when inhaling because they are not compressed or the chest contracted.
- The digestive tract has enough room to function correctly, without being cramped or restricted.
- An even distribution of body weight ensures that the body does not become too tired, nor is too much strain put on any one set of muscles.
- The bones, ligaments and joints are allowed to work fully, without undue effort or the risk of damage.
- The shape and figure looks at its best when the posture is correct, and this, in turn, gives a feeling of confidence and provides a positive mental outlook.

Poor posture results in:

- the lungs not being able to expand fully, as the chest may be restricting their capacity, resulting in poor oxygen levels in all the cells of the body, and lack of oxygen flow to the brain, causing dizziness or headaches

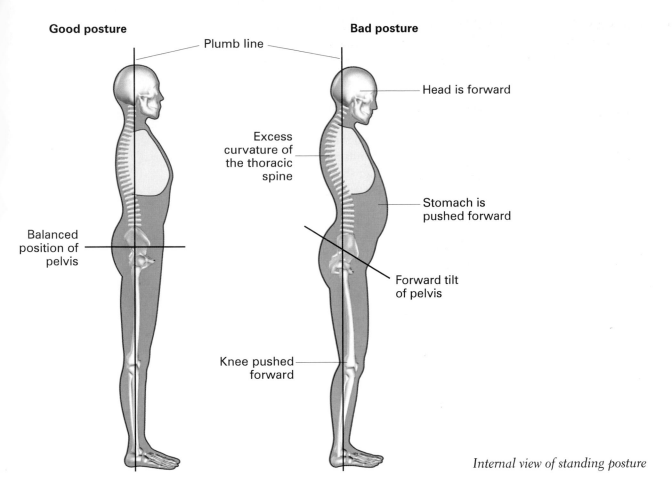

Good posture

Bad posture

Plumb line

Head is forward

Excess curvature of the thoracic spine

Stomach is pushed forward

Balanced position of pelvis

Forward tilt of pelvis

Knee pushed forward

Internal view of standing posture

- digestive problems ranging from indigestion pains or cramps, to wind and reflux, due to pressure on the sphincter muscle which prevents food from coming back up from the stomach
- muscle strain, lower back pain, or backache, because of the poor distribution of weight
- tension headaches caused by tension in the trapezius muscle, if the upper body is hunched over a keyboard or machine, for example, for long periods
- poor blood and lymph flow to the restricted areas, leading to aches and pains, tiredness and pain in the joints and ligaments.

Contributory factors to poor posture

- Poor footwear (throwing the body out of balance).
- Carrying heavy bags.
- Occupational positions (working at a keyboard, etc).
- Eye-strain (leaning over something to see it).
- Ill-fitting clothes.
- Low self-esteem.
- Lack of exercising or stretching (client's sedentary lifestyle).
- Pregnancy, illness or stress.
- The ageing process.

How to assess posture

Ask the client to remove the gown. The client will be in his or her underwear, or if going into the spa or sauna, may be in dry swimwear. Ask the client to stand in a normal, relaxed manner.

1 Observe the natural stance of the client from the front, side view and then from the back.
2 Note the shape of the spine, the level of the shoulder blades and the level of the hips and pelvic tilt. Are they even on both sides? Place your hands on the hips and shoulders to gain a perspective of the balance. If one hip or shoulder is higher than the other, there may be a postural fault, pushing it out of alignment.
3 Mark the scapulae and measure the distance between the vertebral border and the spine – is it the same, or is one further away than the other?
4 Look at the shape of the vertebrae – you should be able to trace with your finger the shape of the spine, along the protruding spinal processes. This will enable you to see and feel if the spine is out of alignment – see below.
5 Fill out the record card accordingly.

What to look for

- The head sits comfortably on the top of the vertebrae, not too far forward or back, with no protruding jaw line or the head being more forward than the pelvis.
- The arms are relaxed at the sides and are even in position and length.
- The shoulders are even and neither droops nor is over-extended.
- The scapula are even and of equal distance away from the spine.
- The spine follows its natural curve and does not force the hips to lie sideways or one higher than the other.
- The abdomen is flat and the waist curves are even and level on both sides.
- The buttocks are sitting naturally, without protruding, and the pelvic tilt looks relaxed, not forced.
- The legs are straight, the knees point forward and are level, and both feet point forward – without the legs being forced into the position or looking unnatural.
- The client is free from any pain in the joints or muscles, and is easily able to maintain the position, while you observe body shape and posture.

Checking the spinal column

The spine is a very unstable structure because it consists of 33 small circular vertebrae, piled on top of one another, with discs of cartilage (acting as shock absorbers) in between. (For further information on the spine, see **Related anatomy and physiology**, page 153.)

Through holes in the middle of the vertebrae, just behind the discs, runs the spinal cord – a column of nerves connecting the brain to the body. To help us move and remain upright, the spine is held rigidly in position by numerous bands of tough muscle and ligament.

Good posture involves holding the body erect so that the concave curvatures of the vertebrae at the neck and the base of the back are not lost. The aim when sitting, walking, driving, standing and even sleeping should be to maintain these natural curves in the back. If the curves are allowed to become convex, the muscles are put under strain and the spine is weakened, leading to the possibility of a prolapsed intervertebral disc (a slipped disc), with severe backache, and sometimes sciatica.

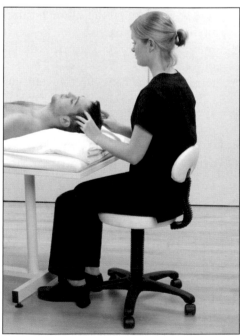

A good sitting posture

Main causes of spinal deformities

- Congenital – present at birth or arising as a direct result of hereditary factors.
- Traumatic – damage resulting from accidents, the most common one being a whiplash injury.
- Environmental – resulting from bad posture, occupation, bad habits. Tall people may stoop to minimise their height.

Curves of the vertebral column

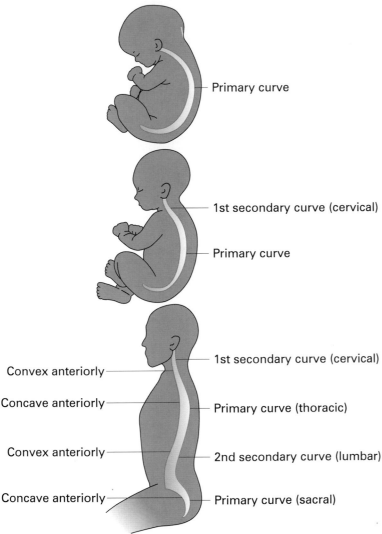

Primary curve

1st secondary curve (cervical)

Primary curve

1st secondary curve (cervical)

Convex anteriorly

Concave anteriorly — Primary curve (thoracic)

Convex anteriorly — 2nd secondary curve (lumbar)

Concave anteriorly — Primary curve (sacral)

Curves of the spine

Remember

Awkward posture when performing demanding physical activities, such as lifting heavy objects, over-strain the spine's muscular supports and may lead to back trouble. (For information on Manual Handling Regulations, see **Professional basics**, page 69; for safe lifting procedures, see **Professional basics**, page 69.)

The primary curve is the first curve to form when the foetus in curled up in the womb. The head and knees are almost touching, because space is a little cramped as the baby develops. The secondary cervical curve develops after birth when the baby has developed sufficient skill and control over the neck muscles to pull the head upright, generally after three months. The secondary lumbar curve develops when the child learns to stand upright and to walk, any time after the first year. The thoracic and sacral primary curves are kept.

This means that all healthy, normal babies have perfect posture, and that poor posture is due to external and environmental influences – poor footwear, diet, psychological factors, poorly fitting clothes or low self-esteem.

There are three types of abnormal curvature of the spine that you will need to check for:

- kyphosis
- lordosis
- scoliosis.

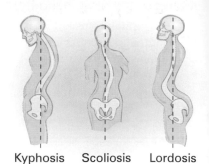

Kyphosis   Scoliosis   Lordosis

Common postural problems

Kyphosis

- A rounded back and rounded shoulders.
- The pectoral muscles on the chest are short and constricted, which restricts breathing and the chest feels tight.
- The thoracic area of the back bows outward as the muscles are over-stretched.
- This results in the abdominal muscles becoming lazy, and the abdomen tends to droop, and the breasts may sag forwards, due to lack of support from the Coopers ligaments and pectoral muscles.
- The condition is common in people who have jobs involving leaning forward, as in driving for long periods, or office workers leaning over a keyboard. It also occurs in girls trying to hide large breasts, or who may be taller than average. Poor carrying techniques of heavy loads also contribute to the development of this condition.

Lordosis

- A hollow lower back, which becomes arched, tight and stiff.
- The muscles in the lower back become short and may cause back ache.
- The pelvis and abdomen are pushed forwards and the gluteal muscles tend to stick out.
- Quite common in the later stages of pregnancy, when the weight of the growing baby pushes out the abdomen, and in men who develop a 'beer belly'. It may also develop from wearing high heels, which alters the centre of gravity and forces the posture to compensate.

Scoliosis

- A sideways pull on the spine, resulting in the curve of the spine going left or right.
- This makes the shoulders uneven, the scapulae being unbalanced, and the leg length may differ on each side, depending upon where the lateral curve is.
- The waistline will be uneven, and a client with scoliosis may walk with a slight roll of the hips.
- Mothers carrying infants on one side at the hip can develop this condition, as can people carrying uneven loads, or standing for long periods of time with all the body weight on one side. It can also be hereditary.

Keys to good practice

Kyphosis, lordosis and scoliosis are recognised medical conditions and a doctor's referral is essential before treating a client – written permission should be sought, and these conditions should be treated as a contra-indication until that happens, even if the client insists you go ahead with treatment.

Treatments which release muscular tension and allow the muscles to relax, such as heat and massage, are often very effective and therapeutic, but the client's doctor's approval is required.

Body types and conditions

Before you can fully conduct your consultation, you will need to be able to recognise the most common body types and conditions, as this will influence your treatment planning. The most common body conditions to look for are:

- cellulite
- poor muscle tone
- sluggish circulation
- blemished/congested skin.

You will need to look at the trunk (the body) and the limbs.

There are three main body types:

- ectomorph
- endomorph
- mesomorph.

Some people are very typical of one body type and are easily classification; often clients are a mixture of types.

The ectomorph

The ectomorph tends to be long, lean and angular. This body type is often tall, as the long bones (the femur), which gives the legs their length, are well developed. Ectomorphs have very little fat, which gives a lack of curves, or breast tissue. They are quite narrow in the hips and shoulders and have small joints. They do not have much muscle bulk and often have a high metabolism, which means they can eat a high quantity of food and not lay it down as body fat.

The endomorph

The endomorph is almost the opposite of the ectomorph. This body type tends to be well-rounded, tending towards heaviness in build, with a high percentage of fat in relation to muscle bulk. Endomorphs easily put on weight, even though they may consider they have a small appetite. Their general frame is solid and the limbs and neck tend to be short, with small hands and feet.

The mesomorph

The mesomorph is usually strong with an even distribution of weight, and is of an athletic build. There are well-developed shoulders, with a slim waist and hips, the muscles are well-defined and there is a low percentage of body fat. While active, this body type remains lean and strong with good muscle tone, but may develop more person fat if the body does not exercise.

Remember

Body shape and size are largely influenced by your genes – the amount of fat cells, your height and colouring are inherited. Although diet and exercise will alter body shape, the fundamental body type remains the same.

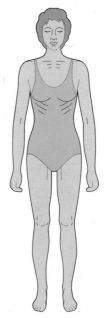

Endomorph

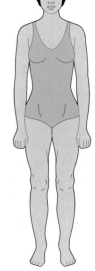

Mesomorph

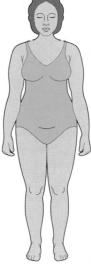

Ectomorph

Body types

Other factors to check in figure diagnosis

After checking the body type, the spinal position and the general posture, work methodically down the body, noting all areas, as they may be relevant to the treatment plan.

Round shoulders

This problem may not be acute enough to cause kyphosis, but can be prominent enough to be noticeable. For example, people with chest problems such as asthma often hunch over and develop round shoulders. Correcting the condition may require heat and massage to release the muscular tension in the pectorals and trapezius muscles, along with stretching exercises and regular postural correction – you may need to physically move the shoulders back into the correct position. The Alexander technique of realignment, Pilates and yoga, all of which stretch the muscles, are very good for this postural fault.

Winged scapulae

This is quite visible from the back, as the vertebral borders of the scapulae protrude outwards and can look a little like wings. This is common with students or back packers who carry heavy rucksacks on their backs – the scapula spread out trying to distribute the weight. It is also common if there is a combination of poor posture and a lack of fat to pad the contours, so it is more noticeable in thinner clients. This needs to be considered when giving massage and using electrical equipment on the back (such as G5 mechanical massage) as it can be quite uncomfortable for the client.

The rib cage

The position of the sternum and rib cage is important, as it tends to dictate the height and angle of the breast position. Thinner clients may have a more noticeably defined shape to the rib cage, and usually with this body type, the breasts have little fat, and are higher up on the rib cage. Note if the client has a slight boxy look to the rib cage or a 'pigeon' or hollow chest – an over expanded rib cage becomes more obvious when the client is lying down, face upwards (supine position).

The breasts

Breast treatments are very popular, and many cosmetic houses and product suppliers make creams especially for the delicate skin found on the breast. The breast has no muscle tissue of its own, and consists of fat and milk ducts, which are stimulated to produce milk by hormones after childbirth.

There are no exercises which affect the breast itself, but size and shape are dictated by weight loss or gain. Surgery can be performed to enhance the size of the breast by implants, or to reduce the fat content in the breast, also affecting its shape. (Males have also been known to have implants under the pectoral muscles to give a better definition to the shape of the chest.)

The breasts are held in place on top of the pectoral muscles by strong ligaments called Coopers ligaments, and as long they remain attached to the breast, then exercise will strengthen the attachment and therefore improve the position of the breast.

Keys to good practice

Some clients may not wish to appear topless, and you should respect their privacy. Others will not mind and may ask if anything can be done to correct their breast shape.

To check if the Coopers ligaments are still attached to the breast and the pectoral wall, ask the client to raise her arms from the side to over the head. If the nipples move higher, and the breast moves, then the Coopers ligaments are attached and can be strengthened through exercise. Diet or surgery are the only two effective methods of altering the breast shape, although creams will help the skin's appearance and tone.

Underwear/clothing

Underwear and clothing, surprisingly perhaps, play a part in poor posture. If the client has gained weight, had a pregnancy or just changed shape, then her underwear size, especially bra size, will have changed too. Clients who develop permanent strap marks and indentations in the skin on top of the shoulder are wearing the wrong size bra, and may be constricting muscles as a result. Check to see if the back of the bra is digging into the flesh, or riding too high up over the shoulder blades. A correctly fitted and sized bra will support the breasts, leave no skin irritation or marks and sit very securely. The cups should encase the entire breast and not give a squashed appearance or large cleavage.

The same applies pants and shoes. Clients suffer because they would rather endure the pain than admit to being a larger size, or wear a slightly lower heel.

Keys to good practice

Tact and diplomacy are essential. You can only suggest to the client that she gets measured correctly, but when you develop a rapport with her, she may be prepared to take your advice. Salon treatments and expensive creams will not correct the problem if the underlying source of discomfort is not corrected.

Abdomen and hips

These tend to be the main areas of fat accumulation, and a majority of treatments are aimed at the tummy, hips and thighs. Look for the amount and type of fat – hard, soft or with cellulite present (see the section on Fat, page 311).

Women tend to accumulate fat in the lower body and men to put weight on in the abdominal area. These figure types are often referred to by their hormonal influences – the male shape may be described as android obesity and the female pear shape can be called gynaecoid obesity.

Remember

When discussing the abdomen, remember to ask about the client's general digestion and diet. Discuss any problems such as irritable bowel syndrome, constipation, diarrhoea, etc. This will indicate the client's stress levels and if the digestion is affected by stress. This will help with the treatment plan – you can offer relaxing treatments.

Stretch marks

Look for stretch marks, often called striations, on the abdomen and hips. Stretch marks appear on the skin as long, faint scars, or wiggly lines in the skin's surface. When they first appear, they can look quite red and angry, and then they diminish into pearly white lines after several years. On black skins, they will appear pink and stand out due to the contrast in skin tones. Stretch marks occur as a result of a breakdown of the skin's connective tissue, which occasionally ruptures. They are most commonly seen on the breast, abdomen, upper arm, inner thighs and hips.

Main causes of stretch marks

- Growth during puberty, especially in growth spurts, and the fluctuation of hormonal influences.
- Increase in body weight.
- Yo-yo dieting where body weight fluctuates.
- Pregnancy.
- When breast feeding, especially on the lateral surface of the breast.
- During toxic or infectious invasion of the body, which alters the elastic tissue and makes it prone to rupture as a result of substantial protein loss affecting the connective tissue content.

Stretch marks can be improved with treatments. They will diminish with microcurrent application and skin treatments to firm the collagen and elastin layers, along with the application of good quality skin-firming creams or oils.

Not every client who is pregnant will develop stretch marks, but pregnant clients, clients with fine skin, or sun-damaged skin should be encouraged to keep the skin supple with regular application of skincare emollients. General massage to the area, in gentle circular motions, with high quality oils will stimulate the blood flow, bringing oxygen and nutrients to the skin, which in turn will help the collagen and elastin fibres become stronger.

Legs and feet

- Check the legs for the presence of cellulite and any surface distortion of the skin, such as varicose veins or inflamed varicose veins, a condition called phlebitis. Phlebitis is easily recognised as the vein becomes painful and tender, and surrounding skin becomes hot and red. It is a contra-indication to treatment, but responds well to medical treatments, such as elastic support for the leg, and medication. Varicose veins commonly develop during pregnancy or with a considerable weight gain.
- Other contra-indications to treatment in this area include broken capillaries, seen as small thread veins on the skin's surface, and broken skin, or cuts on the lower leg caused by shaving rather than waxing the hairs. Small cuts could be covered over, or avoided during massage, but because of a cut's moisture content, an electrical current would be drawn to it. Therefore, it is a contra-indication to electrical treatment.
- Very thin, bony legs are a contra-indication to treatment, as there is little or no adipose tissue to work upon, and the client may bruise if massage movements or heavy mechanical massage were to be carried out.
- Check the legs for knock knees, bow legs and hyper-extended knees:
  - Knock knees (genu valgum) is an abnormal in-curving of the legs, resulting in a gap between the feet when the knees are in contact.
  - Bow legs (genu verum) is an abnormal out-curving of the legs, resulting in a gap between the knees when standing.

Remember

Stretch marks are a contra-indication to some treatments, which may make the condition worse, for example vacuum suction and G5 mechanical massage, or even ski stretching massage movements. A healthy diet and drinking lots of water will also improve the general health of the skin.

Remember

It is not within your role to diagnose any medical condition, and you should refer the client to his or her doctor.

– Hyper-extended knees is an extensive and forceful extension of the knee joint which can affect balance and the ability to stand and may require surgery to correct the condition.

All of these conditions should only be treated after medical approval has been given, as the muscles involved are short and tight and may be damaged if massage or electrical treatments are attempted.

The ankles should be clearly defined and the skin clear. If the ankle is swollen and puffy, there may be fluid retention (oedema). Oedema is an accumulation of tissue fluid, caused when the veins and capillaries become congested, and the fluid is not fully dispersed back via the lymphatic system. This is often caused by pregnancy, when the added weight of the baby puts pressure on the veins in the pelvis so fluid is not drained correctly, or by weight gain. It can also indicate there is a systemic problem in the kidneys. (For more information on the lymphatic system and the functions of the kidneys, see **Related anatomy and physiology**, page 170.)

Feet should be checked for any infections, especially if the client is going into the wet area, as bacteria thrive in warm, moist conditions. (For details of bacterial, viral and fungal infections, see **Professional basics**, page 40.)

Also check on any conditions which may have a bearing upon posture, such as bunions or hallux vulgus – a displacement of the big toe, where it bends towards the other toes. A bunion is a swelling of the joint between the big toe and the first metatarsal bone. A bursa often develops over the site and the big toe becomes displaced towards the others. Bunions are usually caused by ill-fitting shoes and may require surgical treatment. Hallux vulgus can be caused by pressure of footwear, if the client has a broad foot, and is usually associated with a bunion.

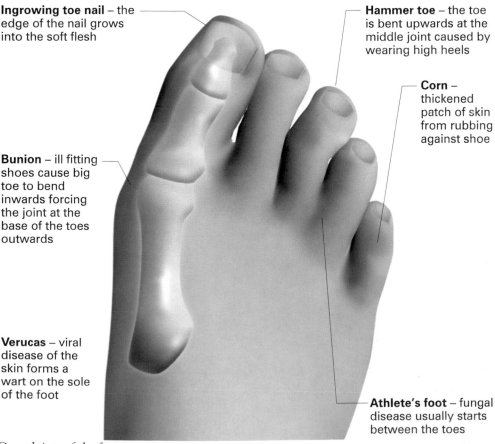

Ingrowing toe nail – the edge of the nail grows into the soft flesh

Hammer toe – the toe is bent upwards at the middle joint caused by wearing high heels

Corn – thickened patch of skin from rubbing against shoe

Bunion – ill fitting shoes cause big toe to bend inwards forcing the joint at the base of the toes outwards

Verucas – viral disease of the skin forms a wart on the sole of the foot

Athlete's foot – fungal disease usually starts between the toes

Complaints of the foot

Manual examination

Manual assessment includes:

- weight
- height
- measuring the body (when carrying out reduction treatments which may not result in body weight loss, but cause a reduction of inches, that is faradic treatments and body wraps)
- blood pressure
- pulse rate
- muscular tone and strength testing
- skin conditions.

Height and weight ratio

Height and weight must be recorded together, to get a true reflection of the size and health of the client.

Keys to good practice
A recording of 102 kg would be of concern if the client was only 1.5 m tall, as this would be considered morbidly obese, but for a man of 1.9 m tall, it might be in the normal range for his body mass index.

Accurate height measurement is important – clients often do not know their height, and people can lose height as they get older through the aging process and spinal shrinkage.

How to measure height accurately

The best way to measure height is to have a fixed ruler on a permanent fixture such as a wall, and ask the client to stand against the wall. With the head held evenly, ask the client to look straight ahead, while the client's body maintains a good, relaxed postural stance. Use a flat surface, such as a book or ruler, to lie flat upon the head, and measure against the ruler on the wall.

Weight

To record the client's weight accurately, all salons should have a good quality set of calibrated digital scales, or a traditional scales with weights sliding across a crossbar scale. Domestic scales with a dial and moving pointer are unreliable as well as being affected by the surface on which they are placed.

Weight needs to be looked at objectively to take into account the client's:

- general build
- height
- body type
- 'spread' of the skeleton.

It is a myth that people can be 'heavy boned', but it is essential to note the client's general frame size. A small woman will have a smaller framework, and weigh less than a large, tall woman with larger feet and hands.

Remember
A height measure attached to a wall is only as accurate as the person who put it there! Often, the metallic strips with centimetres marked on them start at about a metre high, as it is unnecessary for them to reach the floor. However, the person who puts up the strip should make sure the measure is placed at the correct height!

Frame size guide

As a rough guide, measure the wrist at its slimmest point – just below the knob of bone:

- Up to 14 cm = small
- 14 cm–16.5 cm = medium
- 16.5 or more = large.

Muscle tissue

Muscle tissue weighs more than fat, so a body builder with developed muscle bulk would appear to be obese on paper, whereas there will probably not be an ounce of fat on him or her! Clients who work out regularly and have a high proportion of muscle will also have a higher weight reading compared with a client of the same frame who does little exercise.

Body mass index

A body mass index (BMI) reading will enable you to discover if the client has a healthy height–weight ratio. This can be worked out as follows:

$$BMI = \text{weight in kilograms/height in metres}^2$$

To work out your own BMI:

1. Find your weight in kilograms (e.g. 57.2 kg).
2. Find your height in metres (e.g. 1.64 m).
3. Multiply your height reading by itself (e.g. 1.64 m x 1.64 m = 2.69 m).
4. Your BMI is:

57.2 kg/2.69 m = 21.26

Now, check the BMI chart below to see if this is an acceptable reading.

You can also use a height : weight chart to see if your client has a healthy weight.

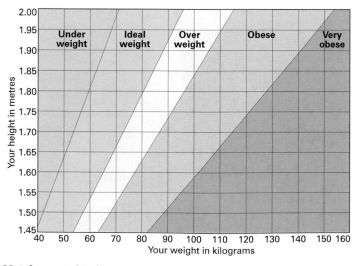

Height : weight chart

BMI reading	What the reading means
Less than 20	Below normal weight
20–24.9	Normal (grade 0)
25–29.9	Overweight (grade i)
30–40	Obese (grade ii)
More than 40	Morbidly obese (grade iii)

BMI readings

Remember

Being either underweight or very overweight may have serious health implications.

Check it out

Are you within the healthy BMI range of 20–25?

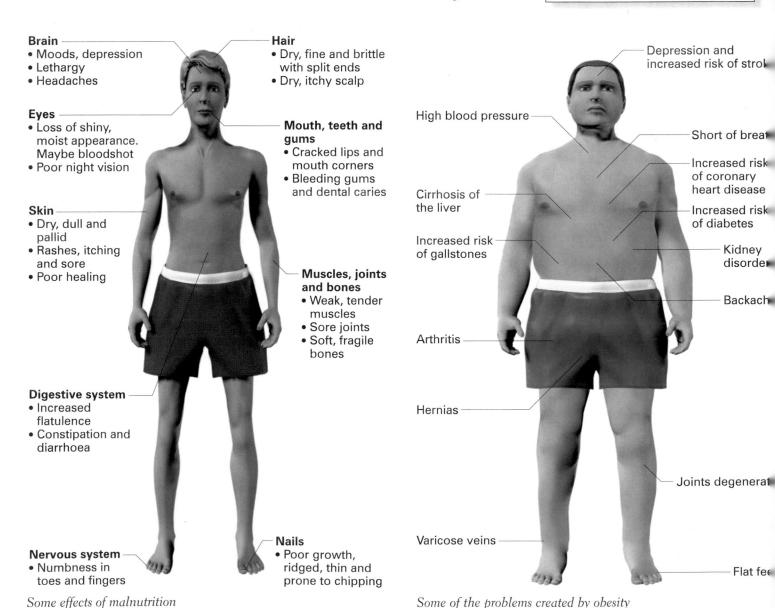

Some effects of malnutrition

Some of the problems created by obesity

Using body fat skin callipers

Some salons use fat callipers to measure body fat. This type of measurement is not as reliable as the body mass index, as it depends upon the client having enough soft fat to pick up. However, callipers still have a place in the consultation when used correctly.

Four sites of the body are measured, using the gauge:

- triceps
- subscapular
- biceps
- supra-iliac.

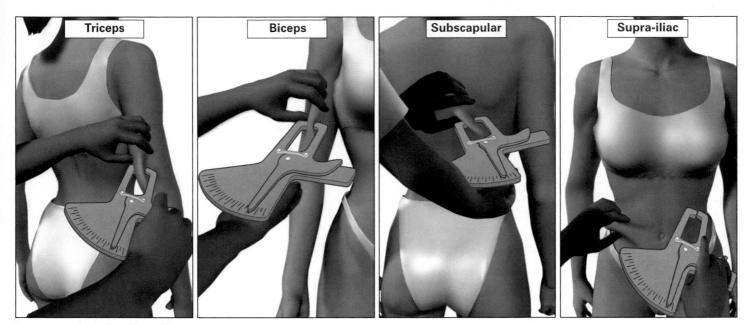

How to use body fat skin callipers

With the client facing away from you:

- Triceps – take the reading from about midway between the shoulder and the elbow joint at the back of the arm, gently pick up the body fat in the callipers, but try to leave out the muscle bulk.
- Sub-scapular – pick up the skin just below the inner angle of the scapula, just above the line of the bra strap.

With the client facing you:

- Supra-iliac – you are aiming to measure just above the line of the iliac crest of the pelvis, but inwards, slightly towards the navel. This is quite difficult to do, and if the client has little body fat, you may have to ask him or her to lean forwards while you pick up the body fat, and then the client can straighten up.
- Biceps – pick up midway between the shoulder and elbow joint on the front of the arm at a right angle to the muscle, rather than in the direction of the muscle. Try to measure with the elbow slightly bent to allow the muscle to soften, although be careful only to pick up body fat.

You should note the four readings, then add them together to get a total figure in millimetres. Using the body fat measurements table on the next page, check the percentage of body fat.

Women		Men	
Total figure (mm)	**Percentage of fat**	**Total figure (mm)**	**Percentage of fat**
8	13	15	5
12	14	20	9
14	15	25	11
18	16	30	13
20	17	35	15
24	18	40	17
26	19	45	18
30	20	50	20
32	21	55	21
34	22	60	22
38	23	65	23
40	24	70	24
42	25	75	25
44	26	80	26
48	27	90	27
50	28	100	28
52	29	110	29
56	30	120	30
58	31	130	31
62	32	140	32
64	33	150	33
68	34	160	34
70	35	175	35
76	37	190	36
80	38	205	37
82	39	220	38
86	40	235	39
88	41	255	40
90	42	275	41
		295	42

Body fat measurements

You can then calculate the acceptability of the body fat percentage using the table below.

	Female	Male
Obese	35%+	32%+
Overweight	29–35%	26–32%
Average	24–29%	21–26%
Lean	19–24%	16–21%
Very lean	Less than 19%	16%+

Body fat percentage

Finally, cross-check your readings against the BMI reading for accuracy.

Why measure the body?

Many body treatments give inch loss reduction, rather than weight loss, so it is a good idea to measure the client before and after treatment, to show a total inch loss reading. A client may simply want a firming treatment such as a course of faradic treatments to tone and firm the muscles, rather than a weight loss treatment. A body wrap is also an effective inch loss treatment.

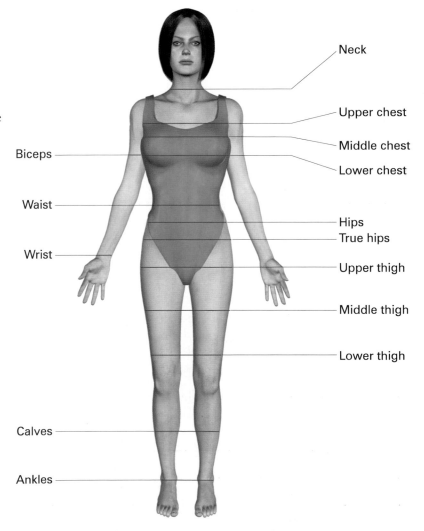

Neck
Upper chest
Middle chest
Lower chest
Biceps
Hips
True hips
Waist
Upper thigh
Wrist
Middle thigh
Lower thigh
Calves
Ankles

Measuring the body

Keys to good practice

When measuring the body, take the readings from approximately the same area, to provide an accurate before and after comparison. Most record cards for body treatments have a little figure drawn on the back, which will help guide you to the right spot. Draw on the diagram exactly where you measured, for example 6 centimetres up from the elbow joint, when doing the bicep measurement. That way, you will know where to return to for the next measurement. Also, it may not be you taking the measurements next time, so a guide will be useful for the next therapist.

Taking measurements at the beginning, middle and end of a course of treatment can be encouraging for the client and if the treatments are combined with a weight loss programme, a chart or graph can be drawn so the client has a record of how well he or she is doing.

Keys to good practice

Another way to work out frame size is to measure the upper chest and true hips, then add the two figures together:

- If this roughly equals height, the client has a medium frame.
- If 6 cm less than height, the client has a small frame.
- If 6 cm more than height, the client has a large frame.

Remember

Most people have a dominant side, usually the right but sometimes the left. This side can be larger by sometimes up to 2.5 centimetres. The foot, hand and breast size can reflect this.

Neck, biceps and calf measurements should be approximately the same to indicate a well-proportioned body shape.

Blood pressure and the pulse

Accurately taking the client's blood pressure is important as high or low blood pressure is a contra-indication to treatment.

It is advisable to take the blood pressure and pulse reading of every client coming to the salon, regardless of the body treatment plan. It will indicate whether the client is suitable for treatment, especially if going into the wet area, as a client with high blood pressure is likely to pass out in the heat.

What is blood pressure?

Blood pressure is the force or pressure which the blood exerts on the walls of the main arteries. Pressure is highest during systole, when the ventricles of the heart are contracting (systolic pressure) and lowest during diastole, when the ventricles are relaxing and refilling (diastolic pressure).

Blood pressure is measured in millimetres of mercury by using a sphygmomanometer at the brachial artery of the arm. This gives a true reading as the blood pressure in the arteries is higher than in the veins.

Blood pressure is affected by and varies with:

- age
- weight
- activity levels
- stress levels
- emotional stability or anxiety
- diet
- smoking
- alcohol intake
- genetic factors.

The condition of the heart and vessels also affects pressure.

High blood pressure

High blood pressure is called hypertension and is a common complaint. The most widespread form of hypertension is associated with arteriosclerosis, a hardening of the arteries, and often leads to strokes and heart attacks. Excess weight, smoking and stress all contribute to raised blood pressure.

Low blood pressure

People with low blood pressure usually have poor circulation, with cold hands and feet. Low blood pressure is less serious than high blood pressure, but in hot weather, during exercise or in the wet area, the client may feel dizzy and need to rest.

This is also important if the client is lying down for a period of time, as in a body massage or an electrical facial treatment. The client will need to be brought back up to a vertical position slowly, to prevent dizziness.

Remember
Both high and low blood pressure are contra-indications to some treatments, but with a medical clearance and adaptation of treatment, it is possible to treat the client.

How to take blood pressure

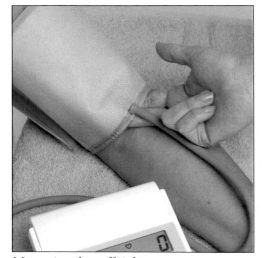

Measuring the cuff tightness

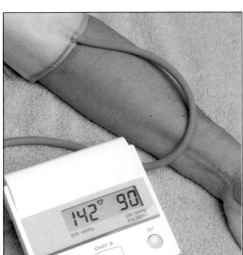

The cuff inflated

Taking the blood pressure

307

Before the reading it is advisable to ask the client to:

- visit the toilet to pass water, and then rest for 10 minutes
- refrain from eating or drinking
- refrain from exercise and try to relax.

Even in these ideal conditions, a person's blood pressure will vary depending on the time, day and season. In general, pressure readings are at their lowest when you are asleep and at their highest when you are at work.

Pressure	Reading
Systolic	High = 150+ Average = 95–150 Low = 95 or less
Diastolic	High = 95+ Average = 60–95 Low = 60 or less

Blood pressure guide

The pulse

The pulse rate is the same as the heart rate, being around 74 beats per minute. The pulse can be felt in arteries because of the expansion and recoil of their walls during each ventricular contraction. The pulse is strongest in the arteries closest to the heart. The pulse is usually taken on the radial artery in the wrist, but can also be taken at the carotid artery in the neck and the brachial artery in the arm.

Feel the pulse by using gentle pressure just to the right side of the wrist, in a direct line under the thumb. Using a watch with a second hand, count the pulse to a 30-second interval, and then multiply by two, to get a minute's reading.

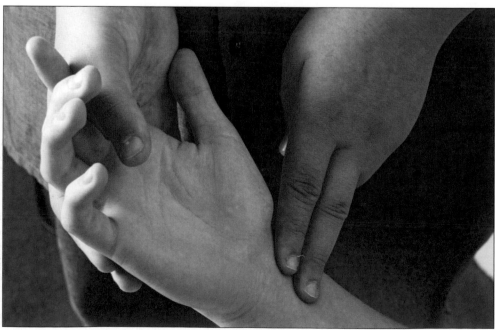

How to take a pulse

Check it out

What are your blood pressure reading and pulse rate? Are they in a healthy range for your age?

Muscular tone and strength testing

When a therapist talks of muscle tone she is discussing the muscle's ability to react and work quickly, how long it can work and how quickly it responds to stimuli from the nerves.

If the muscle:

- is firm to the touch
- is in a state of partial contraction
- contracts quickly
- looks firm and solid

then muscle tone is good.

If the muscle is:

- soft to the touch
- slow to contract
- flabby and loose

then muscle tone is poor.

Some clients come to the salon for muscle toning treatments without needing to lose weight – they want more tone to the muscle to give better shape and definition, especially on the abdomen and hips, legs and arms. One excellent treatment for this is a body faradic treatment (see Unit BT18, Improve body condition using electro-therapy, page 379). As this is a form of passive exercise, because the body is not actually moving, the muscles need to be assessed for suitability for treatment, and the client's flexibility checked.

Flexibility is the ability of the joints to perform a maximum range of movement and the ability of the muscles to support required movement – to be agile and without stiffness. This can be checked by observing the client as he or she walks and gets onto the couch, and by a series of simple exercises, which will help gauge the client's existing muscle tone. The exercises can be performed on the couch, but it is safer to do them on a mat on the floor, with plenty of room for manoeuvre.

Remember

If an elderly, rather stiff client comes into the salon, and has difficulty getting up onto the couch or getting undressed, then his or her flexibility and muscle tone would be so poor that it would be a contra-indication to treatment.

Area to check	Type of exercise
Back	Touching the toes with knees very soft How far the client gets will indicate flexibility Do not perform with the knees locked; movement must not be forced or jerked
Abdominal muscles	Ask the client to breathe in – if muscle tone is good, the abdomen should move upwards and inwards Perform a sit up with knees bent and hands by the forehead Do not perform with the knees locked or hands behind the head
Legs	Leg raises While lying on the back, ask the client to perform individual leg raises, slowly, and ask the client to hold the position in mid air. If the movement is smooth and fluid, muscle tone is good, as is hip mobility
Arms	A resistant movement Ask the client to try to place the right hand on to the right shoulder, while you try to prevent the movement by blocking it at the forearm. If resistance is good, the biceps, triceps and deltoid muscles are in good condition

Exercises to gauge flexibility

Skin conditions

The skin on the body behaves very much like the skin on the face but does not always have the protection of products and make-up, or the pampering that a facial provides.

Skin problems on the body include:

- psoriasis
- eczema
- dry, flaky skin
- oily skin
- congested skin

- scar tissue
- stretch marks
- in-growing hairs
- moles, cysts or pustules.

In most salons, body treatments and related skin problems tend to be seasonal. There is always an increase in demand for waxing, body exfoliation and toning treatments in the salon in the summer, for example. Dry skin tends to be a winter problem, both because the body is encased in winter clothing and because application of nourishing creams tends to be less thorough in the winter. The chest and back tend to be the trouble areas for an oily skin, particularly during the winter months, with congestion or acne occurring, just as it would on the face.

Treat the skin on the body as you would the face. An oily back benefits from exfoliation, steaming, comedone removal and suitable mask application, similar to the face. (See the treatment table on pages 318-322 for suitable treatments and their benefits to the skin.)

Carry out a skin analysis and use the record card to note recommended treatments, which can be combined with the other body treatments of massage, toning or firming treatments. (For information on link selling of products, see Unit G6, Promote additional products or services to clients, page 103.)

In the salon

Shelly had a regular client who enjoyed a full body massage and, as she was going on holiday, had recently been in the salon for some toning treatments.

On the client's return, she booked in for a back massage and toning treatments on the legs. Although the client was very tanned, she complained her skin was very dry and beginning to flake. Shelly began with her normal consultation and then prepared for the back massage, planning to use a rich oil to help with the dryness. She noticed a raised, angry looking patch underneath the bra strap on the client's back. The area was weeping. Shelly asked the client if she was aware of any irritation on her back, and the client said she was. Shelly explained that there was a patch of raised skin, and suggested she go to her doctor to have it checked. As the area was weeping, Shelly decided the treatment was contra-indicated, and went on to the leg treatments.

The client was diagnosed with a skin cancer, which was successfully treated.

- What would have happened if Shelly had ignored the problem?

Fat and fat stores

Many clients will come to you for body treatments because they want to lose weight and burn up their fat stores, tone the muscles and improve their body shape. Many clients will be concerned about cosmetic appearances, but there are also health benefits to being the correct weight for your height. For example, losing just 10 per cent of total body weight increases mobility, eases pressure on the joints and reduces the risk of serious health problems.

To understand how to treat clients with excess fat deposits, you need to know why we have fat stores, and the best ways to treat this problem.

There are three types of fat stores within the body:

- essential fat
- non-essential fat
- brown fat.

Essential fat

Essential fat is essential to the body because it helps to protect vital organs, the central nervous system, the heart, lungs, intestines and even cushions the eyeballs. Essential fat is stored within bone marrow, and released when necessary.

Women have an extra supply of essential fat (four times that of men), which is sex specific. In other words, it creates the female shape – curvy with rounded breasts, etc. The only ones to burn off this essential fat are women with eating disorders, or those in heavy training schedules, such as top athletes. They tend to develop a boyish figure, with little or no breast tissue, and slim hips and shoulders.

Non-essential fat

This type of fat can be rapidly metabolised to produce heat and energy, and is stored in the adipose tissue of most animal species. Men and women alike have this fat, which can be easily shed. Men tend to accumulate fat around the abdomen and women below the waist and on the breasts. Every woman has her own particular pattern of fat deposits, usually governed by heredity, eating patterns and exercise.

Although a lot can be done with a client's basic shape, there is no diet or exercise plan that will enable the client to lose fat from one part of the body rather than another. It will be metabolised from all over the body, but in the long term the client can even lose stubborn fat deposits on, for example, the hips and thighs.

There are a number of variations in the fat cells, both in number and size. Gross obesity occurs when both increase. There can be an excessive number of fat cells, excessively large fat cells, or a combination of the two. Obesity due to an excessive number of fat cells is more difficult to control than obesity due to excessively large fat cells.

Non-essential fat categories

Non-essential fat can be divided into:

- hard fat
- soft fat
- cellulite.

Remember

For clients to benefit fully from salon treatments, you will need to emphasise the importance of eating healthily and taking exercise. Otherwise, the treatments will be a waste of the client's money.

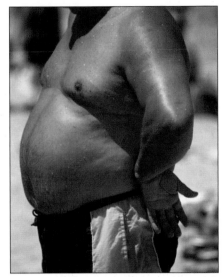

Men tend to accumulate non-essential fat around their stomachs – 'a beer belly'

Check it out

Under consumer protection law, it is illegal to make false claims regarding treatments and the results expected.

If you were to advertise that a course of faradic treatment guarantees a loss of a half a kilogram in weight, under which Act(s) would you be liable for prosecution? (To refresh your memory, turn to 'You, your client and the law' in **Professional basics**.)

Remember

Knowing which type of fat you are dealing with will help you to identify the correct treatment.

Hard fat

Hard fat is usually found in the upper thighs, inner knees, upper arms and deltoid area. Hard fat cells are compact, that is they are firm to the touch and dense. These cells may also be trapped within the muscle fibres and this makes picking up and wringing movements very difficult to do, without picking up most of the muscle bulk. Although overweight on the scales and BMI index, the client with hard fat will be of stocky appearance, without necessarily looking very overweight.

Treatments that involve manipulation of the fat, such as vacuum suction, will not be suitable as the fat cells are not malleable (pliable), and these treatments may be uncomfortable for the client.

Soft fat

This fat is soft to the touch and can be manipulated with massage movements such as wringing and picking up.

Soft fat responds well to salon treatments, and diet and exercise. The fat cells are in the adipose tissue, and not within the muscle fibres. The female client will have soft fat visible in the lower body, hips, buttocks and abdomen, while the male client will have a spread of soft fat around the trunk. Males with a high proportion of soft fat often develop an increased chest size and a bosom shape, as well as a large double chin.

Cellulite

Cellulite is easily identified as an 'orange peel' effect seen under the skin. It is caused by interstitial oedema, initially reversible, attributed to abnormal capillary permeability. Adipose tissue is a network of fibres of connective tissue, known as reticular fibres. They form a delicate supportive meshwork around blood vessels, muscle fibres, glands, nerves, and so on – everything in the dermal layer of the skin. Within the reticular fibres sit the fat cells.

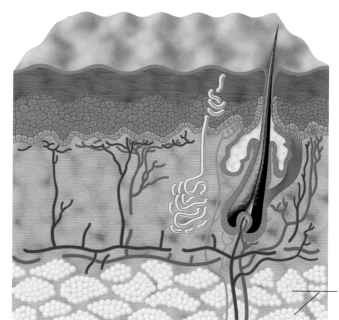

Cellulite

Where cellulite is positioned under the skin

If the fluid between the cells (interstitial fluid) is not drained properly, through the lymphatic system, fluid begins to accumulate between the cells, and over a period of time, will cloak the fat cells, and trap them, rather like a balloon caught in a net. This hinders the blood and lymphatic flow, which slows down causing associated flooding or a pooling effect of the fluid.

As the blood flow slows, the blood balance becomes altered, and plasma, serum and electrolytes, especially sodium, seep into the subcutaneous tissue, further preventing proper functioning. This can cause pain because of pressure on the nerve endings and can reduce the skin's elasticity.

The reticular structure becomes thick and hard, and the mass of fat cells becomes nodular. If this happens to many cells, side by side, then the effect can be seen as irregular patterns on the surface of the skin, as dimples or 'orange peel'.

Cellulite treatments involve stimulating the body's lymphatic system to help internal drainage and include manual lymphatic drainage massage, mechanical massage, vacuum suction, microcurrent and anti-cellulite galvanic application.

As part of the cellulite treatment, the client needs to:

- take part in aerobic exercise
- drink plenty of water
- avoid processed and salty foods
- reduce consumption of alcohol, caffeine and other stimulants
- apply a good quality moisturiser in the area, using brisk massage movements.

Brown fat

Brown fat occurs in the adipose tissue of many animal species and can be rapidly metabolised to produce heat energy.

Metabolism and fat stores

Metabolism is the collective term used for the chemical processes that take place in the body either to break down complex substances into simple ones (catabolism), or when a complex substance is built up from a simple one (anabolism). The thyroid gland in the neck produces hormones for controlling the body's metabolic rate.

The basal metabolic rate (BMR) is the minimum amount of energy used by the body to maintain the vital processes of respiration, circulation, digestion, and so on, even when the body is at rest. Lifestyle and occupation also affect how much energy the body requires, for example a client in a heavy labouring job will require more energy than an office worker.

Using the body's fat stores

Both calorie reduction – dieting – and aerobic exercise, such as walking, cycling or swimming, are required to burn up the body's fat stores. To understand this process, you will need to know how food, or fuel, is stored.

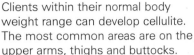

Remember

Clients within their normal body weight range can develop cellulite. The most common areas are on the upper arms, thighs and buttocks.

Remember

Metabolic malfunction will affect the client's ability to lose weight, but it is rare, and comes with other symptoms which will make the client seek medical advice, such as extreme tiredness, feeling the cold, feeling unwell, etc., and in extreme cases loss of sensation and fits. A simple blood test will determine hormone levels in the bloodstream.

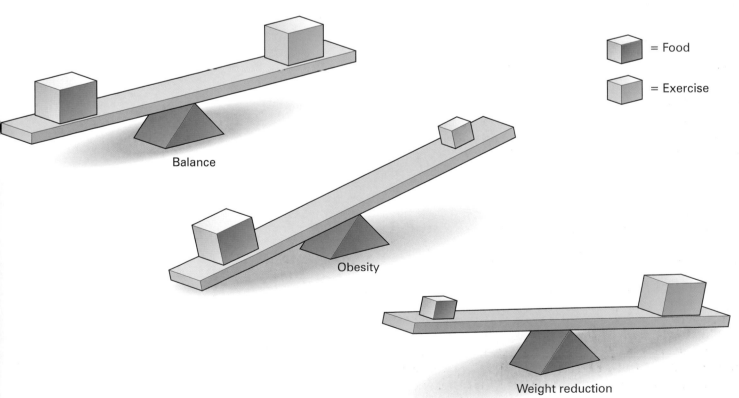

= Food

= Exercise

Balance

Obesity

Weight reduction

A healthy balance of diet and exercise will burn up the body's extra fat

Check it out

Research the various types of diet available to the client, e.g. Atkins, calorie counting, Weightwatchers. Find newspaper and magazine articles that give the pros and cons of each type of diet. Which one would you choose to try, and why would it suit you?

Remember

Burning off excess fat can be a long process, but it is worth persisting.

Weight problems and obesity

Obesity is now a serious problem in the western world. The latest research shows that obese children may be shortening their life expectancy by up to ten years because of the pressures put on the body's systems by being overweight. Obesity is the result of an over-dependence on high-fat and processed foods, which have become increasingly popular in western society, combined with a lack of exercise – without physical activity, the body is unable to burn off the extra calories.

Overweight people may suffer from some or all of the following conditions:

- high blood pressure
- diabetes
- heart conditions
- varicose veins
- hernias
- flat feet
- bronchial disorders
- arthritis
- postural complaints
- snoring and sleep disturbances
- emotional problems.

Besides the health risks, obesity is a burden to the client. It slows the person down physically and makes exercise difficult. The obese client often has very low self-esteem. The combination of these two factors can make the obese person prone to many illnesses and stress.

Causes of obesity
- Poor eating habits.
- Lack of physical activity.
- Psychological factors.
- Genetic factors.
- Internal disorders.
- Medication.
- Age and sex.
- Other factors.

Poor eating habits

The body needs the right balance of nutrients to keep it healthy and functioning properly. A diet of fast foods, take-away meals and processed foods, which generally have a very high salt and sugar content, will not provide those essential nutrients. Snacking between meals on high-carbohydrate foods such as crisps, chips and sweets also leads to poor eating habits.

Changes in physical activity

A sudden drop in physical activity without readjustment of eating habits can easily lead to a weight gain, for example when a person retires or gives up a sporting activity.

Psychological factors

In times of crisis, many people turn to food, hence the term comfort-eating. This often becomes a vicious circle – the more overweight the person becomes, the more he or she eats in an attempt to find consolation. People who give up smoking often find they turn to food as a substitute.

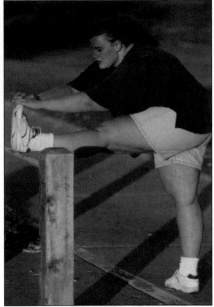

Starting an exercise programme is an important step towards weight loss

Genetic factors

Obesity may run in families, although studies have yet to prove whether this is due to genetics or simply to family customs (poor eating habits, type of foods bought, lack of exercise, and so on).

Internal disorders

Obesity caused by internal disorders is rare. However, there are some genuine cases, particularly those associated with the endocrine system. If you suspect your client has an internal disorder, then you must refer him or her to a doctor as further treatment could be harmful. In most cases, success is achieved with a combination of medical help and advice to the therapist, who may then devise treatments accordingly.

Medication

Certain drugs can cause weight gain, for example many women experience this when they start taking the contraceptive pill. Clients on medication should seek their doctor's advice before treatment is begun. Sometimes, the condition will be temporary.

Age and sex

This often has a bearing on weight gain, either due to hormonal influences, or changes in lifestyle which come with age. The older person is usually more susceptible to weight gain than the younger, more active person. Women are more affected than men, with pregnancy and menopause being two of the common times for weight gain.

Other factors

Research suggests that internal signals tell a person when he or she has eaten enough food. In an overweight person those signals do not work as well as they do in the slimmer person.

An obese person's fat cells have a greater capacity to store body fat and less is used in the body for energy or heat production.

Advice to overweight/obese clients

It is unlikely you will have a child in the salon for treatment, but check with your professional body regarding treating a minor, and always get a doctor's approval.

Adolescents should eat a diet rich in all the nutrients necessary for growth but low in carbohydrates. Encourage participation in exercise (the client might be embarrassed to take part at school in group activities). Advise out-of-school solo activities until the confidence builds up, e.g. exercise to videos in the privacy of the client's own home, jogging/running to burn up extra calories.

Remember

When treating a client who has just had a baby, always wait until she has had her post-pregnancy check-up at six weeks and ask for a doctor's written approval before starting treatment – especially if the client is breast-feeding.

After pregnancy, advice on diet, exercise and salon treatments will help the client to regain her figure. Skincare treatments and massage are also very therapeutic.

- Many women experience fluctuations in weight when they reach the menopause, due to the reduction of female hormones. Once periods have stopped, the body's weight pattern tends to become more stable. Advise a suitable diet, exercise and salon treatments, as necessary. Correct nutrition is vital at this time to compensate for fluctuating hormone levels, leaving the body open to diseases such as osteoporosis. The skin may experience changes, just as it did in adolescence, so treatments can also be included for replenishing the moisture content or redressing the oil balance, depending upon the problem.

Keys to good practice

Some women may experience bouts of depression during the menopause, and this may make them turn to food. It is important for you to be sympathetic, encouraging and understanding.

- As people grow older and retire, they tend to use less energy, but often do not adapt their eating pattern. The basal metabolism decreases, so in order for excess weight not to be gained, they must decrease their food intake. However, it is essential for the correct foods to be eaten, ensuring variety and all necessary nutrients. The appetite does diminish, and the client just needs to ensure that the quality of the food taken is high and full of nutrients.

Fluid retention

As previously mentioned, some clients suffer from fluid retention. This may be hormonal – the breasts feel full and heavy and the waistband may be tighter just before menstruation. After the period, the body returns to normal. If the client has a job which involves being on his or her feet for a long time, then fluid can accumulate around the ankles. Always seek a medical referral before treating a client with fluid retention, no matter how minor. (For more information on oedema, see page 312; for kidney and lymphatic drainage functions, see **Related anatomy and physiology**, page 171.)

Sluggish circulation

Some clients have with very cold hands and feet, even on a warm day, and often the skin is very pale. During the consultation, the client should be asked if the condition is painful, especially as the extremities warm up – this could indicate a condition called Raynaud's disease, and will need a doctor's referral before treatment.

Check it out

Find out more about Raynaud's disease.

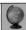

Keys to good practice

Not all cold hands and feet as a result of Raynaud's disease. It could be that the client simply has poor circulation. Once you have established that there is no medical basis for the condition, all stimulating and heating treatments are good for poor circulation, for example the wet area, massage, mechanical massage and paraffin wax application. The skin will suffer if the circulation is poor, so exfoliation treatments and massage are very good to bring blood to the area. The treatment objective is to create an erythema so that oxygen and nutrients are brought to the skin, and waste products are removed efficiently.

The underweight client

A severely underweight client may be suffering from an eating disorder, such as anorexia or bulimia, and should not be treated. Counselling and hospitalisation may be required and medical referral is essential – extreme underweight is a contra-indication to treatment.

However, a client who is perfectly healthy may still be fairly thin, with very little adipose tissue on the body. Careful choice of treatment plans and equipment is essential, as the client will bruise easily and the bony extremities may make some equipment painful. A client with very little underlying body fat may find the G5 mechanical massage too heavy, but will enjoy manual massage, or other skin pampering treatments. The client may have come to increase muscle bulk, and book a course of faradic sessions, which will tone and firm the muscles.

Treatment adaptation is essential on a slim client, and good communication throughout the treatment will ensure the client is comfortable and relaxed.

Equipment used in body treatments

On the following pages is a brief rundown of the equipment used in body treatments, their benefits to the client and the client type most suited to the equipment. (Some of the equipment has already been discussed in **Facial treatments – theory and consultation**, page 220.)

Equipment	Uses and client needs
Hydrotherapy	Any treatment involving water in any physical state, e.g. steam, liquid, water vapour or ice (see below)

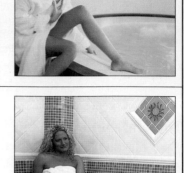

Suitable skin type/body type

Most skin types except where contra-indications present. Timing of treatment can be adjusted to suit skin type

Steaming (facial unit or the wet area cabinet or steam room)	Moist heat – a heating element boils the water, which creates a jet of steam from a nozzle or outlet. Can be used to warm the tissues of the face, upper chest or back when using a facial steaming unit. The whole body is immersed in a steam room. A steam cabinet treats the body only; the face is outside of the cabinet. • Helps open the pores and cleanse the skin. • Warms the muscle fibres and relaxes them, making other treatments after steaming very effective.

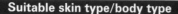

Suitable skin type/body type

Most skin types, except where contra-indications present. Timing of treatment can be adjusted to suit skin types.

Sauna	A pine log cabin, with coals heated over a powerful electric stove. The client adds water to the coals, which increases humidity, reducing the rate of evaporation of the sweat on the skin, felt as a dry heat, causing a rise in body temperature. A communal treatment. The whole body is involved, and it prepares the body for other treatments by softening tissues, relaxing the muscles, cleansing the skin and stimulating glandular activity. There are also individual vibration sauna units. The unit is self-contained, with a vibrating couch to massage the body as it is being heated. Fans and music make the treatment very comfortable for those who do not enjoy communal treatments.

Suitable skin type/body type

Most skin types, except where contra-indications present. Timing of treatment can be adjusted to suit skin types.

Spa	A communal treatment – also called a hot tub or jacuzzi. Water is heated and pumped around a self-contained fibreglass tub, which can hold four, six or eight people, depending on size. Holes in the base of the tub send water jets and/or air bubbles on to the client to massage the tissues, as the body is being heated. Skin is softened, muscles relax and a feeling of well-being is created.

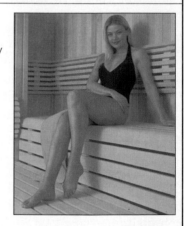

Suitable skin type/body type

Most skin types, except where contra-indications present. Timing of treatment can be adjusted to suit skin types.

(continued on next page)

Prewarming:

Exfoliating treatments:

Equipment	Uses and client needs

Powerjet shower   An impulse or power jet shower has a normal shower head for hot water, from above, and side bars for cold water. The unit is automatically set for alternative water jets onto the client. The cold spray may also have a pump action, which pulses the cold water in a set rhythm to massage the muscles. The treatment is extremely stimulating for the skin and muscles and prepares the body for other treatments.

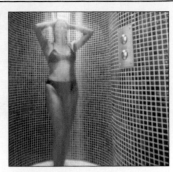

Suitable skin type/body type

Most skin types, except where contra-indications present. Timing of treatment can be adjusted to suit skin types.

Baths   These can be pulsed, foam, wax or muds, with either all the body immersed, or partial immersion to treat a specific area such as the feet or arms. Pulsed and foam baths are rather like a normal domestic bath in shape, with holes in, for the air to be pumped through, creating foam and a massage effect. Products are added, such as seaweed or aromatherapy oils, to enhance the treatment.

Wax or mud baths involve heating up the product, changing it from a solid into a liquid state, and then pasting it onto the body area to be treated. Wrapping the body in plastic or tin foil and cocooning it in blankets keeps in the warmth of the product. The body temperature is then raised, the skin softened and the client is in a relaxed state.

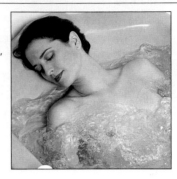

Suitable skin type/body type

Most skin types, except where contra-indications present. Timing of treatment can be adjusted to suit skin types.

Infrared lamp   See **Facial treatments – theory and consultation**, page 227.

Suitable skin type/body type

Most skin types, except where contra-indications present. Timing of treatment can be adjusted to suit skin types.

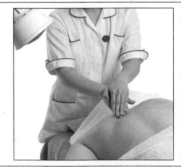

Brush cleansing   See **Facial treatments – theory and consultation**, page 227.

Suitable skin type/body type

Most skin types, except where contra-indications present. Product use will be determined by skin type or problem

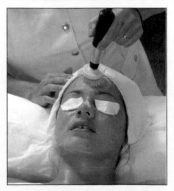

(continued on next page)

Exfoliating treatments:

Equipment	Uses and client needs
Body scrub with mitts	An exfoliant can be used prior to a fake tan application – the product can be applied using just the hands, with buffer mitts worn, to accelerate the product use.

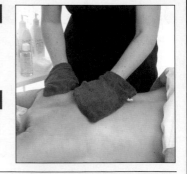

Suitable skin type/body type

Most skin types, except where contra-indications present. Timing of treatment can be adjusted to suit skin types.

Massaging treatments:

Manual massage	Used on the full body. See **Facial treatments – theory and consultation**, page 228.

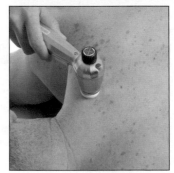

Suitable skin type/body type

Most skin types, except where contra-indications are present. Product use willl be determined by skin type or problem

Audio-sonic	Most popular on the upper back/shoulder region, legs, or around a joint. See **Facial treatments – theory and consultation**, page 228.

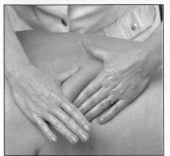

Suitable skin type/body type

Most skin types, except where contra-indications present. Not suitable on very thin, bony clients with very little muscle bulk – it may be uncomfortable

G5	An upright machine on a free-standing base, with a motor which makes a hand-held rubber head revolve. Various detachable heads available, depending upon the effect required – ranging from a soft head for effleurage to a multi-pronged head for stimulating movements. Gives a penetrating vibration massage, which is labour saving for the therapist, and can be used on either the full body or just the back. Creates a strong erythema and is useful for desquamation of the skin, stimulating for the muscle fibres and increased metabolic functions.

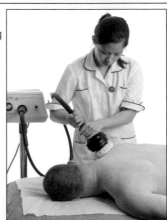

Suitable skin type/body type

Most skin types except where contra-indications present. Not suitable on very thin, bony clients with very little muscle bulk – it may be uncomfortable. Very suitable on large muscle bulk, and therefore large male clients

Percussion Vibrators	See **Facial treatments – theory and consultation**, page 228.

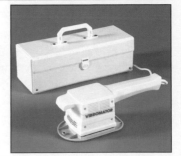

Suitable skin type/body type

Most skin types, except where contra-indications present

(continued on next page)

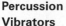

Massaging treatments:

Electrical treatments (for skin and contour improvement):

Equipment	Uses and client needs
Vacuum suction	This machine uses a pump to create a vacuum within an attached cup, which picks up the tissue. Can be used either: • to glide to the lymphatic nodes, in a single movement, or • to create a pulse within the vacuum, for extra stimulation. There is also a multi-cup static vacuum suction machine for use with up to six cups at a time, but the cups remain static on the body, rather than used with a gliding movement. This is suitable for treating larger areas in one treatment such as the buttocks and upper thighs. Both types promote the body's lymphatic and circulatory systems, thus helping the removal of toxins from the body. It is desquamating; it stimulates glandular activity and improves the general skin texture.

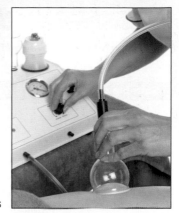

Suitable skin type/body type

Check for contra-indications, as treatment will not be suitable for all skin types, especially thin or fine skin with a tendency to bruise easily. Also, will not be comfortable on thin, bony clients or clients with older, crêpey skin

Indirect high frequency	See **Facial treatments – theory and consultation**, page 228. Can be used within a full body massage routine. Most frequently used on a dry face or back massage, but does create warmth in the lower legs and feet, so could be incorporated into a pedicure.

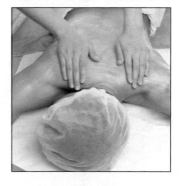

Suitable skin type/body type

Most commonly used on dry or fine skins, as the medium used is oil which will help the glide of the treatment and lubricate the skin

Direct high frequency	See **Facial treatments – theory and consultation**, page 229.

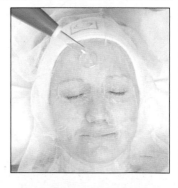

Suitable skin type/body type

Most commonly used on oily, congested or acne skin types, to the face, back or chest area

Galvanic	See **Facial treatments – theory and consultation**, page 229.

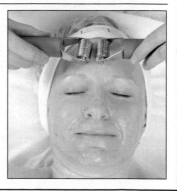

Suitable skin type/body type

Most skin types, except where contra-indications present. Desincrustation – for oily skins or skins in need of a deep cleanse; iontophoresis – for a dry skin or as an anti-cellulite treatment

(continued on next page)

Electrical treatments (for skin and contour improvement):

Equipment	Uses and client needs
Microcurrent	See **Facial treatments – theory and consultation,** page 229. Can be used on its own for lifting body contours.

Suitable skin type/body type

Most skin types, except where contra-indications present

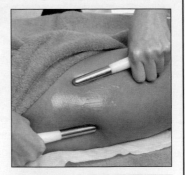

Faradic	See **Facial treatments – theory and consultation,** page 229. Ideal for the abdomen, thighs, buttocks, chest and arms.

Suitable skin type/body type

Most skin types, except where contra-indications present

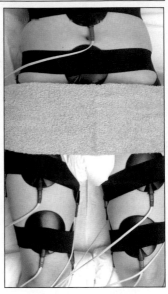

Provide head and body massage treatments

Unit BT17

Body massage is a satisfying treatment to give and receive. It is the stepping stone towards other qualifications within holistic treatments – aromatherapy, sports massage and remedial massage all require a recognised body massage certificate as a condition of entry. Successfully completing this unit could be the start of an exciting career path, using an ancient art form in manual massage techniques, leading into mechanical massage using equipment.

Swedish massage is the term most commonly associated with massage. It relates to the use of hands, rather than mechanical massage, and refers to the nationality of the man who developed the movements we still use today – Heinrich Ling. However, the Swedes were not the first people to recognise the benefits of massage. Long before, the Romans introduced massage to Europe. So massage has been with us for a long time – the term massage is thought to come from Greek meaning 'to knead'.

Within this unit you will cover the following outcomes:

BT17.1 **Consult with the client**
BT17.2 **Plan the treatment**
BT17.3 **Prepare for the treatment**
BT17.4 **Massage client head and body using suitable massage techniques**
BT17.5 **Perform mechanical massage treatments**
BT17.6 **Complete the treatment**

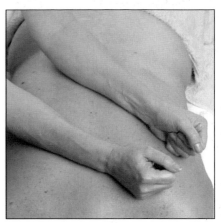

Manual massage is rewarding for both you and your client

Remember

Throughout your massage course, you must uphold the professional image that all therapists involved in massage treatments have worked hard to maintain. Massage is a personal treatment and, unfortunately, has suffered from a sleazy reputation. However, a fully trained masseuse/masseur will have worked hard to achieve a recognised qualification.

Keys to good practice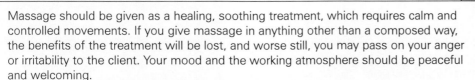

Massage should be given as a healing, soothing treatment, which requires calm and controlled movements. If you give massage in anything other than a composed way, the benefits of the treatment will be lost, and worse still, you may pass on your anger or irritability to the client. Your mood and the working atmosphere should be peaceful and welcoming.

Before beginning a body massage treatment, you will need to refer closely to the **Professional basics** section and **Body treatments – theory and consultation**.

Consult with the client

BT17.1

> ### In this outcome you will learn about
>
> - observation
> - manual examination
>
> - the record card.

As with all other treatments, it is essential to carry out a full consultation. Clients' body massage requirements will vary, as will the necessary depth of pressure due to tissue density and differing body weight distribution. An athletic female client with lean tissue and little adipose tissue will require something different from a male client with poor muscle tone and quite a proportion of fat.

To refresh your memory on all aspects of the consultation process, look back at the **Professional basics** section and **Body treatments – theory and consultation**.

Observation

Your observation of the client should be subtle and tactful. For example, if the client is obese, make sure you have plenty of large towels to keep the client warm and comfortable.

The size of the client also directly relates to the amount of massage medium used – the larger the client, the more medium will be required. Massage depth and pressure will also need to be adjusted to penetrate into the muscular layer.

Manual examination

The observation should include a manual examination to assess the skin for texture, pigmentation, moles and other irregularities. This requires a keen eye and sensitive fingers.

Any condition that could be made worse through massage is contra-indicated. For example, a skin infection could spread not only to other areas of the client's body but also to yourself as the therapist and then from you to other clients. If the client had a condition such as infected varicose veins, stimulation of the blood flow in the area could make the condition worse, or be uncomfortable.

Often, the treatment can be modified and adapted, for example a pregnant client may prefer lying on her side during back massage, and the abdomen would be avoided. An ordinary varicose vein could simply be avoided and a protruding mole could be massaged around.

The record card

A record card is the linchpin to the whole treatment, as it contains all the information you will need to plan for the client's treatment and protection (for more information on record cards, see **Professional basics**, page 37; and **Body treatments – theory and consultation**, page 287).

Contra-indications

Below is a checklist of all contra-indications to massage.

Contra-indications to massage

More visible contra-indications:

- Skin which is thin or papery, or damaged.
- Infectious skin diseases, e.g. scabies. There is a risk of cross-infection.
- Any fungal or viral disease, e.g. athlete's foot, warts, or verrucas.
- Non-infectious skin disorders, e.g. eczema, dermatitis.
- Bruises, sepsis, spots, boils. Avoid the area as there is a risk of cross-infection, the treatment might spread or worsen the condition, and the client will experience discomfort.
- Recent sunburn.
- Varicose veins, phlebitis (inflammation of a vein). Avoid the area as massage worsens the condition, and the client will experience discomfort.
- Tumours, unrecognisable lumps, bumps and swellings of either skin or the joints or painful areas.
- Any damaged muscles or tissue, e.g. sprains. Avoid the area as massage worsens the condition, and the client will experience discomfort.
- Any form of acute joint disease, e.g. rheumatoid arthritis.
- Broken bones and recent fractures. Treatment might cause client discomfort. If the area is in plaster, you will be unable to treat it.
- Postural deformities, e.g. scoliosis or spastic conditions.
- Avoid tapotement on extremely thin or elderly clients.

Less visible- contra-indications (obtain a doctor's approval before treating):

- Clients with chronic diabetes tend to have thin, papery skin that bruises easily.
- Clients with haemophilia may have no clotting capacity and could bleed.
- Clients with epilepsy.
- Clients with asthma or a lung condition. The treatment may require adaptation.
- Clients with a cardiac condition, high or low blood pressure, including clients who have had a stroke or suffer from thrombosis. People with low blood pressure can feel faint when suddenly sitting up from a lying position.
- High temperature.
- During menstruation, avoid the abdomen. Some clients may feel discomfort and the treatment could increase the flow.
- Immediately before or after operations, e.g. hysterectomy.
- In cases of stomach complaints, e.g. diarrhoea.
- In pregnancy, ensure the client never lies on the stomach. After birth, always wait until the post-natal check-up.
- Cuts/abrasions. Cover with waterproof dressing, and avoid area due to risk of cross-infection and client discomfort.
- Allergies. Select appropriate massage medium; carry out a patch test, if necessary.
- Medication. If a client is on medication for a health condition that could be affected by massage treatment, a doctor's approval will be needed.

Remember

An easy way to remember the contra-indications to massage is to visualise the body from the outside, going inwards. Start with the skin and problems you can actually see, then work through the underlying anatomy of muscles, bones, blood and the organs.

Remember

A contra-action is different from a contra-indication. A contra-indication prevents the massage from being carried out, or means that the area should be avoided during massage. A contra-action is a reaction that occurs during the treatment.

Special considerations for certain conditions

You will need to give special consideration to clients with the following conditions:

- diabetes
- epilepsy
- heart disease
- high or low blood pressure.
- pregnancy.

The elderly and clients who have recently had surgery will also require special attention.

Diabetes

Clients with diabetes have delicate skins, with a tendency to bruise easily. Their circulation may also may be impaired if it has been a long-term condition, with the consequence of poor healing if an infection has been present. Many people with diabetes have regular foot treatments from a qualified chiropodist, to avoid developing ingrown toenails or nail infection. Therefore, the lower legs and feet are delicate areas, and although foot massage helps improve the circulation, you should be on the lookout for infection in the area. Heavy massage movements can further damage the skin, so avoid these.

Check that the client has had enough to eat prior to the massage. Although a heavy meal would normally be a contra-indication, there is a risk that the blood sugar level will drop dangerously low if the client has not eaten recently. Then avoid the abdomen during the massage.

Epilepsy

Most epilepsy is controlled by regular medication, and although clients may not have had a seizure for many years, care must still be taken. Never leave the client unattended on the couch, and be careful that the client does not have a bright light shining into the eyes, as this is a known to be a trigger.

In some young people, the risk of a seizure is most likely as the person is waking up and brain activity is beginning. Since the client may fall asleep during a soothing massage, a doctor's approval for treatment is necessary.

High or low blood pressure, heart disease

Clients with high or low blood pressure and/or a heart condition should also be reviewed on an individual basis. The sufferer of low blood pressure may experience dizziness on getting up from a massage (as the blood flow is slower to the brain). The solution is to have the head raised slightly higher than normal, but be careful when turning the client over to massage the back, as it may be uncomfortable not to be lying flat out.

High blood pressure sufferers should also avoid being laid flat, and while massage has a calming, sedative effect, you are still stimulating the circulation, so again avoid any heavier movements. Keeping the head higher than the heart will ensure that palpations are avoided and prevent the client hearing the blood pressure in the ears, which can be disruptive to the massage.

Pregnancy

Pregnant clients gain real value from massage, providing the correct support is provided. Use a covered towel under the tummy, and ensure the client is not laid flat on her abdomen. When she is face up, use props to support the knees and head.

Some clients may not wish to reveal their body during pregnancy. If so, the neck and shoulder, face and scalp can be massaged with the client in a chair, but the real benefit is a massage to the lower back, where the muscles are put under strain to support the extra weight of the baby. Never massage a client who is pregnant directly over the abdomen. Be guided by your client – she knows what is best for her.

The elderly

The elderly also gain great benefit from massage. However, their skin may lack elasticity, have a tendency to bruise and be slightly drier in texture. Use plenty of oil, and avoid dragging the skin and heavy movements.

Recent surgery

Clients who have undergone surgery recently are unlikely to attend a massage appointment without a doctor's approval, but massage is recognised as very beneficial, as it improves the blood supply and so aids the healing process. Be careful to use light circular movements and avoid the area if the client prefers – you can show the client how to massage the area to promote the healing process.

Scar tissue and keloid tissue which has hardened can be visibly softened and minimised with massage.

The healing crisis

As well as talking through the contra-indications to treatment and the possible contra-actions, you should tell the client about other likely reactions to massage – often referred to as a 'healing crisis'. Massage has both a physiological and psychological effect on the client.

Physically, as the muscular tension is released, and the build-up of lactic acid in the muscle is dispersed, along with other toxins, the work of the lymphatic system is increased, filtering the lymphatic fluid through each of the nodes. This may result in a feeling of tiredness and aching in the groin, abdomen and underarms, where the nodes are situated. Instead of feeling uplifted, the client may experience flu-like symptoms. He or she might also suffer from a headache and slight nausea. Psychologically, the client may feel emotional, especially if he or she has been feeling very stressed.

All these symptoms are short lived. They show that the massage has worked and is stimulating the body to heal itself.

Plan the treatment/Prepare for the treatment

BT17.2/BT17.3

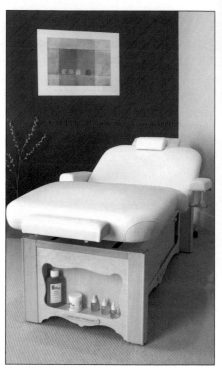

Prepare your treatment area before the client arrives

The working area

The working environment should meet all legal, hygienic and treatment requirements – these are covered in **Professional basics**, which also looks at your professional appearance and personal responsibilities.

The working area – the treatment room, couch and trolley – should be fully prepared shortly before the client arrives. This will allow you to give the client your total attention during the consultation.

Keys to good practice

Both a full body massage and a back massage require clients to remove clothing, which may make them feel vulnerable, so along with equipment preparation, make sure you have either screens, a curtained area or a separate cubicle which will allow the client to undress in privacy, and be certain of confidentiality.

Room temperature

Consider the atmosphere of the area – too stuffy and the client may develop a headache and feel claustrophobic; too hot and the client may become overheated and faint, or end up with clammy skin, which is not comfortable to massage.

If the temperature drops too low, the client will automatically tense up, the muscles will be stiff and not easily massaged, and the relaxing benefits of the massage will be lost. So an even temperature should be maintained, with a good flow of air circulating, but without the draught from an open window.

Lighting

The most effective type of lighting is wall lighting, as it gives a soft glow of light, will not shine directly into the client's eyes and creates a warm feel, while providing enough light for you to work by.

Music

Soothing background music will create a calm ambience, but choice of music is personal – find out the client's preferences. Some clients dislike having the radio on during a massage as the chatter of the presenter may be disruptive. Always be guided by the client's wishes.

The treatment room

This needs to be clean, tidy and hygienic – wipe all surfaces with a suitable disinfectant to ensure no cross-infection takes place. (See **Professional basics**, page 47, for sterilisation methods.)

The couch

Height, width and type

The height, width and type of couch are very important both to the client and you, the therapist. The client needs to feel secure and comfortable lying on a base that does not feel as though it will collapse at any second, and offers support and firmness. You will need to ensure that the height of the couch is not too low, ideally at hip/low waist height, to avoid stooping. Equally, the couch should not be so high that your movements are inhibited. Correct posture is vital for the working therapist – after all, you may carry out several massage treatments in the course of a day, and poor posture will lead to backache, neck strain and hip problems.

Working at the correct couch height will also ensure that the correct depth of pressure can be achieved to meet the client's requirements.

Preparing the couch

After wiping the vinyl cover of the unmade couch, fresh bed linen should be put on. This varies from salon to salon – the base of the couch is usually covered with a fitted sheet, but some salons use a quilt, with a cover, to create a feeling of getting into bed. However, it can be costly to keep washing the quilt covers and not always suitable in hot weather. Other salons favour open-weave blankets and towels, layering the towels over the blanket so that the blanket is protected and does not need to be changed after every client. Be guided by your training establishment.

Finally, place a layer of couch roll over the blanket and towels. The couch roll can be replaced after each treatment and will offer additional hygiene protection for clients. In some establishments, therapists put a split layer of couch roll along the length of the couch, ensuring all towels are protected. Others opt for just the head and foot areas to be covered. Care must be taken if the whole length of the bed is covered in couch roll as it is easily picked up within the massage movements, gets covered in oil and ends up sticking to the therapist's hands, again detracting from the massage movements.

The bedding set-up needs to be ready for the client to slip into and for you to cover the client. Most establishments or training centres have their own uniform format for bed layout, so check this with your lecturer or trainer.

Massage stools or chairs

There are many adapted massage stools and chairs available from suppliers, if the treatment is not a full body massage. They provide support for head and shoulder massage, Indian head massage and foot massage.

The floor area

Couch roll should be placed on the floor for the client to stand on once he or she has removed shoes and tights or socks. This prevents cross-contamination from the floor covering and can be disposed of after the treatment has finished.

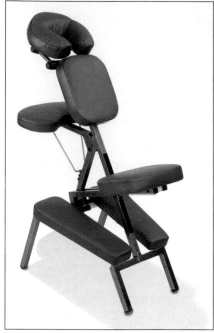

A massage stool

Keys to good practice

Before choosing equipment, try it out for your comfort and size, as well as the comfort of the client. Always buy from a reputable manufacturer and ask probing questions about the repair and maintenance service offered.

Trolley layout

At this stage, you may not know the client's skin type, personal preferences or body type, which will affect the choice of massage medium, so ensure you have talc, oil and cream available, although the client may provide his or her own massage medium, particularly if the client has any known allergies, or preferences.

Before setting out the trolley, wash the surfaces of each tier, and line each tier with a single sheet of couch roll if your training establishment recommends this.

Remember

All equipment must be to hand, so that you do not leave the client unattended, except to wash your hands, before and after treatment.

Remember

Some massage oils, almond for example, have a nut base and are not suitable for clients with nut allergies.

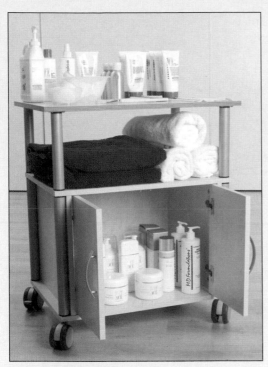

A suggested trolley layout

First tier:
- Talc, oil and cream, gel
- Medium-sized bowl to decant talc or cream into
- Large bowl for cotton wool squares
- Bowl or tub for tissues and spatulas
- Turban or headband (if not doing head massage)
- Client record card, if an existing client; blank one for a new client
- Pen
- Alcohol steriliser/hibitane and surgical spirit, or your preferred anti-bacterial wipe for the feet

- Eau de cologne, or similar, to remove any residue of oil after treatment
- Modesty towel. This is provided in health farms and spas, when the client has come from the sauna or steam room and has no clothing on. It is a long, small hand towel, covered in couch roll, which the client lies on, and then pulls up between the legs and over the pubic bone, allowing access to the upper thigh and buttocks, while maintaining client modesty. It can, however, be bulky to lie on. Most training colleges strongly recommend that female clients keep on their lower underwear or wear dry bikini bottoms and male clients wear boxer shorts or briefs. Be guided by your training establishment, but be prepared in industry for modesty towels or disposable pants to be provided.

Second tier:
- 2 small hand towels
- Support props (these may be required to support the knees during leg massage, or to go under the ankles, taking the strain off the abdominal muscles)
- Bowl for the client's jewellery
- Space for the client's belongings, e.g. handbag
- Dressing gown or towelling robe

Third tier:
Leave empty to store client's clothing, or store any spare products or equipment you may need

Massage mediums

Skin type

For a detailed description of skin types, see **You and the skin**.

If the skin is dry, oil is the best medium to choose, as it will help to nourish and moisturise the skin during treatment. A greasy/oily skin does not respond well to having more oil added to it, so cream or talc is more beneficial. When your massage techniques are perfected you may try a completely dry massage, with no lubrication on the skin, which is effective, especially if doing a pressure point massage; but clients would normally expect some products to be used.

Which one to choose?

Which medium you choose will depend on:

- the client's skin type
- the client's preference
- the client's allergies
- the client's contra-actions in previous treatments
- the area to be treated
- the desired effect
- other treatments combined with massage.

Prop
1. Fold small towel in half lengthways

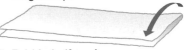

2. Fold in half again

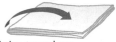

3. Roll the towel up

4. Place on a single sheet of tissue

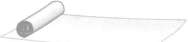

5. Roll the paper around the towel

6. Tuck in as you roll

7. Tuck ends of paper in

Modesty towel
1. Place towel over tissue

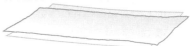

2. Fold towel into centre, followed by tissue

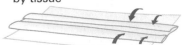

3. Fold it in half again

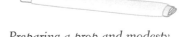

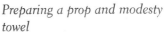

Preparing a prop and modesty towel

Some skin conditions may not be contra-indicated to treatment, but need additional attention when choosing the massage medium. For example, mild eczema sufferers may be suitable for massage, but you should use a light aqueous (water-based) cream which will help the condition. Some clients will bring their own cream for you to use.

Keys to good practice

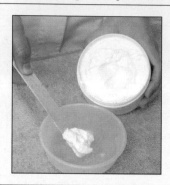

To avoid cross infection, always decant products from salon-size containers into bowls and use a spatula for application. Never pour unused product back into the container as it will contaminate the remaining product. With experience, you will be able to judge the amount required, and not waste any. If you find you have product left over, decant it into a small jar and give it to the client to use at home.

Decant products into a small bowl using a spatula

The client's preference

This needs to be discussed during the consultation, as some clients do not like the feel of oil on the skin, others prefer cream and some will bring their own products.

Keys to good practice

Be careful when using pre-blended aromatherapy oils should the client bring such a product. At this stage of your training, you are not trained or insured as an aromatherapist, and even diluted oils can be toxic, with potential to harm the client, especially if she is pregnant and does not yet know it.

Allergies and contra-actions

Allergies can occur at any time, from any source, and the client may develop a reaction to a product he or she has been using for years. The most common visible skin reaction is itching, red irritation in the area, developing into swelling or heat. Lanolin is found in some massage creams, and can cause problems, as can perfume additives and some colourings. A client with a known nut allergy should always inform the therapist during consultation, as the reaction caused may be life threatening (see **You and the skin**, page 199).

If the client develops an irritation caused by the medium during the massage, remove it immediately. Calm the area with a cool compress – a hand towel dampened in cool water should reduce the irritation immediately.

Area to be treated

Skin texture and conditions vary in different parts of the body. It is possible to use two mediums in the same massage. For example, the client may have an oily, slightly spotty back, requiring cream, but very dry legs, which require the richness of oil. This is perfectly acceptable and proves you are able to adapt to client requirements. (It also covers two ranges on the one assessment!)

Remember

If the client has a history of reactions or irritability to products, do a small patch test. Place a small amount of product to be used in the inner elbow 24 hours before the treatment and ask the client to monitor the skin reaction.

Desired effect

During the consultation discuss the outcome of the treatment and the client's expectations, as these will also influence the choice of medium. If the client wants a soothing, relaxing massage to aid stress, then pick oil as it is designed to be smooth and flowing over the skin's surface, helping you achieve the right effect. Should the client want a heavier massage for muscular problems, when more vigorous movements are employed, use talc or cream. Many sports therapists prefer to massage with talc.

The client's schedule after the treatment should also be considered. Will the client be able to shower to remove any excess oil? Does the client need to return to work and therefore to be oil-free, or has the client come in loose clothing with the intention of leaving the oil on the skin to maximise the benefits?

Types of massage medium

Massage creams

Massage creams contain a mixture of wax, oil and water, and the consistency is determined by the ratio of ingredients. A cream that is too sloppy will drip off the skin and be irritating to the client, so most professional creams are of a whipped cream consistency, that is they will not fall off the spatula as you decant the product.

The oil used is usually white soft paraffin, lanolin and mineral oil. The wax is white beeswax. These are mixed with water and an emulsifying agent is added to prevent the oil and water separating.

Oils and waxes condition and improve the skin's natural water barrier and some oils, like jojoba, can help prevent water loss.

Massage oils

Most types of oil make a suitable medium for massage. Vegetable oils such as olive oil, corn oil, sunflower or peanut oil can be used, although olive oil may be expensive in large quantities.

Mineral oil is a by-product of the oil-refining business and is inexpensive to purchase, so it is useful when you are first practising, although it is not used commercially.

Talc

Talc is a dry powder which provides slip and smoothness if applied to a dry skin. Talc consists of magnesium silicate ground into a very fine dust. Corn starch is another common ingredient and iron oxides are added – quantities vary between products.

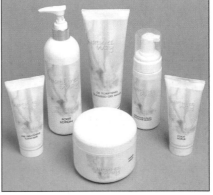
Massage creams

Remember

Vegetable oil goes off after a time, so do not buy in large quantities.

Keys to good practice

Should you open a new jar of cream and find the ingredients have separated, return it to the supplier, as the product may be old stock and will have deteriorated.

Talc	Ideal for combination or oily skins, skins with spots, and skins with a perspiration problem
Cream	Used for normal or dry skin. Suitable for clients who do not like the feel of oil on their skin
Oil	Can be used on most skins, ideally suited to a dry skin and lots must be used on a client with a hairy body

When to choose talc, cream or oil

COSHH considerations for each medium

- All ingredients are commonly used in cosmetic products.
- Non-hazardous.
- Non-inflammable.
- If ingested, drink milk or water.
- If in contact with eyes, wash well with water; if irritation occurs, seek medical advice.
- If spilled, use absorbent towels to clean the area, wash with detergent and water to avoid slippery floors.
- No special handling and storage precautions necessary.
- Avoid breathing talc deeply into the lungs; the fine particles if inhaled over a long period are known to cause lung damage.
- Store creams and oils in a cool, dark cupboard.

The benefits of massage

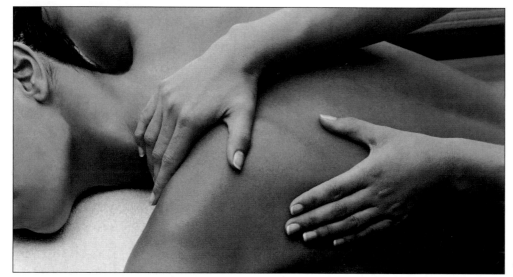

The benefits of massage

Massage has both physical and physiological benefits.

What benefits?	How the body benefits
Skin	• It gains moisture from the medium used, so becomes softer in texture
	• The sebaceous glands are stimulated by the pressure on the skin from the hands and so sebum is produced, helping keep skin lubricated
	• The pressure also helps the old dead cells come away easily (desquamation), allowing fresh cells to come to the surface. This gives the skin a clean, bright look
	• The blood supply to the skin is improved bringing food and oxygen to the cells, while taking away the waste products and carbon dioxide. This can be seen as a reddening in the area (erythema)
	• The stroking actions within the massage help soothe the sensory nerve endings
	• The motor nerve endings are stimulated and also receive a surge of blood to feed them, making them work effectively
	• Cellular functions are improved due to the stimulation
	• Small lesions or fibrous growths in the skin can be reduced
	• Dispersal of milia formation
	• Warming of the skin brings a small rise in body temperature, and the blood comes to the skin's surface (erythema)

(continued on next page)

What benefits?	How the body benefits
Muscles	• Blood flow is increased to the muscles bringing oxygen and nutrients, while removing carbon dioxide and waste products such as lactic acid • The heat generated within the muscle fibres and the stretching action of massage allows the fibres to soften and relax, so eliminating bands of tension • Muscle tone is improved due to relaxation of fibres • Muscular performance is improved so that the muscle can perform to maximum potential • Muscular pain and tension is relieved • Tension headaches can be relieved through massage to the muscles at the top of the neck
Body systems	• As massage is always performed in the direction of the lymphatic flow, the lymph system is stimulated and therefore removal of waste and toxins is improved • The central nervous system is either relaxed or stimulated, depending upon the type of massage movements used. Slow stroking movements will help relaxation and sleep, vigorous movements will stimulate – both help the nerve endings and improve their functioning • General circulation is improved. The pressure on the superficial arteries helps aid the transportation of food and oxygen to all parts of the body, and veins are stimulated to bring back the deoxygenated blood to the heart faster. This promotes healing and regeneration of cells all over the body • Biochemical healing takes place not only by alleviating anxiety but also stimulating the production of antibodies, especially immunoglobulin, so enhancing the immune system • The systolic and diastolic blood pressure and heart rate are slowed down during massage and a cumulative effect of regular massage is beneficial to clients with blood pressure problems

What happens within the body, and what you see during massage

What happens in the mind during massage?

- The stroking movements have a restful, relaxing effect.
- The client feels soothed and pampered.
- The rhythmic movements have a sedative effect on the brain and the client may feel drowsy or drift off to sleep.
- Accumulated emotional stress can be dispersed or put into perspective.
- Stress and fatigue are diminished, and a general feeling of well-being takes over.
- A healthier outlook can be adopted, both mentally and physically, as the client is encouraged to look after himself or herself better.
- The self-esteem of the client may be improved.
- Sleep patterns improve, bringing a sense of calm, as sleep allows the brain to rest and process the day's information.
- The stress hormone, cortisol, has been shown to drop after a massage.

Preparing the client for massage treatment

Explain to the client what the first part of the procedure involves – removal of clothing except pants/boxer shorts, etc., then putting on the robe provided, which will be found on the trolley. There may be a locker or hanger provided for clothing, and coats should be left at reception. If not, ask the client to place clothing on the third tier of the trolley along with handbag, briefcase, and so on. Assure the client of privacy while changing. You will be waiting outside the treatment room or cubicle and the client should call out when ready.

When you re-enter the cubicle, you may need to tidy away any remaining clothes or shoes. Ask the client to remove any jewellery, to prevent damage from the massage

> **Remember**
>
> Body massage not only benefits the client, it also has a relaxing effect on the therapist. Once the movements become automatic to you, the calming rhythm of your hands will bring down your blood pressure and you to will enjoy the stress-relieving benefits of the treatment.

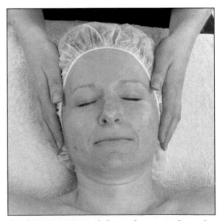

A client prepared for a face, neck and scalp massage

medium, and place it in the bowl provided. If long, the client's hair should be restrained in a turban or headband, again to prevent oil or cream spilling on it, but also to stop your hands becoming entangled in it!

Next, sit the client on the bed, with the robe closed, but not underneath the client. Hold a large towel in front of the client as he or she disrobes. Take the robe, fold it, put it away on the trolley, and then cover up the client.

Some establishments provide a modesty towel for the bust area, which the client holds in place with one hand while you help her with the robe. In this case, be guided by your training establishment.

At this point, you are ready to wipe the feet with a suitable cleanser, using one pad of cotton wool per foot, to avoid contamination, and then wash your hands.

If the client is booked in for facial massage, you will need to remove her make-up with suitable cleansers. If there is a cut or abrasion on the skin, it should be covered with a plaster, and the area avoided.

Some clients will have showered prior to coming to the salon, while other salons are able to offer the facility of a shower before the treatment.

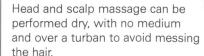

Remember

Head and scalp massage can be performed dry, with no medium and over a turban to avoid messing the hair.

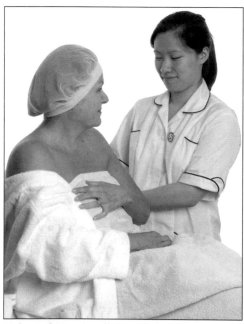

Taking the gown off the client

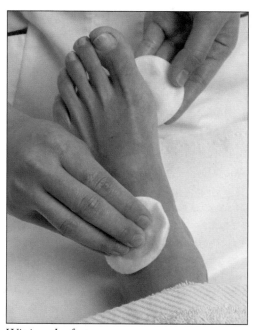

Wiping the feet

Massage client head and body using suitable massage techniques

BT17.4

In this outcome you will learn about

- the therapist's posture during treatment
- the client's position during treatment
- massage movements
- pre-warming treatment for massage
- suggested massage routine
- massage procedure.

Basic massage movements are easily recognised and should be linked together in a continuous flowing rhythm. The actual routine followed is an individual choice, providing it meets client needs and makes sense. As you become more experienced (and qualified) and watch other professionals at work, you may adapt your massage routine, including particular movements used, say, in aromatherapy, and missing out the odd movement that you do not feel totally comfortable with. Most therapists would agree that they have not stuck rigidly with the routine they learned in training, but to start with it is a good idea to use the routine you have been taught until you develop enough skill and experience to change.

Remember

Learning massage is like any other motor skill – you would not expect to play the piano in a day, nor drive a car. These are skills that require practice and supervision, so do not be despondent if you cannot do all the massage movements right away.

Keys to good practice

Your tools are your hands. Examine them, feel them, and rub your fingertips together. How do they feel? To give a good treatment your hands will need to be soft, supple and smooth. Long nails may scratch the client, so keep your nails short. A good rule to follow is: if you can see the free edge over the end of the fingertip, when your palm is facing you, your nails are too long. Start applying a hand cream at night to improve the texture, and a manicure will remove any jagged hangnails or rough cuticles which may catch on the client's skin. Later in this unit some hand exercises are given which will improve the flexibility of your hands and help with the massage movements – practise them regularly.

The therapist's posture during treatment

Your lecturer will demonstrate the correct posture to use during massage. This will save your back and shoulders from aching, particularly as you will be doing more than one full body massage in the course of a busy salon day. It will also help you develop the right pressure, using your whole body, rather than all the pressure coming from your shoulders and upper back.

Keys to good practice

Students often say that initial use of the correct stance during massage treatments does not feel natural, but you must persevere, as this will prevent muscular damage and strain.

There are only two ways of standing for massage:

- walk standing
- stride standing.

Walk standing

Walk standing is usually used when working down the length of a muscle, with the feet, hands, hips and shoulders, all facing in the same direction! The leg farthest away from the couch is placed in a walking position, slightly in front of the other one. Do not take a great big step, as if going hiking, just a gentle walking step in your natural pace is ideal.

This allows plenty of manoeuvring when massaging a long leg or back area. The body weight can be rocked from one foot to the other, without the need to shuffle or stretch. Do not be tempted to use the inner leg closest to the couch as you will then be working across your own body, which is awkward, and then if you have to come backwards, say from the top of the thigh, to the toes, there is a real risk of falling over!

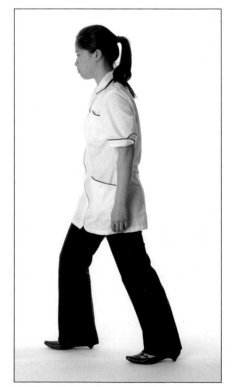

Walk standing

Stride standing

Stride standing is used when working across the muscle bulk. The feet are evenly spaced apart, side by side, again in your normal comfortable stride, and the fingers, hips, toes and shoulders all face the same way.

Good posture	Poor posture
Upright spine	Bending at the waist
Shoulders gently back	Hunching over at the shoulders
Hips above knees and feet	Twisting at the hip
Soft knees	Poking a hip out and balancing all body weight on it
Body weight evenly spread	Locked knees

Massage posture – dos and don'ts

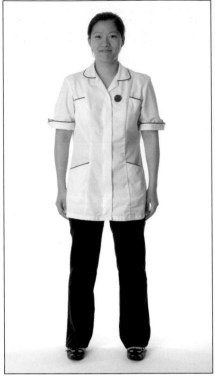

Stride standing

The client's position during treatment

There are two ways in which the client can lie on the couch:

- in the **supine** position – face upwards
- in the **prone** position – face downwards.

Massage movements

Massage movements are divided into five main categories:

- effleurage
- petrissage
- tapotement
- vibrations
- frictions.

The table below lists the main massage movements and identifies the categories within each movement. All movements can be altered or varied by using differing pressure, direction, rate and rhythm.

Remember

A quick way to remember supine is to think of the s(u)pine touching the couch.

Movement	Description	Categories within the movement	Reasons for use
Effleurage	• A stroking movement • The whole hand is in contact with the skin • Slight pressure in the palm with deeper effleurage	Superficial and deep	• Introduces medium to the skin • Soothing first touch of the skin • Links movements together
Petrissage	• Compression • Deeper and firm kneading of the tissues	Kneading – palmar, thumb, digital; ironing or reinforced stroking; wringing; skin rolling; picking up; pinchment; knuckling	• Aids lymphatic and blood circulation • Helps release muscle fibres, so eases tension knots • Increases venous return to the heart

(continued on next page)

Movement	Description	Categories within the movement	Reasons for use
Tapotement	• Often called percussion movements • Heavy, stimulating movements	Clapping; cupping; beating; pounding	• Stimulates blood flow • Stimulates sensory nerve endings • Improves skin texture through erythema
Vibrations	• Literally, vibration of the fingertips or thumb, or the whole palmar surface can be used	Static and running vibrations	Relieve tension along the nerve path either side of the spine When used along the path of the digestive tract, aid digestion
Frictions	• Regular, even pressure applied to areas of tension or fibrous build-up	Thumb or finger frictions	Aid relaxation Relieve tight nodules in muscle fibres Increase lymphatic return and circulation to the area, creating heat

The five main massage movements

Effleurage

There are two types of effleurage:

• superficial
• deep.

Superficial effleurage

This is a light flowing pressure used at the beginning and the end of most treatments. It introduces the therapist's hands on to the client and spreads the massage medium but is also a linking movement to help the massage flow. It heralds the start of the massage, so the rate and tempo of the massage are established from the beginning – if you start off in a rush, you will continue in that hurried fashion and possibly be under time for the treatment (therefore short changing the client out of the full hour's body massage).

If you are applying the massage medium to the skin, use superficial effleurage. You can tell the client what you are doing, and that you may have to remove your hands to apply more oil, especially if the skin is dry and soaks up the medium. Once you are satisfied that both you and the client have sufficient medium to keep you going throughout the entire routine for that area, then make a definite statement of touch that you have started.

Try not to use a light, feathery touch, and never remove the hands – the client will not know if you have started!

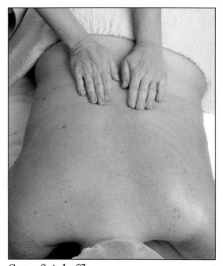

Superficial effleurage

So how do I do it?

Glide the hand onto the skin, starting with the fingertips, so that the whole hand is in contact with skin. Try to keep the fingers relaxed. Your hands should feel as if they are moulded to the part of the body you are working on.

Use the entire palmar surface of the hands, keeping the fingers together, and still soft, with the thumb either close into the side of the hand, or open and out of the way. Depending upon the area being massaged, all or part of the palmar surface should cover it. Pressure should be light and even, with good contact with the skin, and the hands warm and relaxed.

Superficial effleurage does not normally affect the circulation, as it is not a deep movement, and theoretically it can be used in any direction. However, massage should always be directed towards the heart (often referred to as centripetally) to aid the natural flow of blood back to the heart, from the limbs and trunk.

As effleurage can be used to link other movements, it will knit the routine together.

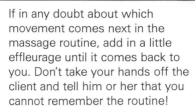

Remember

If in any doubt about which movement comes next in the massage routine, add in a little effleurage until it comes back to you. Don't take your hands off the client and tell him or her that you cannot remember the routine!

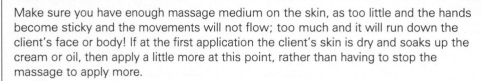

Keys to good practice

Make sure you have enough massage medium on the skin, as too little and the hands become sticky and the movements will not flow; too much and it will run down the client's face or body! If at the first application the client's skin is dry and soaks up the cream or oil, then apply a little more at this point, rather than having to stop the massage to apply more.

Benefits of superficial effleurage

- Relaxes tense muscle fibres.
- Gives a general feeling of relaxation.
- Stimulates sensory nerve endings and gives a feeling of pleasure.
- Introduces the massage medium and cream on to the skin.
- Soothes and calms.

Deep effleurage

This is the same type of movement as superficial effleurage but with more pressure applied – not too much to make the sensation uncomfortable, but enough to encourage muscular relaxation and for you to feel the tension knots.

Maintaining contact with the skin helps avoid over-stimulation of the nerve endings. Otherwise, when contact is broken and then re-established, this sets up a reflex response in the nerve endings which prevents the muscles from relaxing. It can produce a very disjointed feel to the massage.

Benefits of deep effleurage

- Aids venous return and increases lymphatic flow within the area.
- Creates an erythema as the blood flow comes to the skin's surface.
- Stimulates glandular activity, helping a dry skin receive more sebum from the sebaceous glands.
- Aids arterial circulation by removal of congestion from veins.
- Aids desquamation.
- Has a relaxing effect.
- Can begin to generate heat in the muscle fibre and help disperse tension.

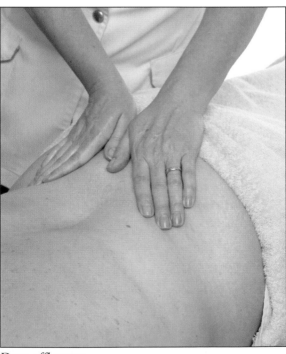

Deep effleurage

Petrissage

Petrissage is divided into the following categories:

- kneading
- ironing
- wringing – mostly used on body
- skin rolling – mostly used on body
- picking up
- pinchment
- knuckling.

Petrissage *always follows* effleurage.

> **Remember**
>
> A petrissage movement requires the client to have a good covering of muscle and underlying tissue to be effective. It can be quite painful on an underweight, bony or elderly client, so would be considered a contra-indication.
>
> Too much pressure may result in damage to the skin – so adapt to suit the client's needs.

So how do I do it?

Petrissage involves compression movements, performed using intermittent pressure with either one or both hands using different parts. It requires practice and good hand mobility, to mould around the muscle for good manipulation. Most petrissage movements work on all or parts of a muscle and it is important that as a muscle is slowly released from application, pressure is reduced.

Petrissage movements must be applied rhythmically and in a repetitive pattern, not in a hurried way.

Petrissage movements

Kneading

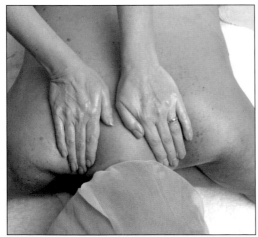

Palmar kneading of the trapezius

Kneading uses small circular movements, with the whole hand in contact with the skin, but the pressure is coming from the heel of the palm – the fleshy part at the base of the thumb. The general pattern and direction should follow the direction of effleurage, but instead of big sweeping movements, these are smaller circles, going outwards and upwards.

It can be used with both hands in larger areas, such as the back, or single-handed on smaller areas like petite arms and legs, with the other hand offering support to the limb.

If when working the area, you find a tension knot, intersperse palmar kneading with some thumb or finger kneading to disperse the tension. Again, use small circular rotations, remembering not to press too hard.

Ironing

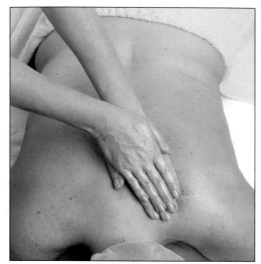

Reinforced ironing

Ironing, or reinforced stroking, is a deeper form of kneading. Place one hand on top of the other, and follow the direction of the kneading routine. It can be used along the length of the muscle, or across the muscle fibres, or in a figure of eight around the shoulder blades. This is a deep movement, so avoid using on a thin or bony client.

Wringing

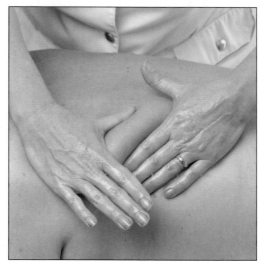

Wringing

Wringing is a very effective movement, but one which requires practice. The tissue is lifted away from the body and compressed between the hands – rather like wringing out a towel. The flow of tissue goes from the fingers of one hand to the thumb of the other, so that the movement forms an S-shape. This is continued along the perimeters of the back, and again, goes towards the heart. It is more difficult on the back, if there is little tissue to wring, so may be left out, but it is an excellent movement on limbs. Avoid pinching the tissue between the fingers and thumbs of the same hand, as this hurts!

Keys to good practice

Try practising wringing on a rolled-up towel and create an S-shape with your hands.

Skin rolling

Skin rolling, as the name suggests, involves rolling the tissue by pulling it away from the skeleton, towards your body, using all the fingers, in a flat formation and then rolling the tissue back down with the thumbs. It works best on fleshy parts of the body, such as the perimeters of the back and the neck.

Keep a steady pace, work in the direction of your effleurage movements, and repeat as necessary. It is much easier to perform this movement on the opposite side of the client to you, as you are rolling the skin towards your body. When doing the side closer to you, take a small step back from the client, bend at the knee, and perform the roll in reverse, that is the tissue is rolled down and then pushed up by the thumbs.

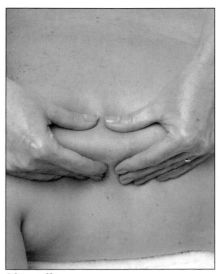

Skin rolling

Picking up

Picking up can be carried out with either or both hands, depending upon the area and the amount of tissue present. The tissue is grasped firmly between the index finger and thumb, with the hand forming a U shape. Using the whole hand, with fingers together, and flexion at the wrist, scoop up the tissue, squeeze and release. The index finger and thumb should be kept apart – if they come together, you will end up pinching the client's skin. Move along the length of the back and limbs towards the heart.

Double-handed picking up is performed on larger muscle bulk, such as the upper thigh, and single-handed picking up on less muscular areas, such as the arms.

Pinchment

Pinchment tends to be used in facial massage only, and involves the skin and tissue being gently pinched between the index finger and thumb. A small compression is used and then the hands glide along towards the next pinchment. It is most effective along the length of the eyebrows and jaw line to remove tension and works very well on small muscles.

Knuckling

Knuckling is a form of circular kneading, but instead of using the ends of the fingers or thumbs, make the hand into a loose fist and use the knuckles. The circular movements can come from the wrist, so the whole hand is rotating over the area of tension, but also, with practice, the fingers can be rotated individually. This helps to break down tension nodules. Knuckling can be used on the face, in a light form, and on the body with more pressure.

Benefits of petrissage
- Relaxes aching, hard muscles, helping to prevent tension modules forming.
- Stimulates skin regeneration.
- Tones muscle tissue.
- Helps eliminate muscular fatigue by aiding the removal of lactic acid.
- Helps remove waste products and improves lymphatic flow.
- Increases circulation to the area.
- Helps to relax the client.

Tapotement

Tapotement (drumming or tapping) comprises a stimulating set of movements which bring blood flow to the area very quickly. These include:

- hacking
- cupping
- pounding or beating.

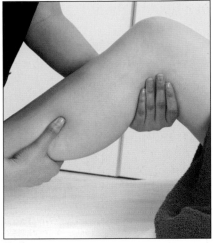
Picking up

Remember

Always use effleurage to link petrissage movements.

Remember

Some clients may believe that as you compress and knead the tissue, with quite firm pressure, this will 'burn off' their fatty deposits and make them slimmer. This is not the case – only diet and exercise can burn off fat. Never promote the idea that massage can help clients lose weight as it is unlawful to provide misleading information about goods and services (see the Trade Descriptions Act, **Professional basics**, page 77).

Keys to good practice

If the client wants a relaxing massage, you should use minimal tapotement, or leave it out altogether.

So how do I do it?

If done incorrectly, tapotement can leave the skin bruised and sore. The client also needs to have enough underlying tissue to absorb the movements – thin, bony clients would be contra-indicated.

Tapotement movements

Hacking

Hacking uses the outside edge of the middle, ring and little fingers of both hands. As the little finger makes contact with the skin, so the wrist is rotated and the outer ridge of the ring finger and then the middle finger make contact. The hand is loose and the palm slightly opens, so that the movement is firm, but does not produce a chopping movement – the key is keeping the wrists relaxed, which allows the hands to turn outwards as you complete the movement. Rigid, stiff hands will produce a chop using only the outer side of the little finger and hand, which will be painful for the client. The movement you are trying to achieve is a quick springy flick, not a dull heavy blow.

Hacking can be light or deep, depending upon where you are working and the amount of underlying tissue present. Light hacking uses only the ends of the fingers and has a tapping effect on the skin – deeper hacking, such as on the buttocks, can be performed using the whole hand and wrist, with a heavier force used. Light hacking on the face and neck are often referred to as point or digital hacking, as only the lightest of touches is suitable.

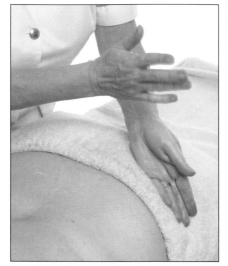
Hacking

Keys to good practice

Practise hacking on a hard surface such as a kitchen work surface or desk. Start slowly and keep the hands relaxed, rotate the wrists so that all fingers come in contact with the hard surface. Try to produce an even rhythm and do not go too quickly – speed will come later; you should be able to see your fingers touching the surface. If you hurt yourself, you are doing it too hard, or chopping when you should be rolling the wrist.

Cupping

Cupping uses the whole hand, held in a cup shape (hence the name!) with the thumb tucked over the forefinger joint. The fingers are closed and the wrists are soft and flexible. As the cup shape strikes the skin, a slight vacuum is created, and a hollow, cupping sound is heard. The hands cup alternately onto the area, and they should be light and springy. If the sound created is more like a slap, then the hand is not cupped enough, and the client will feel as though he or she has been slapped.

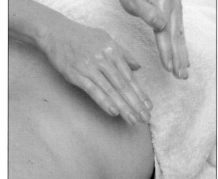
Cupping

Keys to good practice

Practise on a pillow or towel to get the cupping sound correct.

Pounding/beating

Pounding uses loosely clenched fists and performs the same rotation of the wrist that is used in hacking. The soft pounding as skin contact is made is followed by a flick of the wrist, so it almost becomes a flick of the skin.

Beating follows the same hand position, but the fists are dropped more heavily, and there is no flick of the wrist to remove the hand.

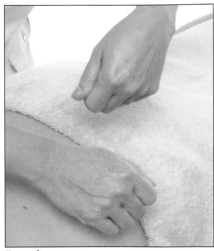

Pounding

Benefits of tapotement

- Increases localised blood supply, bringing erythema to the skin's surface and causing a rise in local body temperature.
- Increases nervous response due to stimulation. If hacking is completed across the muscle fibres, it can cause them to have a momentary mini-contraction, as if responding to stimuli. Nerve paths can be cleared and therefore muscle performance and tone are improved.
- Stimulates the blood supply and produces a tingling and revived sensation in the skin.
- Light hacking aids digestion if it is done over the abdominal area – it should follow the direction of the digestive tract where stimulation will occur. It stimulates the wave of the gut as food passes through (peristalsis).

Keys to good practice

With all tapotement movements look very closely at the tissue you are working on, and if an erythema occurs quickly, move on to the next movement, or interlink some effleurage to soothe the area – do not over-stimulate or keep working the same area, as you may cause bruising.

Vibrations

Vibrations are fine trembling movements performed on or along a nerve path by the fingers. They can be static or running, and you can use either the fingertips or the whole hand.

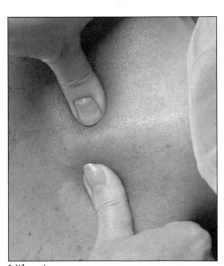

Vibrations

So how do I do it?

The muscles of the therapist's forearm are continually contracted and relaxed to produce a fine tremble or vibration, which runs to the fingertips. The tremor can run along the muscle length or side to side, depending on the size of the muscle bulk and the client's needs. The easiest way is to place one hand on top of the other, and tap the bottom hand with the top hand, using the fingertips, so that the vibration passes through to the other hand and then to the body below.

Benefits of vibrations

- Used at occipital region in facial massage.
- Can relieve pain and relax client due to its sedative effect.
- Soothes the nerve paths after stimulation.

Frictions

Frictions are often classified within the petrissage group, but their purpose differs. Friction movements will loosen adherent skin, loosen scars and aid in absorption of fluid around the joints.

So how do I do it?

These are stationary, concentrated pressure manipulations, exerting deep force on a small area at a time, with a gradual increase in pressure as you work along the muscle. This maximises the movements. Pressure is firm and the movement is usually applied in circular directions, with a regular pressure, On the face, fingertips or thumbs are mostly used. On large bulky muscle areas, one palm does the friction movement, reinforced by the other hand.

Keys to good practice
Try not to over-extend the fingers when performing frictions. As the pressure needs to be constant and firm, there is a danger of damaging your knuckle joints.

Benefits of frictions

- Frees adhesions in the muscle.
- Creates warmth in the area, as blood is brought to the skin's surface.
- Stretches and loosens scar tissue.
- Aids relaxation.
- Helps break down the tight nodules found in stiff muscles (particularly useful on the trapezius).
- Stimulates lymphatic and blood flow in the area.
- Spinal frictions produce a tingling sensation – stimulates all nerves attached to the spine.
- Releases fluid trapped around the joints – make sure medical approval is sought first, and the swelling, or oedema, has no medical systemic origin, e.g. a kidney problem. If it is a swelling caused by poor circulation or tiredness, then relief can be given with frictions.

Keys to good practice
Adjust the pressure and rhythm of the massage sequence to meet the client's individual needs. Not all massage movements will be appropriate for every client. Continue to monitor the effectiveness of the massage throughout the treatment – if the client falls asleep, you know it has been a success!

Pre-warming treatment for massage

Warming the muscles and tissue before starting the massage doubles the effectiveness of the massage movements and makes the tissue soft and more malleable to work with. If the client does not enjoy or does not have time for a spa or sauna, an infrared lamp is an invaluable form of pre-heating treatment. It is portable and gives out a warm deep heat. (See Unit BT30, Provide UV tanning treatments, for a full explanation of infrared and its place in the electro-magnetic spectrum.) Any area of the body (and face) can be treated, although usually it is the back. It may also be used before electro-therapy (electro-muscular stimulation, galvanic, vacuum, etc.).

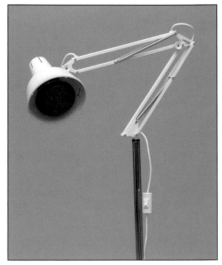
Frictions

Remember
Most awarding bodies do not dictate the order of these movements, so do not worry if you cannot remember the procedure without looking at your notes when you first start. As you become more practised and confident, so the routine will become second nature – your hands will automatically take over! Make each class of movements clear and recognisable – an assessment will depend upon your assessor being able to identify which movement is which.

Infrared lamp

Contra-indications

- Circulatory problems, e.g. fluid retention, swelling, varicose veins (if treating the legs).
- Skin disorders – dermatitis, eczema.
- Diabetes – because of less efficient circulation and lessened sensitivity to heat.
- Respiratory problems and illnesses – congestion of the lungs, e.g. bronchitis.
- Metal pins and plates.
- Conditions requiring medical attention/approval prior to treatment.
- Very low blood pressure.
- Heart/artery problems.
- Inflammation of any kind.
- Remove contact lenses – these act rather like a magnifying glass and intensify the heat.
- No oil or lubrication must be on the skin, as this intensifies the treatment.
- Loss of skin sensation, or lack of response to the skin sensitivity test, which should always be carried out before starting the treatment.
- Claustrophobia – especially when used on the face.
- Hypersensitive skin.
- Cuts, wounds or bruises in the area to be treated.
- The nervous or highly strung client.

When to use heat radiation treatment

Relief of pain

The mild heating will have a sedative effect and assist general aches and pains associated with muscular tension, poor posture, and so on.

Muscular relaxation

Muscles relax most readily when warm and aches and pains can be relieved and hopefully avoided. Heat treatment is particularly good after exercise. Any muscle spasms or tension or tightness can often be alleviated.

Fibrous accumulations usually respond well to gentle heating and rapidly disperse, particularly when massage is applied afterwards. These accumulations are commonly found in the trapezius muscle of the back.

Regular heat radiation treatment should maintain beneficial preventative effects.

Physical and physiological effects of heat radiation treatments

- Circulation is stimulated – an erythema is produced. The improvement in circulation means that there is an increase of oxygen and nutrients being brought to the tissues under treatment and increased removal of waste.
- There is a local rise in skin temperature which is warming and relaxing. There may be a general rise in temperature with a more prolonged or extensive treatment. This should not exceed 0.5–1°C.
- As muscles become warmed and circulation is aided, the muscle tissue relaxes, enabling fibres to relax and contract more easily. The efficiency of muscle action is improved. Any tension should be relieved and stiff and aching muscles should ease.
- Mild heating has a sedative and calming effect on the sensory nerve endings. Intense heating, however, has an irritating effect.

- The higher temperature increases the rate of metabolism. Repairs to damaged tissues are speeded up and there will also be an increase in waste removal such as lactic acid and carbon dioxide.
- Sweating is induced as the blood in the treatment area is warmed and circulates. Temperature regulation centres in the brain are eventually affected and gentle perspiration occurs which will have a cleansing action on the skin.
- The capacity of the skin to absorb oils and creams is greatly enhanced by the effects of warming, thereby increasing the effectiveness of subsequent treatments such as massage.

Keys to good practice

Therapists should only use infrared treatment for muscular aches or pains, unless given a doctor's consent. Heat does not help all pain, for example heating a sprained ankle will lead to vasodilation and causes bleeding. A cold compress, for instance, would be more suitable.

Use and storage of heating equipment

- Check plug and leads are intact.
- Check apparatus to ensure reflective surfaces are clean and free from dents, or 'hot spots' will result.
- Check the tightness of the angle-poise joints. They must hold the lamp in position and not allow it to fall on to the client. Tighten if necessary.
- Always ensure the client's and therapist's eyes are protected from the infrared rays. Wear goggles if necessary.
- If the lamp's outer casing becomes hot when in use, do not touch it. Use a towel if the lamp needs to be repositioned during treatment – this will reduce the risk of the therapist being burned.
- Do not move the lamp when it is turned on.
- Keep flammable material away from the lamp.
- Always ensure the client cannot touch the lamp or move closer to it during treatment.
- Never place the lamp directly over the client due to the risk of the lamp being accidentally knocked or the bulb shattering.
- Protect the working area – use a screen so others cannot accidentally walk into the lamp while it is on.
- Never leave the client or treatment area unattended.
- Never exceed treatment times – always gauge client responses carefully.
- When leaving the lamp to cool down, ensure it is left somewhere safe and protected with a sign to show that it is still warm. Similarly, if the lamp requires a warming-up period, ensure this is done in a safe and controlled manner. Never leave the lamp heating over a couch, for example, which might become hot and eventually burn.
- Store the lamp carefully – bulbs are delicate and easily damaged!

Remember

Elderly clients should have a skin sensitivity test because their skin sensation may have become impaired.

Step-by-step

Application of heat treatment

1 Check the lamp for safe, correct working order.

2 Ensure the couch is prepared in readiness for the client's arrival.

3 Carry out a consultation, checking carefully for contra-indications.

4 Instruct the client to remove as much clothing as is necessary, depending on the treatment area, and make him or her comfortable on the couch.

5 To ensure the client is suitable for treatment, carry out a skin sensitivity test at the treatment site. If the client is unable to tell the difference between hot and cold and hard and soft, then the treatment is contra-indicated.

6 The area to be treated must be completely clean and free from any products, e.g. liniments. To avoid any possible reactions, e.g. burning, wash the area with warm, soapy water.

7 Ensure the client removes any jewellery that could get hot and burn at the treatment site.

8 Position the client so that he or she cannot move closer to the lamp or touch it. Heat radiation is commonly applied to the back so a good position is to have the client lying on the side supported by pillows.

9 Only expose the area to be treated and ensure the client is warmly covered.

10 Position a white reflective towel across the back of the client's neck and drape it in such a way that the eyes are shielded.

11 Explain the effects of the lamp and treatment to the client.

12 Position the lamp so that the rays strike the area at 90°, thus allowing maximum absorption. The lamp should never, at any time, be directly placed over the client. The treatment area should then be made into a 'safety zone' by placing a screen or something similar around it.

13 The lamp's distance from the client is usually 45–90 cm and the heat is applied for 5–20 minutes. However, it is essential to follow the manufacturer's instructions as lamps can vary considerably in their intensity and output. Guessing distances is dangerous, so always use a tape measure. The client should experience only a mild, gentle heating effect with the resultant therapeutic erythema.

If the client's tolerance of the heat is poor, the therapist must apply the inverse square law (ISL) which governs intensity of heat in relation to distance (see next page).

14 During treatment, closely monitor the client's reaction by watching the area under treatment and also by obtaining feedback from the client.

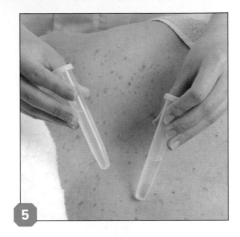

5

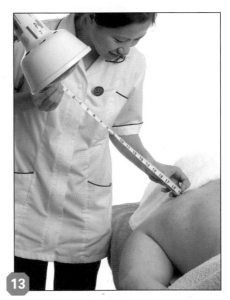

13

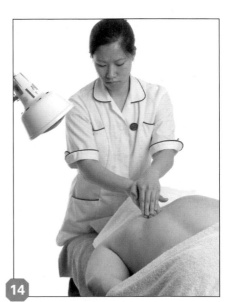

14

Step-by-step (cont.)

15 If the lamp needs to be repositioned during treatment, handle the lamp carefully – use a towel.

16 When the treatment is complete, switch off the lamp and unplug it. The outer casing is likely to be very hot, so place a towel over the head of the lamp and then move it into a safe, screened area to cool down.

17 Reposition the client as necessary in readiness to perform subsequent treatment(s). If the client is not having another treatment, then assist the client into a sitting position before getting down from the couch. This is to avoid the dizzy feeling associated with the fall in blood pressure levels often accompanying a treatment of this type.

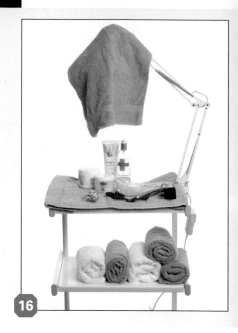

16

Inverse square law

The law states that the intensity from the source – the lamp – varies with the square of the distance from the point of source. In other words:

- If the distance increases, the intensity decreases by the square of the distance.
- If the distance decreases, the intensity increases by the square of the distance.
- If the distance is doubled, the intensity is quartered.
- If the distance is halved, the intensity will increase four times.

So if you double the distance, multiply the time by four. For example, if the original distance is 45 cm and treatment time is 5 minutes, after applying the inverse square law, if you double the distance to 90 cm you can multiply the treatment time by four to 20 minutes.

In this way the client will receive the same amount of radiation, but more slowly and gently.

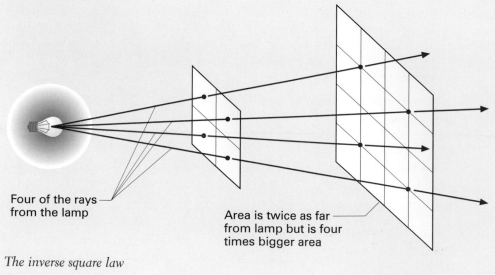

Four of the rays from the lamp

Area is twice as far from lamp but is four times bigger area

The inverse square law

Identify the hazard	What is the risk?
Infection spreading	Low
Burning of the skin of client and therapist	High
Postural problems for the therapist	Low
Eye damage	High
Bulb falling onto the client's body	High
Allergic/sensitive reaction to the heat	High
Migraine	High
Fire	Low

What should I do to prevent the hazard from becoming a risk?

Follow full consultation and contra-indication checklist
Carry out thermal sensitivity testing
Measure the distance of the lamp from the body
Provide goggles
Time the treatment
Never leave the client unattended
Monitor for any developing contra-actions
Keep flammable substances away from the direct heat
Remove jewellery which will get hot
Position the lamp parallel to the body, never directly over the client
Cover the client's neck with a towel
Move the head of the lamp with a towel over the hand
Check posture and couch height

Risk assessment for infrared treatment

Suggested massage routine

The massage procedure is as follows:

Client in a supine (face-up) position

1   front of right leg
2   right arm
3   left arm
4   front of left leg
5   abdomen
6   neck and chest.

Client in a prone (face-down) position:

1   back of right leg and buttock
2   back of left leg and buttock
3   back massage.

This standard procedure ensures minimum discomfort for the client, as he or she only has to turn over once. The procedure will vary, depending upon your training establishment's preferences.

Variations on the theme

- Some therapists complete a leg massage from the front and do not treat the back of the leg separately.
- Buttocks are an option for massage. Some training establishments only do the top of the buttock and include it within the back massage routine; others fully expose the buttock for massage. (The latter option does not cater for the client's privacy, but some health spas would expect full gluteal massage to be part of the routine.) Commonly, one half of the buttock is exposed at a time, both for client comfort and to stop the muscle from getting cold.
- If you are left-handed, you may wish to start on the left-hand side of the body – most students find they have a 'better' side, where they feel more comfortable, especially with posture corrections, and that is acceptable, too.
- Male massage will require adjustments within the routine – the upper thigh and abdomen areas are usually omitted, and more time given to the back and shoulder area, but most male clients would expect the back of legs to be part of the routine. If you progress to sports massage, the upper thigh would be included for pre-sport warm-up to maximise the muscle's performance.

To begin with, you will practise massage movements on fellow students. It is good to swap around the class, rotating whom you work upon, as a variety of body shapes and variation in tissue will provide invaluable experience.

When initially learning massage, it is best to begin on the back as it is a large area on which to practise, although you would not start the full treatment with the back massage. The client is prone so that eye contact is avoided, allowing you to concentrate on the massage.

Massage procedure

Arm massage

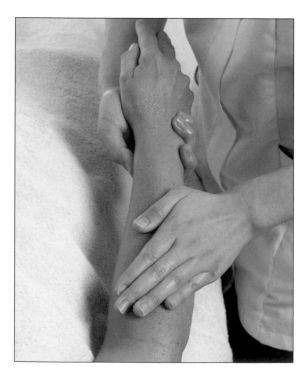

Check it out

Each lecturer or therapist develops his or her own particular massage movements, through years of experience. Why not volunteer to be a model for another class being taught body massage? The fundamentals will be the same, but some of the massage techniques may be different. You will learn something new, and the students will be pleased to have a model on whom to perform an assessment. It's extremely useful to play the role of client in a different class, where you are not known, so you realise how vulnerable or nervous a client can feel.

The client's arm positioned for massage

Step-by-step

Arm massage

Therapist in walk standing – outer leg in a comfortable forward position.

1 Effleurage to whole arm. Support at the wrist and supinate the arm for inner access so that the posterior and anterior aspects are covered. (×3)

2 Lock into the client's elbow with one hand for support and massage with the other.

3 Palmar kneading – single-handed to the deltoid, triceps and bicep muscles. (×3)

4 Picking up – single-handed to the deltoid, triceps and bicep muscles. (×3)

5 Thumb kneading to the deltoid muscle insertion on the humerus. (×1)

6 Light hacking to upper arm with one hand followed by effleurage. (×1)

7 Deep stroking to elbow joint. (×1)

8 Thumb kneading to elbow joint. (×1)

9 Deep stroking to the flexors and extensors of the forearm, supporting at the wrist, supinating for inner access. (×3)

10 Thumb kneading as above using one or both hands. (×3)

11 Thumb frictions to carpals. (×1)

12 Manipulations to carpals – flexion, extension and rotation at wrist. (×2)

13 Thumb kneading between metacarpals. (×2)

14 Thumb stroking to palms. (×3)

15 Effleurage to whole arm to finish arm massage. (×3)

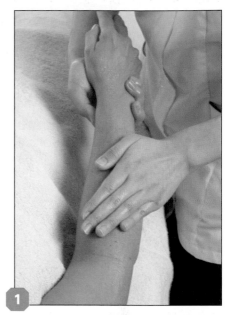

1

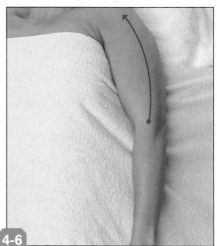

4-6

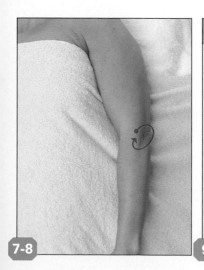

7-8

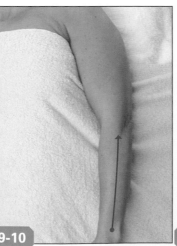

9-10

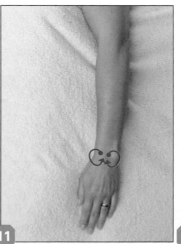

11

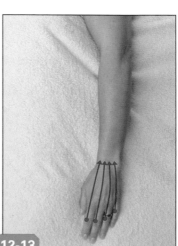

12-13

Step-by-step

Front of leg massage

Therapist in **walk standing** – outer leg in a comfortable forward position. Client fully covered, except the exposed leg. Prop at the ready. This massage covers the front and the back of the leg, all from the front.

1 Superficial effleurage to the whole leg from toes to thigh, with slight pressure in the groin to finish the movement. (×3)

Thigh only

2 Superficial effleurage to thigh only. (×3)

3 Palmar kneading – single-handed, to the outer, central and inner thigh (avoid going too high on the inner thigh). Support the limb with your free hand. (×3)

4 Picking up – to outer, central and inner thigh. (×3)

5 Wringing – to outer, central and inner thigh. (×3)

6 Alternate palmar kneading to outer and inner thigh. (×3)

7 Alternate palmar kneading to top and under the thigh (quadriceps and hamstring muscles). (×1)

8 Tapotement to all of thigh (depending upon client's needs). (×1)

Knee only (with support prop, if desired)

9 Effleurage around the knee joint. (×3)

10 Palmar kneading either side of the knee. (×3)

11 Thumb kneading around the knee joint – fingers supporting around the back of the knee. (×3)

12 Effleurage around the knee joint to finish. (×3)

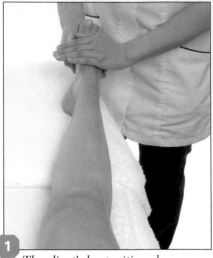

1

The client's leg positioned for massage

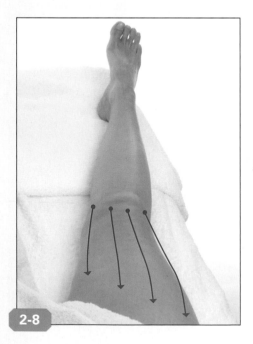

2-8

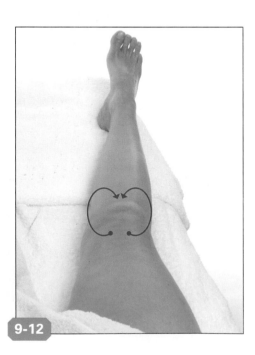

9-12

Lower limb – support under the knee and bend the leg so that the sole of the foot is flat to the bed, and hold up the leg in this position with one hand at the ankle.

13 Superficial effleurage to the calf (gastrocnemius). (×3)

14 Deep palmar kneading to calf. (×3)

15 Picking up of calf. (×3)

16 Thumb kneading along the length of the outer aspect from ankle bone upwards (tibialis anterior). (×1)

Place leg back down onto the couch (you may use your pedicure routine as massage to the foot, but be careful with timing)

17 Effleurage to whole foot. (×3)

18 Thumb kneading to foot – top and sole. (×3)

19 Palmar stroking to sole of foot. (×3)

20 Scissor movements using thumbs, across sole. (×3)

21 Snatching/grabbing of toes. (×1)

22 Superficial effleurage to whole leg, as in the beginning of the leg massage. (×3)

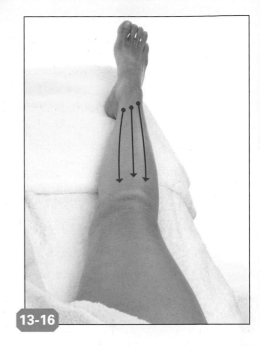

13-16

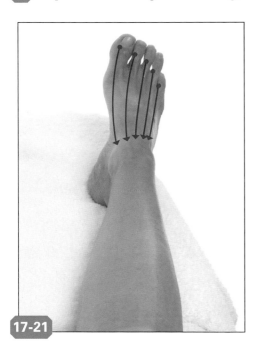

17-21

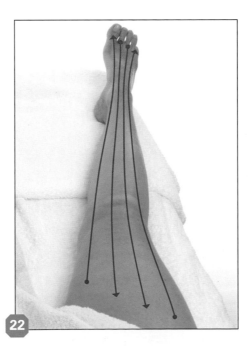

22

Step-by-step

Back of leg massage

Should the client prefer it, or your client is a male who is quite sporty and would like or needs a firm massage to the back of the leg, below is an alternative to the leg massage from the front. Adjust your time on the front of the leg massage, so that you have enough time to do the back of the leg and the top of the buttock. Keep only the limb you are working on uncovered, the one resting should be covered and warm. Do the same movements in the sequence above for the back, but avoid the back of the knee joint. The client will feel most comfortable with a prop under the ankle.

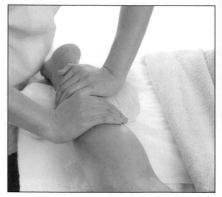

The client's leg positioned for massage

Walk standing The hamstring muscle (all x3)

1 Superficial and deep effleurage with light effleurage back down.

   Deep kneading following same pattern.

2 Alternate palmar kneading.

3 Ironing.

4 Thumb rotations.

Stride standing The gastrocnemius muscle (all x3)

5 Superficial and deep effleurage with light effleurage back down.

   Deep kneading.

6 Alternate palmar kneading.

   Thumb rotations.

7 Foot massage.

   Light stroking.

   Thumb kneading.

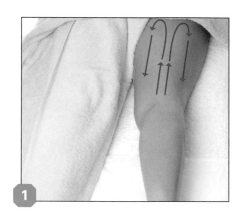

1

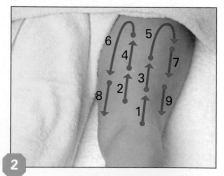

2

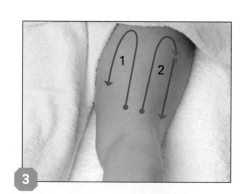

3

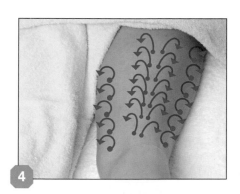

4

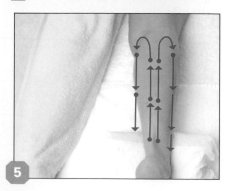

5

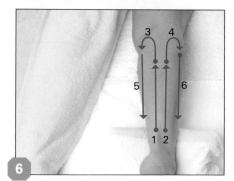

6

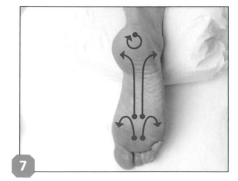

7

Step-by-step

Chest and neck massage

1 **Stride standing behind the head**
Superficial effleurage down the sides of the neck from chin, across chest, out to finish shoulders. (×3)

Deep effleurage down the sides of the neck from chin, across chest, out to finish shoulders. (×3)

Stroking down the sides of the neck from chin, across chest, out to finish shoulders. (×3)

2 Deep kneading fingers following the same direction as previous movements encircling the deltoid, depressing slightly and continuing over the trapezius towards the spine, and with hands together, lift the occipital slightly to street the atlas and axis of spine. (×3)

3 Ironing over chest, going from shoulder to shoulder, using circular motions. (×3)

4 Knuckling, in circles, from chin, down neck, out to shoulders and return. (×3)

5 Picking up trapezius from shoulders towards spine. (×3)

6 Return to effleurage as No.1 to finish. (×3)

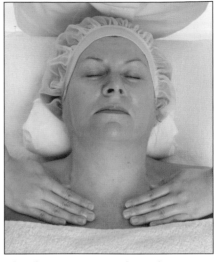

The client in position for a chest massage

1

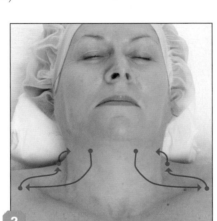

2

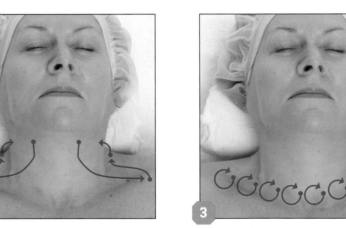

3

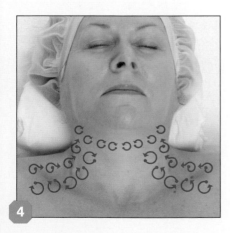

4

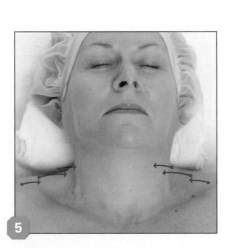

5

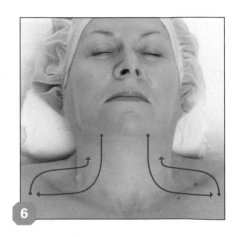

6

Step-by-step

Abdomen massage

The abdomen should only be included if the therapist is sure that it is appropriate. A specific contra-indication is early pregnancy.

Ask the client if she would like a prop placed under the knees to relax the abdominal muscles, and keep the pressure light at all times.

The client should have been given the opportunity to empty her bladder before starting the whole massage.

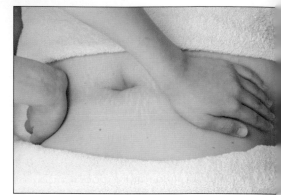

The client in position for an abdomen massage

Walk standing parallel to the client's hip

1. Superficial effleurage from the pubis, up to the bottom of the sternum, out to the sides and then up over the iliac crest to the starting position.

2. Deep stroking following the same direction, pulling in slightly at the waist.

3. Circular kneading or ironing following the direction of the colon.

4. Wringing around the sides and front of the abdomen.

5. Picking up the perimeters – where possible.

6. Vibrations and light hacking – following the digestive tract.

7. Stroking\effleurage as for No. 1 to finish.

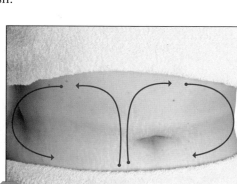

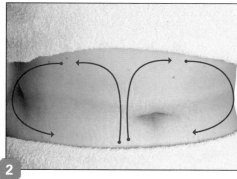

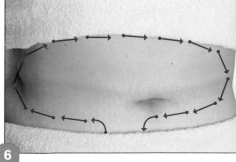

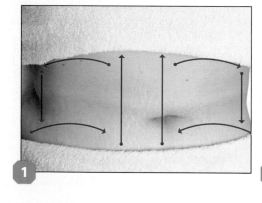

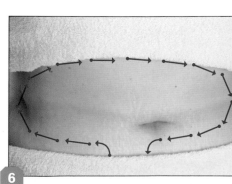

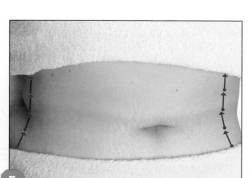

Step-by-step

Back massage   Walk standing

Superficial effleurage – to cover the whole back three linked sequences are required

1 Working from the sacrum to the trapezius, either side of the vertebral column, with light effleurage back down.

2 Work from sacrum to over the deltoid to cover the middle of the back.

3 Work from sacrum to under arms covering the perimeters of the back.

These three movements cover all of the back and the pattern is continued for the other back movements.

4 Palmar kneading following the same direction as photos 1–3.

5 Alternate palmar kneading following pattern of 1–3.

6 Circular kneading to scapula and thumb\digital kneading where necessary, following an upward flow towards the clavicle lymph nodes.

7&8 Reinforced ironing, starting at sacrum and covering all of the back. Use a figure-of-eight over the scapulae.

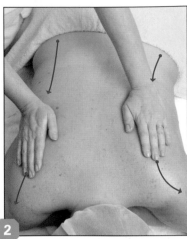

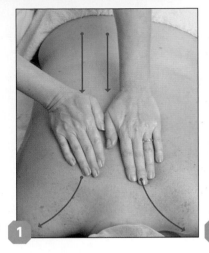

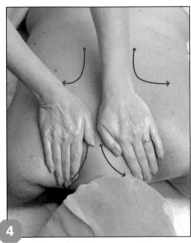

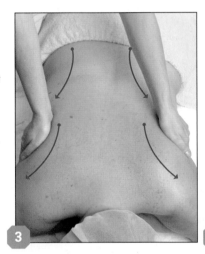

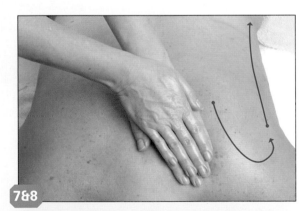

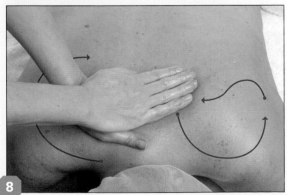

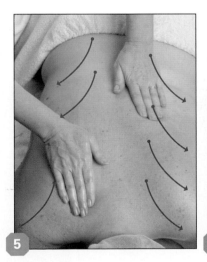

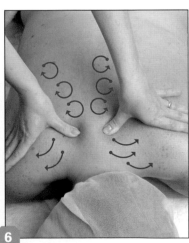

Step-by-step

9 Wringing following perimeters of body, where possible.

10 Picking up perimeters, where possible.

11 Skin rolling of perimeters, where possible.

Walk standing

12 Thumb kneading either side of spine from sacrum to occipital bone.

13 Spinal frictions following same pattern.

Stride standing

14 Scissor movement up and down the back with light effleurage strokes.

15 Superficial effleurage to the top of the gluteals group.

16 Deep effleurage to the top of the gluteals group.

17 Re-enforced ironing to the top of the gluteals group (figure of eight).

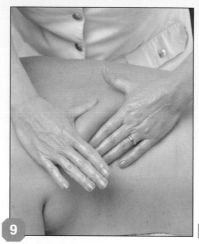
9

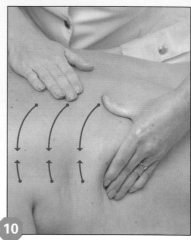
10

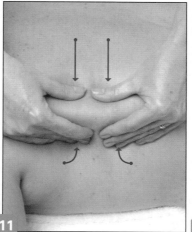
11

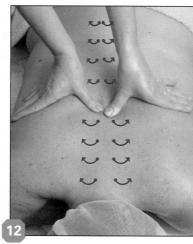
12

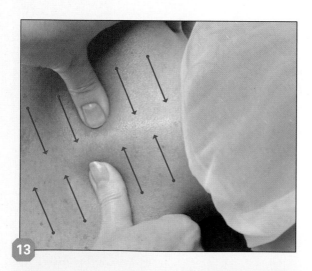
13

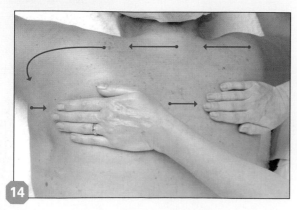
14

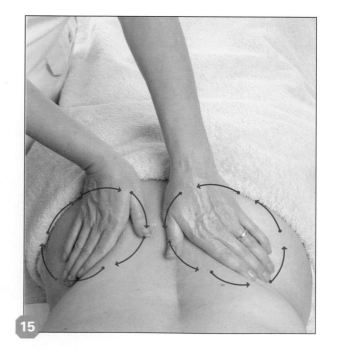
15

Step-by-step

18 Tapotment to the top of the gluteals group, depending on client size.

Hacking

19 Beating.

20 Pounding.

21 Cupping.

22 Hacking to the whole back, or just trapezius area, depending on client size and amount of tissue present.

23 Light effleurage all over the back.

24 Reverse light stroking from head to sacrum to finish the massage.

25 Stretch the tissue out using the forearms.

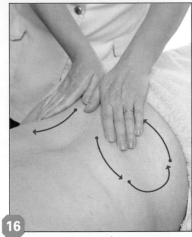

16

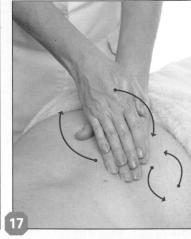

17

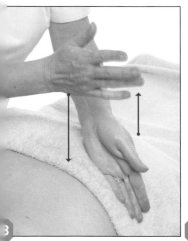

3

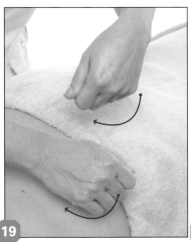

19

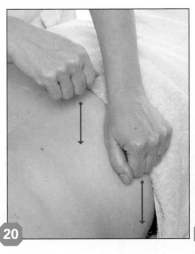

20

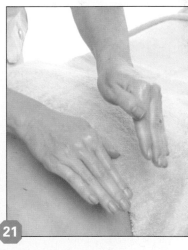

21

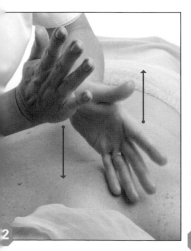

2

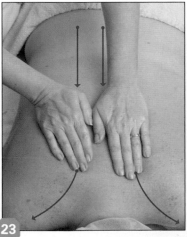

23

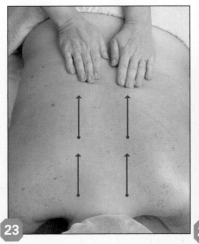

23

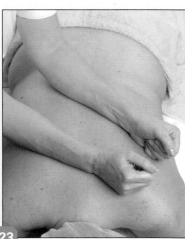

23

Remember

Although the routine is started on the front of the body, finishing on the back, it is easier to teach massage on the back, so you may start there, to get used to the different movements.

Head and scalp massage

You can simply adapt your facial massage routine and add scalp massage movements. There are no set rules for scalp massage, but this is neither an Indian head massage routine (which is quite stimulating) nor an aromatherapy massage.

Step-by-step

Face and neck massage

After a full consultation, prepare the client for a facial massage using your usual cleansing routine.

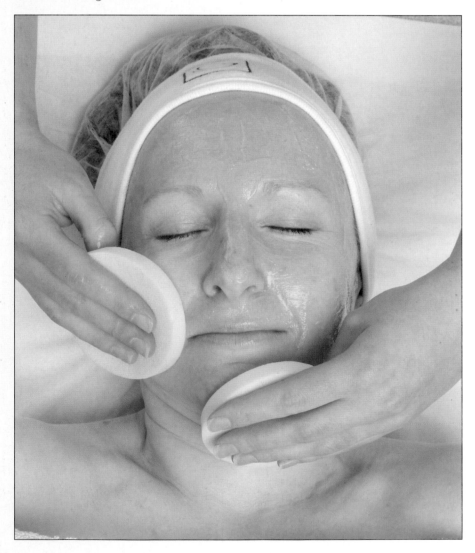

Step-by-step

1 Using both hands with a light pressure allow your breathing to marry up with your client's and pace your breathing to theirs, with your hands on the chest area.

Follow this action on the jaw line, cheek areas and forehead.

2 Do a sweeping effleurage movement to encompass the forehead, neck, deltoid and pectorals.

3 One hand on the forehead, the other cupping the chin.

4 Effleurage to the left eye area, and repeat on the other eye.

5 Rotation to the temples.

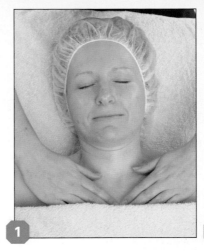
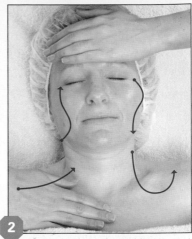

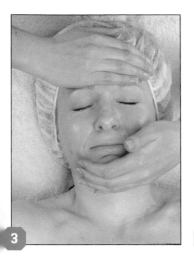
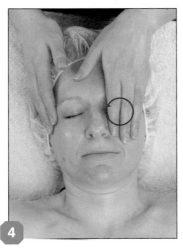
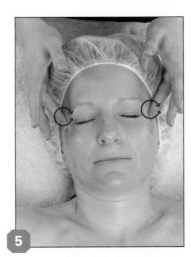
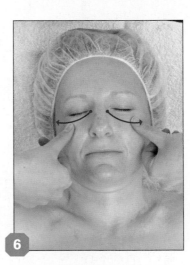

6 Using the thumbs carry out drainage to the eye socket and brow area.

7 Carry that through to the brows.

8 Alternate hand effleurage.

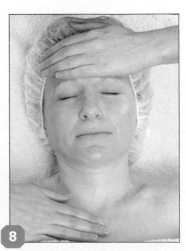
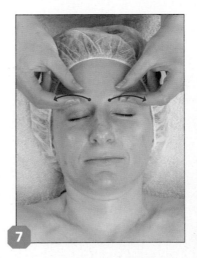

Step-by-step (cont.)

9 Effleurage to trapezium.

10 Effleurage pressure to cranium.

11 Thumb kneading around the hairline.

12 Pressures to temporals.

13 Thumb pressures to hair line to crown and return.

14 Digital pressures, some rotation.

15 Effleurage to finish.

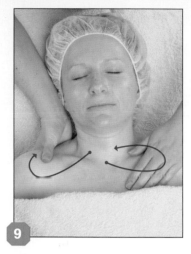
9

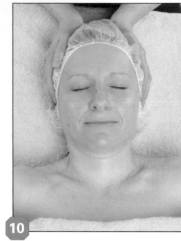
10

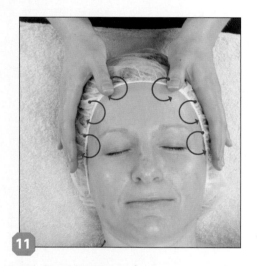
11

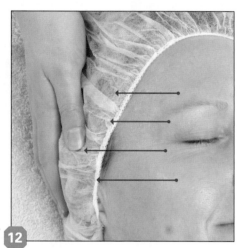
12

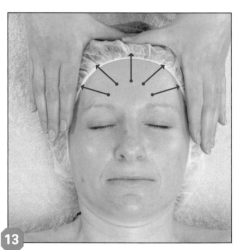
13

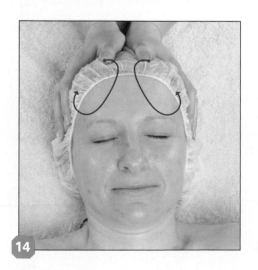
14

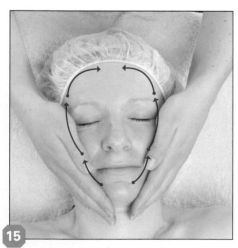
15

Contra-actions to body massage

A contra-action may occur randomly. For example, it might be caused by a product that the client has used for years with no ill effects, which suddenly causes a reaction. This is more likely if the client has changed regular medication or in a woman's case, is particularly hormonal, because of the contraceptive pill, or changes occurring in the menopause, or the early stages of pregnancy. The client should be advised that this may occur and what action she should take.

Erythema

This may occur after a treatment and is a by-product of vigorous tapotement. It should subside after treatment.

Skin reactions

A skin reaction is not common in massage, but sometimes the client may suddenly develop an allergy (for allergic reactions, see **You and the skin**, page 199). The reaction should stop naturally, but ask the client to monitor the area for 24 hours and refer to the doctor if the reaction does not subside.

> **Remember**
>
> A contra-action is a reaction which may occur during treatment.

> **Remember**
>
> Record details of the medium used on the client's record card and note if a reaction occurs.

Identify the hazard	What is the risk?
Infection spreading	Low
Bruising to the skin	High
Spillage of products	Low
Scratching of skin through jewellery or long nails	High
Dragging of the skin	High
Falling getting on and off the couch	High
Slipping in the wet area	High
Postural problems for the therapist	High
Allergic/sensitive reaction to the massage medium	High

What should I do to prevent the hazard from becoming a risk?

Follow full consultation and contra-indication checklist
Carry out a patch test 24 hours before treatment. Ask clients to provide their own hypoallergenic creams if this is a known problem.
Adjust massage movements to suit depth of tissue and client preference
Never carry out tapotement over bony areas
Cut nails so that with the palm facing you, no free edge is visible over the fingertips
Have sufficient product on the skin to keep it well lubricated
Monitor for any developing contra-actions
Provide suitable floor covering, e.g. woven matting or shower mats for wet area. Never allow the client into the wet area with bare feet
Decant products prior to use, and mop up any spillage immediately
Remove all jewellery
Provide a suitable step for the client to use when getting on the couch, not a chair
Check posture and couch height to ensure good posture when massaging

Risk assessment for body massage

Perform mechanical massage treatments

BT17.5

In this outcome you will learn about
• audio-sonic treatment.

Mechanical treatments tend to have a superficial effect on the skin, rather like ripples in the water spreading outwards when a stone is thrown into a pond. Audio-sonic does not behave in this way on the tissue – it penetrates downwards rather than outwards.

Audio-sonic is not strictly a mechanical treatment, but as it is motor-driven (by electricity), it is included within this unit. The G5 treatment is covered in Unit BT18, Improve body condition using electro-therapy.

Audio-sonic treatment

The audio-sonic machine creates sound waves of 100–10,000 Hertz (in the range of human hearing) which cause all body tissue under treatment to vibrate simultaneously, resulting in nerve stimulation. Working like a tuning fork, the sound waves are transferred deep into the tissues up to around 6 cm. When applied to painful areas, for example tension in the shoulders, audio-sonic treatment speeds up the healing process through increased blood supply.

Hand-held audio-sonic has different applicator heads, ranging from a flat disc to a round knob and hedgehog type, depending on the machine you are using.

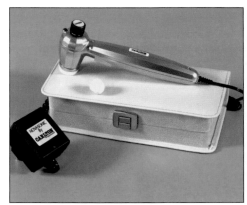

The audio-sonic machine

Contra-indications to audio-sonic

- Inflammation, sepsis, skin irritation.
- Recent scar tissue.
- Skin infections.
- Extreme vascular skin conditions, dilated capillaries.
- Sinus blockage – causes extreme discomfort.
- Very bony areas – due to deeper penetration of audio-sonic. On less bony areas, audio-sonic may be used over the therapist's hands or fingers – the hands absorb some of the sound waves and this makes the treatment less penetrating and more comfortable for the client.
- Crepey skin (percussion type only).

When to use audio-sonic treatment

- Any skin condition where stimulation is required but surface irritation needs to be avoided, e.g. sensitive skin, as little erythema is produced.
- To increase cellular function, improve sebaceous secretions in normal, dry or dehydrated skin.
- If manual manipulations cause discomfort, audio-sonic can be used, e.g. stiffness to aid relaxation of tense muscle fibres.
- Most used on the body, rather than the face, for dealing with 'trapped fat' and is used with vacuum suction for reducing 'hard fat' in spot reduction.

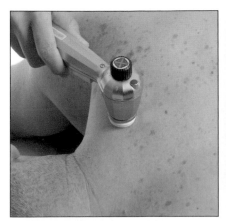

Audio-sonic treatment on the trapezium muscle

Care of the machine

- As the equipment is motor driven, avoid lengthy, continuous use – about 15 minutes to avoid overheating.
- Keep applicator heads clean and sterilised with a suitable antiseptic anti-bacterial solution.
- Remove all traces of medium used from rubber applicator heads to avoid perishing.

> **Keys to good practice**
>
> As an audio-sonic machine is small, it is most suited to treating specific areas of tension and is not cost-effective for a full body massage – it would take far too much time. It is a low-maintenance, portable piece of equipment particularly suitable for the mobile therapist.

> **Remember**
>
> Some areas of pain require a doctor's approval before being treated by a beauty therapist. If in doubt, ask the client to seek medical advice before treating.

Guidelines to method of treatment

1 Normal application time: 5–15 minutes.
2 Best to use with manual massage, as on its own the treatment may appear too mechanical for some clients.
3 Can be used with either talc, cream or oil as a medium to cut down on friction and increase smoothness of application. Oil will benefit dehydrated skin.
4 Adjust the speed in rhythm with the machine, if possible, or use the indirect method (over your hand/fingers) on bony areas.
5 Alternate straight and circular patterns for client interest.
6 Follow the natural contours of the muscle in a general upward direction.

> **Remember**
>
> There is no need for a risk assessment when using audio-sonic as the machine has little potential for harm.

Complete the treatment

BT17.6

> **In this outcome you will learn about**
>
> - aftercare
> - using your time cost-effectively.

Aftercare

Immediately after the treatment

- The client will be drowsy, or even asleep. Allow time to wake fully.
- Gently prop the client in a semi-reclining position on the couch.
- The client will not be sufficiently alert to take in details of aftercare – give the client a leaflet explaining long-term aftercare which he or she can read later.

Precautions after massage

- There is a risk that the client will become dizzy or light-headed if he or she gets off the couch too quickly. You may wish to help the client off the couch.
- Offer the client a glass of water to prevent dehydration.

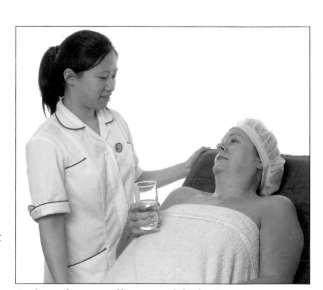

A glass of water will prevent dehydration

- Allow time for the client to get dressed in a warm cubicle – rushing the client will undo the relaxation created by the massage. It is also important that the muscles stay warm, so suggest to clients that they wear loose, warm clothing, e.g. a track suit.
- You may find that the client's reflexes are very slow after massage, almost as if he or she has been sedated, so check to make sure the client is capable of driving.
- While not always possible, the client should avoid being thrown back immediately into the stresses of working – that is why an evening appointment is so beneficial. The client has time to rest and sleep, so will be more able to cope with everyday pressures at work.

Aftercare advice

- Recommend the client drink eight glasses of water a day for healthy functioning of cells, to improve the skin and aid digestion.
- Eat a light diet for 24–48 hours after the treatment. Avoid over-refined and processed foods, curries or other spicy foods.
- Avoid stimulants such as alcohol, tea and coffee. Try a herbal tea, hot lemon juice or fruit juice.
- If the client smokes, recommend giving up.
- Take regular gentle exercise to help keep muscles flexible – encourage the client to join an exercise class, or take a gentle walk three times a week, or recommend a swim which keeps joints supple.
- Suggest the client sets aside time to relax.
- Try relaxation techniques and breathing exercises. The client may find that visualising a relaxing scene with eyes closed at times of stress will help keep the tension at bay, in between appointments with you.
- Any form of heat is very relaxing for tense, tired muscles, so a warm bath, a hot-water bottle on the shoulders or a heat lamp will soothe aches and pains.

Home care

As well as aftercare advice, you should recommend suitable products for the client to use at home.

Body scrub or exfoliation

This should be used weekly to prevent a build-up of dead skin cells so that the skin is kept smooth. Products contain finely ground olive stones, nuts, oatmeal or tiny synthetic micro-beads.

Body moisturiser lotion

Moisturisers are oil and water emulsions which help retain the moisture balance of the skin, keep the surface soft and smooth, prevent cracking and give some protection to the skin from the external environment. They should be applied morning and night for best results.

Loofah or body brushing

A variety of loofahs (body brushes) are available. They tend to be used in the shower when the skin is slightly damp, to remove dead skin cells and improve circulation and skin texture. Many cosmetic houses also produce abrasive gloves, which can be worn in the shower for really good exfoliation.

Reviewing the treatment

It is essential to review the massage treatment with the client to find out if the objectives of giving a relaxing massage and creating a sense of well-being were met. Is there any aspect of the massage that the client would like to change? Was he or she comfortable at all times? Did he or she like the massage medium and all of the movements? Write down this information on the record card so that you will be able to improve and enhance the service next time.

Using your time cost-effectively

As well as posture, hand movements and foot positions to consider, you also have to be cost-effective and time the massage treatment – both for assessment criteria and for commercial viability. You will need to ensure the massage does not feel rushed to the client, but that you are within your time limit and ready for the next appointment.

Massage area	Time allowed (minutes)
Arm	10 (5 per arm)
Leg	20 (10 per leg)
Neck and chest	5
Back*	20
Abdomen	5
Total time allowance	60

Suggested massage timings
*Buttocks optional – tops of gluteals are often included within the back massage time allowance.

If massaging the back of the legs and buttocks separately from the front of the legs, as in male massage, then split the leg time in half, that is 5 minutes only for the front, allowing 5 minutes for the back. As you will not be completing an abdominal massage, you can use those 5 minutes too.

There will be times when the client's needs will require you to adapt the routine. For example, if the client is menstruating, she may not wish her abdominal area to be touched. Adjust the timing to allow for this, and perhaps spend more time on an area with lots of tension such as the upper or lower back, or the neck and chest.

As well as a full hour's body massage, you will need to allow time for the consultation, the client undressing and getting on the couch, followed by waking the client, re-dressing, aftercare advice and review consultation.

If you have another client waiting, and you need to prepare the area, this could be a problem. Health spas and saunas have rest lounges, with easy chairs and recliners where the client can relax, have a drink and perhaps continue dozing, which leaves your working cubicle free to prepare. The client does not then feel rushed.

> **Remember**
>
> Standard salon practice is one hour for the massage routine.

Improve body condition using electro-therapy

Unit BT18

Unlike facial electrical treatments, body treatments do not offer instant results although the skin will be improved almost immediately. Body treatments often require a course of six, eight or ten sessions alongside a commitment from clients to adjust their lifestyle, diet and exercise routines, which may contribute to their particular problem areas. Choosing a suitable treatment plan for the client, and using the equipment in a safe and appropriate way, is the focus of this unit.

Body treatments aim to:

- improve the skin and body condition
- improve muscle condition and the contours of the body
- improve lymphatic drainage of the body
- aid in relaxation, both physically and mentally.

Using equipment safely and with confidence is essential, and it is very important that you follow the manufacturer's instructions for the machine you are using, since these will vary. Products used, treatment times and the dials showing strength of current will differ from one make of machine to another. The only way to be totally safe and competent for your assessments is to understand each machine thoroughly and know its capabilities. This will provide you with the confidence to treat clients in a professional manner, which in turn will instil the client with confidence in your abilities.

Within this unit you will cover the following outcomes:

BT18.1 Prepare for the body treatment
BT18.2 Consult and plan the treatment with the client
BT18.3 Perform electro-therapy treatments
BT18.4 Complete the treatment

You will learn how to achieve all of these outcomes using:

- a high frequency unit
- a galvanic unit
- a faradic unit
- a microcurrent unit
- gyratory massager
- vacuum suction.

Before beginning a body treatment, you will need to refer closely to the **Professional basics** section, **You and the skin**, **Body treatments – theory and consultation** and Unit BT19, Improve face and skin condition using electro-therapy.

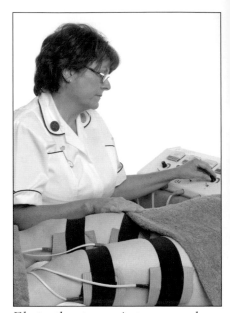

Electro-therapy can improve muscle condition

Remember

Always maintain client modesty when giving body treatments. Make sure you have plenty of big towels available, and only expose the part of the body to be worked upon. Keep the rest of the body warm, and then when you have finished on one particular area, keep that warm too. This will reinforce the relaxation of the muscle fibres and heat generated in the tissue.

Keys to good practice

When learning to use a piece of equipment, it is important that you, too, have experienced the treatment. You are then able to describe the sensation of the current to the client and you can fully understand the importance of client modesty.

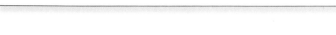

In this unit you will learn about

- preparing the skin for treatment
- high frequency
- vacuum suction
- galvanism

- faradism
- microcurrent
- gyratory vibration.

Preparing the skin for treatment

Let's assume that the body consultation has gone smoothly, the client has no contra-indications, the chosen treatment can go ahead and the client is in a suitable position for treatment, and you are ready to use your chosen electrical equipment. The skin has been cleansed and is grease free. It is still essential to further prepare the skin to be receptive to the electrical treatment you are about to perform.

Ideally, before the treatment, the client should have taken a relaxing sauna, steam bath or jacuzzi treatment, finishing with a shower. This both prepares the skin and warms the tissues, making the body very receptive to the current and the treatment easier to perform.

The skin can be prepared for treatment by:

- cleansing
- exfoliation
- pre-heat treatments.

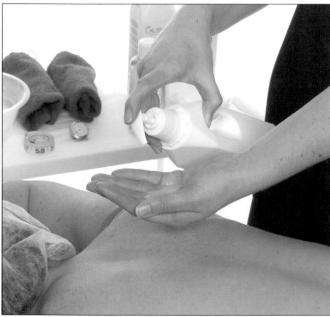

Application of exfoliant to back

Cleansing/exfoliants

If the client does not have time for a shower, using the wet area or an infrared treatment, the best way to prepare the skin is to use exfoliants, to slough off any remaining dead skin cells from the surface of the epidermis, which may hinder the benefits of the treatment. (For further information on exfoliation ingredients and their application and removal, see Unit BT19, Improve face and skin condition using electro-therapy, page 236).

Pre-heating treatments

These include:

- infrared lamp (see Unit BT17, Provide head and body massage treatments, page 323)
- sauna, steam cabinet or spa (see Unit BT29, Provide specialist spa treatments, page 439)
- manual massage (see Unit BT17, Provide head and body massage treatments, page 323)
- hot shower (see Unit BT29, Provide specialist spa treatments, page 439)
- brush cleansing.

These options require a certain amount of time in order to be effective, which the client may not have. If not, then treat the skin as if you were doing a facial treatment. Choose an appropriate cleanser, with a superficial and deep cleanse, using effleurage movements. This especially applies to a congested back, which can be treated exactly as the skin on the face, although you will need to use slightly more product, because of the larger surface area. Feet can be wiped over with an appropriate cleanser.

If the client has applied body lotion, and you feel that the grease on the skin is going to interfere with the treatment, if no other treatment is available (and the client cannot shower), then wash the area to be treated with warm soapy water and pat dry with a towel.

Keys to good practice

Whichever pieces of equipment you choose as the most suitable for the client's treatment plan, always follow the five golden rules – see **Facial treatments – theory and consultation**, page 230.

Remember

The different types of electrical currents have various effects on the body. Most of them will warm the skin and muscles through the increase in circulation to the area; lymphatic drainage is stimulated by using the equipment in the direction of the nodes; and the nerve endings are soothed by the heat generated. Only the faradic current is used to cause muscular contractions, and no electrical currents have an effect on the skeleton.

High frequency

Refresh your memory of the application of high frequency and its theory from Unit BT19, Improve face and skin condition using electro-therapy, page 236. The benefits and effects on the skin, safety precautions and contra-actions apply in the same way to the body as to the face.

Remember

Carry out thermal and sensitivity testing on the area to be treated.

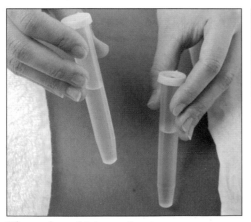

Thermal sensitivity testing to area

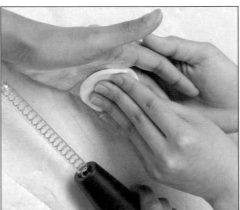

Talc hand that will hold saturator

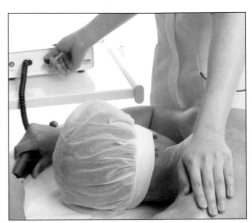

Make contact prior to switching machine on

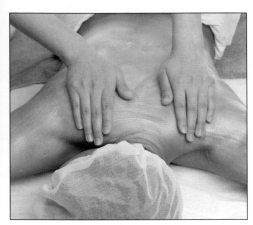

Begin massage avoiding tapotement movements

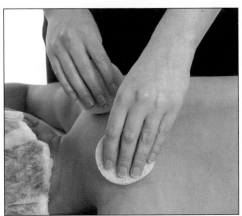

Turn equipment off before removing product

Remember

Avoid tapotement-type movement within the indirect massage as you will break contact.

What to consider when using high frequency treatment

- Follow the same procedure as facial application.
- The main areas for direct high frequency use are on a congested back or chest, with no need to follow a particular direction – just ensure the whole area is covered.
- Indirect high frequency can be used to warm the body and give a deep body massage – follow manual massage directions of stroke, avoiding breaking contact.
- More oxygenating gel may be required for a body than a face, and your salon may find this is not cost-effective when treating a large back or congested chest. Some manufacturers are quite happy for direct high frequency to be applied with a light dusting of talc on the back, as it conducts electricity well, but check with your awarding body. Remember to decant the product, apply on cotton wool and avoid inhalation.
- Gauze is not required when applying direct high frequency with ozone cream to the back, as the client is lying flat in the prone position so the cream is very unlikely to slip off the contours of the body.
- When applying high frequency to the body, avoid trailing the lead across the skin. To keep it off the client, try wrapping the coiled wire around your wrist once.
- The larger roller applicator works well on the back, as does the larger mushroom electrode. Avoid using the smaller ones – it will take too long for the treatment and this is not a cost-effective use of your time.
- Try to avoid your hip or abdomen making contact with the couch as you work across the back – it will draw the current to you instead of the client's skin.
- Always make contact with the skin before turning on the current, or turning it up. You will find clients can tolerate a slighter higher current on the body than on the face as there is more adipose tissue to absorb it.
- The noise of the high frequency unit is less of a worry to clients if they are not having the treatment on the face.
- If carrying out an indirect massage to the body, keep an eye on the hand which is holding the saturator, as the client can become so relaxed that he or she loosens the hand, breaks contact and the saturator drops on the floor. Breaking contact may also be uncomfortable for both client and therapist.

Indirect high frequency

> Used on dry skin with suitable massage medium.

> Used in place of normal manual massage.

> Indirect contact – client holds saturator in a talced hand.

> Make contact with the skin before turning on the machine.

> All dials at zero to start.

> No tapotement movements.

> After massage is completed, remove one hand and turn off machine before removing other hand.

Direct high frequency

> Drying, germicidal effect, often used with oxygenating cream or talc.

> Place saturator on to the skin before switching on.

> Use small circular movements – avoid breaking contact.

> Switch off before removing the saturator from the skin.

> Often done after galvanic to finish treatment.

Vacuum suction

The application of vacuum suction to the body is the same as the facial procedure except that the cups are bigger and the lymph nodes you work towards are positioned differently (for positioning of lymph nodes, see **Related anatomy and physiology**, page 170; and for the facial procedure, see Unit BT19, Improve face and skin condition using electro-therapy, page 242).

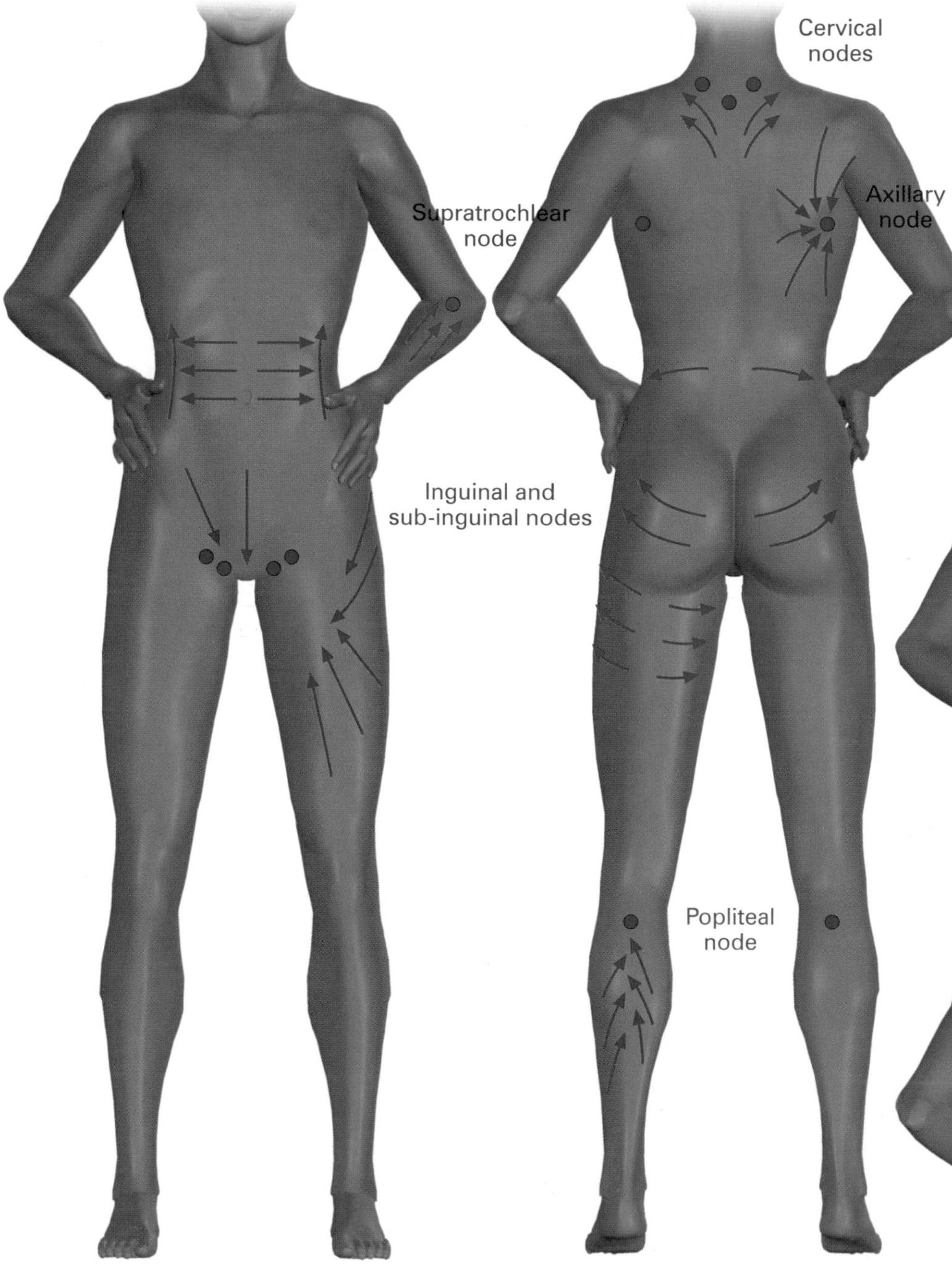

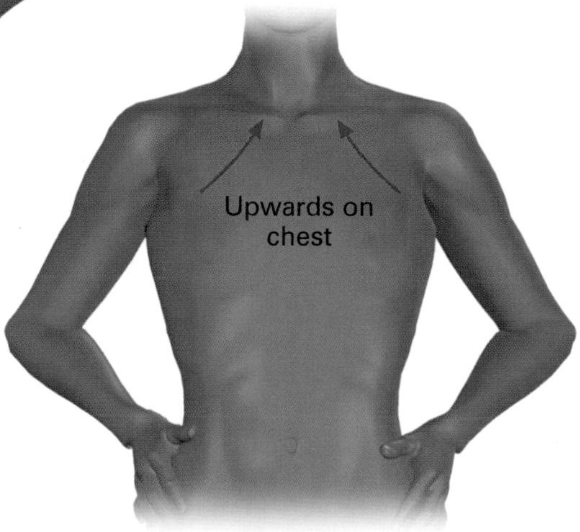

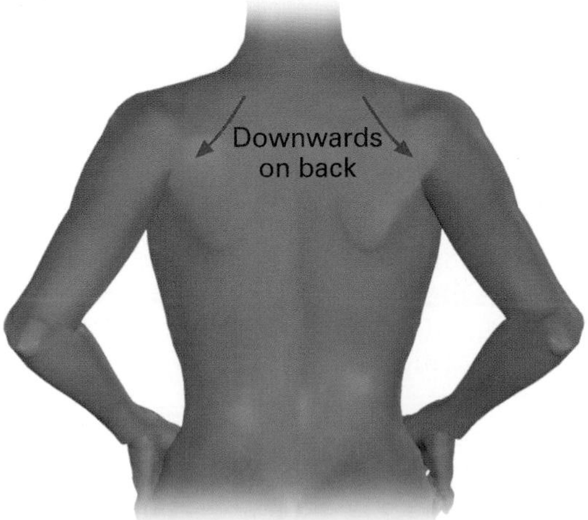

Vacuum suction movements

Remember

Carry out a thermal sensitivity test on the area.

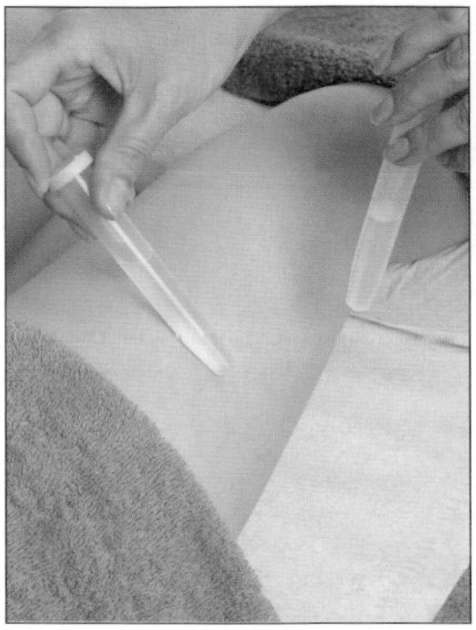

Thermal sensitivity test for vacuum suction

Cervical nodes

Supratrochlear node

Axillary node

Inguinal and sub-inguinal nodes

Popliteal node

Upwards on chest

Downwards on back

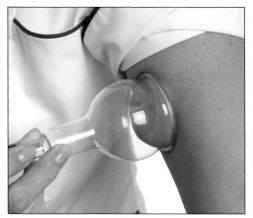

Test equipment on self

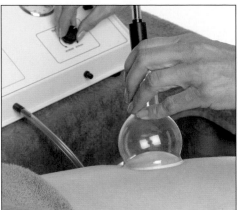

Don't fill the cup move than 20%

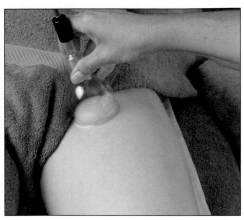

Work towards lymph nodes (see pages 170–1)

What to consider when using vacuum suction treatment

- Although very hairy areas on male clients are not contra-indicated, the treatment may not be very comfortable for the client – a lot more oil is required.
- Almond oil is fine oil suitable for the face, but it is quite expensive so is not cost-effective for body treatments – use the usual massage oil instead.
- All contra-indications apply as for the facial application, but remember to avoid varicose veins on the legs.
- The treatment makes a very good deep lymphatic drainage massage, especially after body faradic treatments where there may be a build-up of lactic acid in the skin.
- If the client is using anti-cellulite treatments (galvanic, diet and exercise), then vacuum suction is very effective, but if the fat is solid and hard, there may not be enough tissue to get comfortably into the cup (20 per cent fill only). Avoid treatment if the legs have hard fat – the golden rule is that if you can do petrissage movements of wringing and picking up on the tissue, then there is enough soft fat to use a vacuum machine.

Care of body glass applicators

After each treatment, place the glass applicator into warm, soapy water with a little antiseptic solution, clean thoroughly and dry. Place in a sanitiser or store in the facility provided in the back of the machine.

> **Remember**
>
> Always work towards the major lymph nodes in the body.

> **Keys to good practice**
>
> Never force the cup into the tubing as it is made of glass and will break. However, most companies manufacture a set of four plexiglass body cups together with an adaptor handle vacuum tube as an option.

Atomiser spray

Some machines have an atomiser spray for easy application of the body oil to the area. To operate:

1 Unscrew the white top from the atomiser spray and fill the container with the product to be used.
2 Screw on the white top and insert the metal prong into the spray tube.
3 Set the main switch to the on position.

4   Hold the atomiser bottle 20–25 cm from the area to be treated.

5   To spray, place your finger over the air bleed hole on the top of the atomiser.

Body cups

There are two sizes of cups available for body work – small (40 mm) and large (52 mm). The size of cup selected will depend on the amount of fatty tissue present.

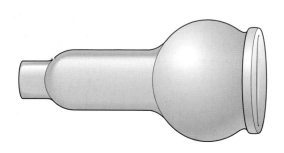

Small – 40 mm

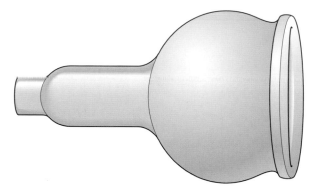

Large – 50 mm

Body cups

For other skin recommendations, see **You and the skin**, page 188; for aftercare, see Unit BT19, Improve face and skin condition using electro-therapy, page 236.

Galvanism

Refresh your memory of the theory of electrical treatments from Unit BT19, Improve face and skin condition using electro-therapy, page 236.

The galvanic current – both desincrustaton and iontophoresis – can be used on the body for:

*   skin correction
*   anti-cellulite treatment

Skin correction

If the client has skin problems on the back, then treat the area as you would for a facial treatment – using the rollers, complete a desincrustation to cleanse the area, with the client holding the indifferent electrode, and then perform iontophoresis to rebalance the skin. A back also benefits from a steam prior to treatment or a brush cleanse, and a face mask with direct high frequency to finish the treatment.

Anti-cellulite treatment

This uses iontophoresis only. The galvanic unit for the body behaves exactly as in a facial treatment, but instead of rollers and an indifferent pad forming a circuit, the pads are the same size and go across the limbs, forming a circuit. The principle of iontophoresis is exactly the same – instead of using moisturising products to keep moisture in the skin, use diuretic anti-cellulite gels to help with the retention of fluids.

Vacuum suction

Choose correct cup size to start treatment.

Cover the hole at the side of the ventouse to create the vacuum.

Place ventouse on client before turning up intensity.

Put on plenty of product to lubricate the gliding movements.

Work towards the lymph nodes in the area.

Remove ventouse by breaking the vacuum – release your finger from the hole.

Never flick or pull the ventouse from the skin.

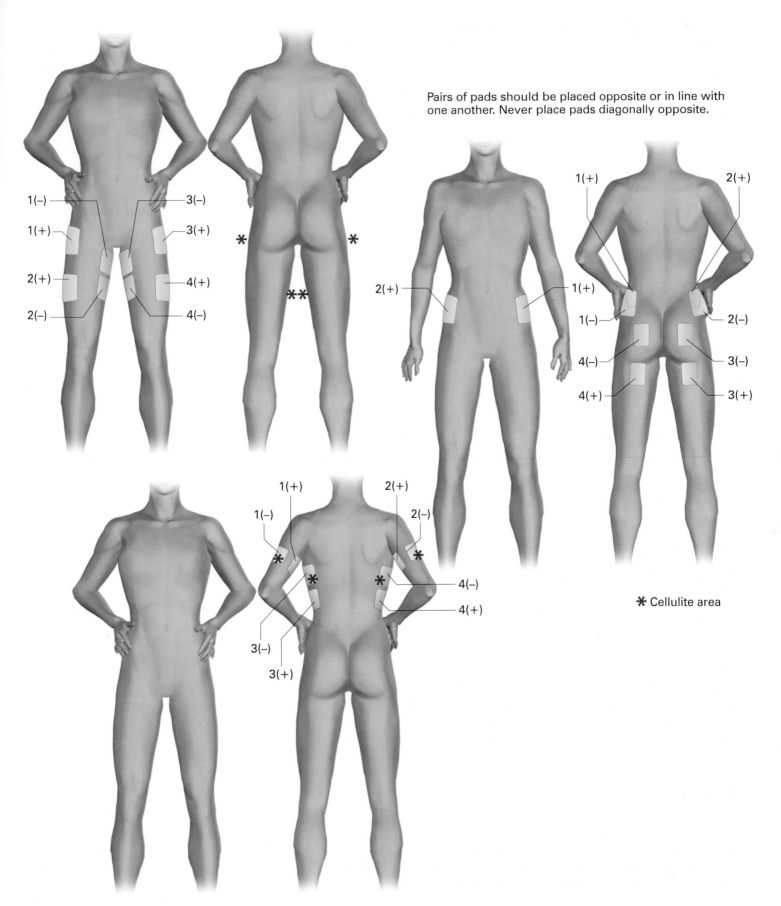

Pairs of pads should be placed opposite or in line with one another. Never place pads diagonally opposite.

1(−)
1(+)
2(+)
2(−)

3(−)
3(+)
4(+)
4(−)

*
*
**

2(+)
1(+)

1(+)
2(+)
1(−)
2(−)
4(−)
3(−)
4(+)
3(+)

1(+)
1(−)
2(+)
2(−)
*
*
*
3(−)
3(+)
4(−)
4(+)

* Cellulite area

Galvanic padding

What to consider when using galvanic treatment

- The skin's resistance to the current is broken down more quickly if the area is pre-warmed by manual massage, a shower or infrared treatment.
- The skin must be grease-free and clean to allow the gels to penetrate the skin.
- The electrodes must be fully covered in damp sponges, otherwise a galvanic burn will result – refer to the manufacturer's instructions.
- Only place the anti-cellulite gel under the active electrode, that is where the treatment is taking place – paste it on like buttering a piece of bread to ensure even coverage.
- The pads are held in place with Velcro strips, so ensure the size is correct for the body part – too loose and the contact will be insufficient to penetrate the skin, and a galvanic burn may be the result of uneven contact with the skin; too tight and you will stop the circulation in the area (the Velcro strips act like a tourniquet) or the strips may come undone half way through the treatment.
- Never exceed the recommended time or milliamps recommended by the instructions, usually a maximum of 3.0 mAs for no more than 20 minutes.
- Time the treatment and never leave the client unattended.
- Always turn the current off before removing the pads.
- There will be an obvious erythema under the active pad. This is perfectly normal, and shows

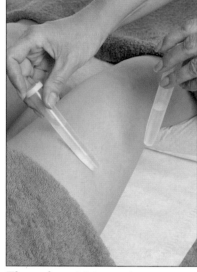

Thermal sensitivity testing to area

the treatment has worked. Some manufacturers recommend reversing the polarity for 3–5 minutes of the treatment to reduce the erythema effect. Do this by turning down and then off, and then switch polarity on the machine – you do not have to adjust or swap over the pads.

Remember

A diuretic substance causes an increase in the flow of urine, so one of the effects of using anti-cellulite gels is that for a day or so after treatment, the client will be urinating more frequently than usual. Reassure the client that this is part of the treatment working. Therefore, specific contra-indications to a body galvanic treatment are:

- kidney problems
- urinary tract infections
- fluid retention, which may indicate kidney problems (for information on how to spot fluid retention, see **Body treatments – theory and consultation**).

Remember

The cream/gel should be the same polarity as the active pad, so that they repel, and the ions in the cream are drawn towards the indifferent electrode opposite.

Remember

It is vitally important to carry out a thermal sensitivity test for **each** area you are treating.

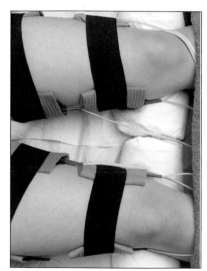

Pads are usually placed in pairs opposite each other

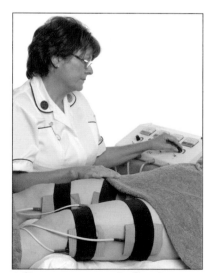

Adjust current to suit client's tolerance

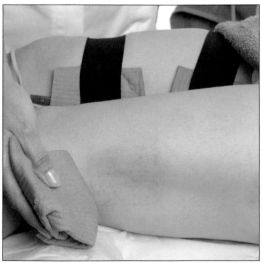

Clients often develop an erythema under the active pad

- Finish with lymphatic drainage, either manually or with vacuum suction, but be careful not to over-stimulate the area, as it already has an erythema. Some manufacturers also recommend G5 massage or faradic after galvanic.
- A course of treatment is most beneficial and can be recommended for three times a week, up to 12 sessions. The treatment responds well to good home care – diet and exercise play a big part in aiding the dispersal of pockets of cellulite.

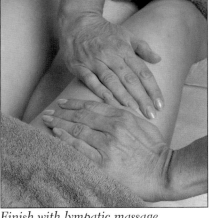

Finish with lympatic massage

Keys to good practice

Explain to the client that there will be a slight itching sensation under the active pad, especially as the product/current is beginning to break down the skin's resistance. If the itchiness is severe, or is accompanied by a burning sensation, then the client is having a reaction to the gel and the current should be turned off, the pads removed and the products removed at once. A cold compress should be sufficient to calm down the area.

Remember

The first treatment should not exceed 10 minutes and the maximum treatment time is 20 minutes.

Remember

Leave the equipment as you would wish to find it! Wash the sponge covers in warm, soapy water to remove any gel, and leave them to dry as naturally as possible – drying them over a heater or radiator will cause the sponges to dry out and crack, which causes uneven concentration of current and a galvanic burn.

Faradism

A faradic treatment to the body is carried out along the same principles as the face, except the settings are altered to be more suitable for larger muscles groups and the pads are bigger and come in pairs, rather than together in one unit, like the facial box.

Faradic, passive exercise of specific muscle groups is very effective in creating tone and muscle definition, and if used in conjunction with a healthy diet and regular exercise, can visibly reduce inches. Be careful about stating that a faradic treatment can help the client lose weight – if you are increasing the muscle bulk, then muscle weighs more than fat, so the client may find he or she gains a little weight, but it is lean muscle tissue rather than fat.

Galvanic treatment

Check product polarity needed for anti-cellulite gel and choose the correct polarity.

⬇

Check electrodes are covered with damp sponge covers or sleeves.

⬇

Active pad and cream/gel must be the same – only place gel on the active sponge, not on both.

⬇

Check active electrode is over area of cellulite.

⬇

Turn up current gradually, and never exceed 3 mAs.

⬇

Time treatment and reverse polarity for final 3–5 minutes.

⬇

Turn current off, remove pads and remove any residue of the gel.

⬇

Carry out other treatments which encourage lymphatic drainage such as manual massage, G5 or vacuum suction.

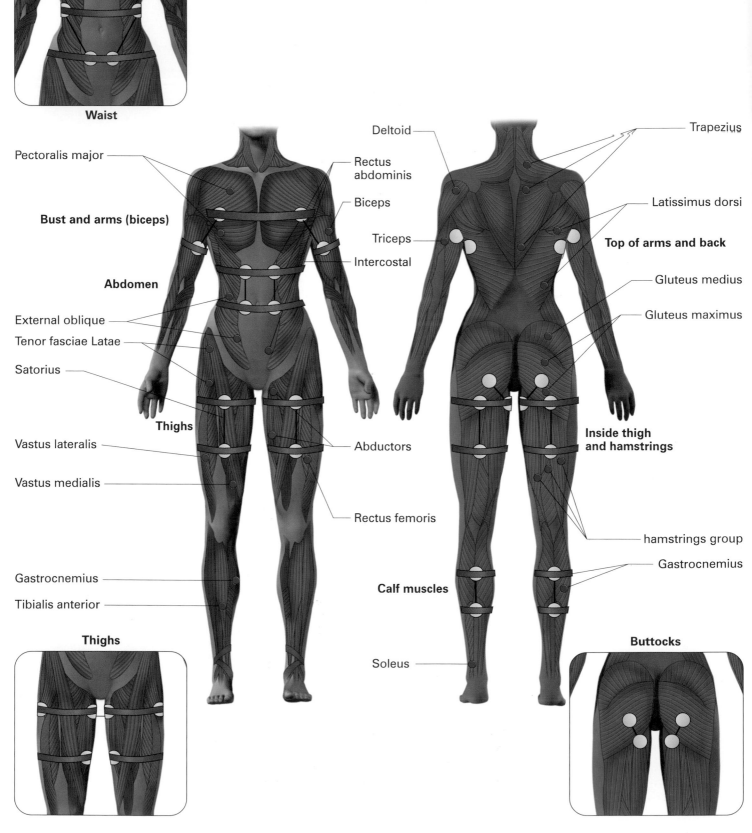

Waist

Deltoid

Trapezius

Pectoralis major

Rectus abdominis

Biceps

Bust and arms (biceps)

Triceps

Latissimus dorsi

Intercostal

Top of arms and back

Abdomen

Gluteus medius

External oblique

Gluteus maximus

Tenor fasciae Latae

Satorius

Thighs

Inside thigh and hamstrings

Vastus lateralis

Abductors

Vastus medialis

Rectus femoris

hamstrings group

Gastrocnemius

Calf muscles

Gastrocnemius

Tibialis anterior

Thighs

Buttocks

Soleus

Padding layouts and motor points for faradic treatment

380

What to consider when using faradic treatment

- Ensure that all leads are firmly inserted into the faradic unit.
- Black and red pads should be inserted into corresponding mini plugs.
- Ensure the unit is off and all intensity dials are in the off position.

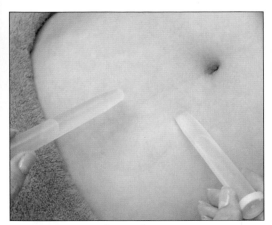

- Carry out a thermal sensitivity test.

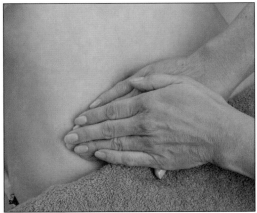

- Pre-warm muscles in the area with massage or infrared treatment.

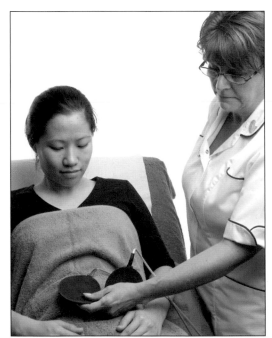

- Dampen the rough side of the faradic pads with warm water and test on yourself prior to treatment.

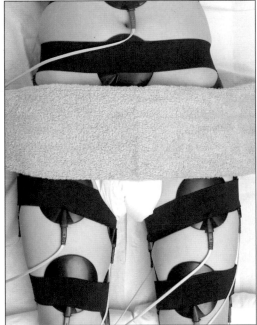

- Place the pads on to selected muscles. Secure into place with Velcro faradic straps ensuring good, firm contact with the skin. Select the required pulse sequence.

- Ensure that contraction and relaxation dials are at minimum.
- Select the required frequency and pulse width.
- Switch on the unit by turning the minute timer clockwise and press the yellow reset button. The alarm will sound until the reset button is pressed (alarm on/off switch) at the back of the unit.
- Turn up each individual intensity control slowly until the desired muscle contraction is obtained.

- Increase the contraction and relaxation settings as required.
- Turn the minute timer to the required treatment length, that is 30–40 minutes.
- Cover the client to ensure warmth and muscle relaxation.
- Give the client the panic button and instructions on its use. After 5–10 minutes, check the contraction intensity and increase as necessary. The pulse width may now be adjusted to ensure maximum comfort of the muscle contraction.
- After the treatment time has elapsed, the unit will automatically switch off. Turn all intensity controls to the off position and switch off the unit. Remove the straps and pads.

	Frequency settings	Pulse width settings
Normal body work	80–100 Hz	160 μs
Deep muscle work	60 Hz	240 μs

Settings for body work

Preparation of pads

The pads must be clean. After every client, wash with warm, soapy water, or follow manufacturer's instructions to remove grease and wipe with a suitable antiseptic preparation. Any grease on the pads will act as a barrier to the current.

Ensure the pads are thoroughly wet with solution and warm on their working surface before being applied to the skin. This breaks down the skin resistance and allows the free flow of current. Lack of moisture on pads can cause a faradic burn.

It is essential the pads are all held firmly against the body by the straps.

Reinforced padding should be used when the load or resistance that the muscle has to carry is excessive and contractions will be difficult to get, for example a pair of pads on each thigh for the rectus fermoris muscle will produce a good result – it needs more than one pair of pads as it is a big band of muscle. A slim, well-toned person will produce contractions with very few pads and low levels of intensity as there is little resistance. A larger person presents more resistance, a larger load and padding must reflect this.

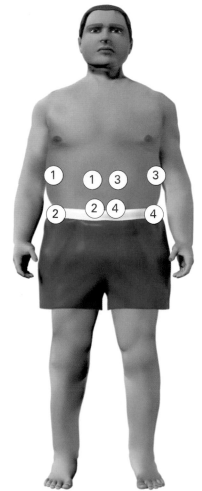

The size of the client will affect the number of pads required

Following natural movement

The natural movements of the muscles should be considered and pads placed to copy these movements as much as possible. If the muscles of an area normally work together to produce a movement, they should be padded and exercised as a group. It is not natural for each segment to work independently, for example the quadriceps.

Muscles must never be made to work against each other. As natural antagonists, the back and front of the body should not be worked together, as the body cannot lean forwards and bend backwards at the same time, and should not be asked to do so artificially. Anything which does not produce a natural movement will not be helping the body back to natural strength and tone in its muscles. For example, it would be unnatural for the buttocks to contract one side at a time – they should always be artificially stimulated so both sides work evenly at the same time. The trapezius muscle works evenly along both sides of its spine attachments for most movements, and this is how it should be exercised. The quadriceps and hamstrings work as a group and not separately.

Types of padding

Longitudinal padding

Originally, the term longitudinal padding referred to the padding of the origin and insertion of a muscle where the current had to flow via the motor point to bring about a contraction. Modern longitudinal padding usually refers to the placing of the electrodes onto a muscle with two motor points.

Modern longitudinal padding involves placing the pads towards the top and bottom motor points of the same muscle, for example rectus abdominus, triceps, rectus fermoris, etc., bringing about a smoother, even contraction. It is essential that there is no movement, so you must not place the pads right over the origin and insertion as these would run over joints, causing movement.

Dual or duplicate padding

This type of padding involves using a pair of pads on one or two muscles on one side of the body and then mirroring the placement of another pair on the adjacent muscle group, for example the oblique muscles, rectus abdominus, adductors, abductors, etc.

Split padding

With this type of padding, one pair of pads is split and placed on the same muscle group on opposite sides of the body, for example gluteus maximus, pectorals, etc.

> ### Remember
>
> Faradic treatments are like any exercise – a regular course of treatments, say twice a week for six weeks, is far more effective than just one treatment, and results will be increased if the client also does the home care exercises and has a good diet.

Keys to good practice

Only turn up the contraction intensity when the block is in contact with the skin, and the contraction light is on. This will ensure you do not exceed the client's tolerance. If turned up in a relaxation phase, the client may have too strong a sensation, and it will be uncomfortable and may even hurt.

Remember

If the client wishes, you could offer her another treatment while she is lying on the couch, e.g. a facial, eyebrow tidy, eyelash tint or similar, but make sure you do not have water near the machine. Some clients just prefer to rest quietly.

Microcurrent

Refresh your memory of microcurrent treatments from Unit BT19, Improve face and skin condition using electro-therapy, page 236.

The body-lifting effect of a microcurrent offers very good results for the client but requires the therapist to have a firm hand as the movements are firm and controlled. Body lifting works on the first four programs of the face-lifting routine. Instead of rollers, there are two bar electrodes to move along the skin. They do not need a sponge cover – as microcurrent is such a low frequency, there is no risk of a burn to the client.

A course of treatments is recommended. Most parts of the body can be lifted, but the treatment is especially popular on the thighs, abdomen, hips, buttocks and breasts. Older clients like to have their arms lifted, so that the biceps are firmer.

Microcurrent

Remove all grease from the skin and any jewellery.

⬇

Set up Velcro straps and pads – choose the most suitable for the muscle group.

⬇

Adjust pulse sequence, frequency and pulse width settings as required (see suggested settings). Check that all intensity dials are in the off position.

⬇

Switch on the minute timer and press the reset button.

⬇

Dampen the body electrodes and place onto selected muscles.

⬇

Turn up the intensity control and set timer – depending upon the number of treatments the client has had.

⬇

Never leave the client unattended, and check for client comfort.

Thighs

Programme 1: Circulation

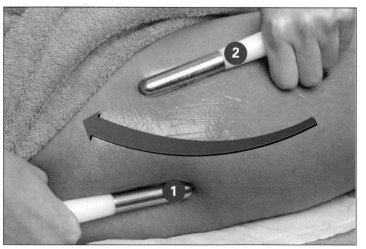

Light pressure. Hold one fixed electrode ❶ at the top of the thigh. Move the other probe ❷ from just above the knee slowly towards the fixed electrode. Move from one side of the thigh to the other, concentrating on the inner thigh.

Programme 2: Tightening

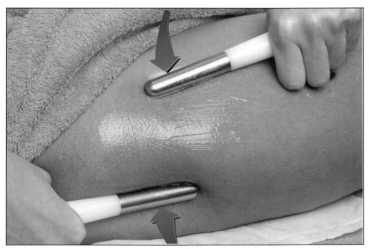

Firm pressure. With adductors stretched (knee straight), leg outwards, pinch the lateral edges of the muscle with the tips of the probes and hold, moving down each muscle on the thigh (quadriceps), concentrating on the inner thigh. Hold movements for 8 seconds.

Programme 3: Tightening

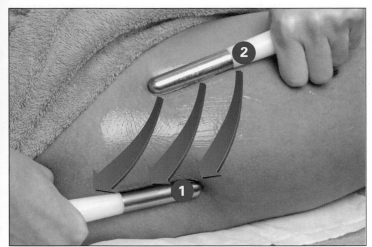

Firm pressure. Hold a fixed probe on ❶ the upper outer thigh. Push the other probe ❷ from the inner thigh, diagonally up to meet the fixed probe, slowly and firmly, and then hold. Work across the thigh.

Programme 4: Firming

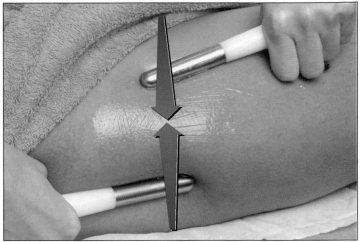

Very firm pressure. The hip and knee should be bent. Allow the knee to fall outwards (approximately 45 degrees – the adductor magnus is then stretched). Active contraction is now needed to prevent the knee falling outwards. Place the probes at each end of the adductor magnus muscle and press as if to move them together but without slipping. Hold movements for 8 seconds.

Upper arms

Programme 1: Circulation

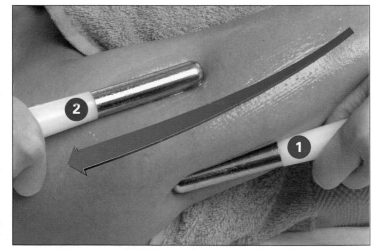

Light pressure. Place one probe just under the shoulder ❶ (at the top of the biceps for the front or the triceps for the back). The other probe ❷ is pushed up over the front and back faces of the arm, from the elbow towards the fixed probe. (The flat edge or the tips of the probe may be used.)

Programme 2: Tightening

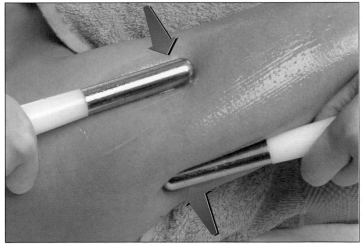

Firm pressure. Biceps stretched, elbow straight for the front. Triceps stretched, elbow bent for the back. The lateral edges of the muscle are pinched with the tips of the probes moving towards the shoulder. Hold movements for 8 seconds.

Programme 3: Tightening

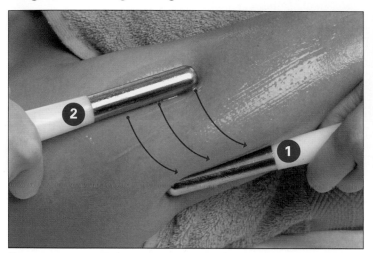

Strong pressure. Repeat programme 1 but with more pressure.

Programme 4: Firming

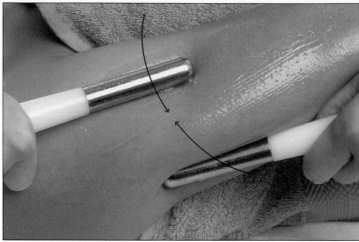

Firm pressure. Biceps stretched, elbow straight for the front, with static contraction of the biceps. Triceps – stretched, elbow bent for the back, with static contraction of the triceps. The probes are placed at both ends of the muscle (biceps or triceps) and pressure is exerted as if together but without slipping. Hold movements for 8 seconds.

Breasts

Programme 1: Circulation

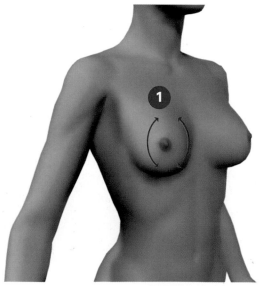

Light pressure. Start at the bottom of the breast, follow the direction of the arrows using the tips of the probes, up then down.

Programme 2: Tightening

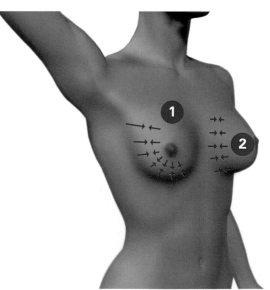

Firm pressure. With the arm behind the head, elbow bent, start at the top of the pectoralis muscle under the collar bone. Hold one probe fixed and lift the other probe to meet it. Work around and down each side of the breast. Hold movements for 8 seconds.

Change the values to the following settings:

- 400 FIz
- 400 μa sine waveform
- duration: 5 minutes

Programme 3: Tightening

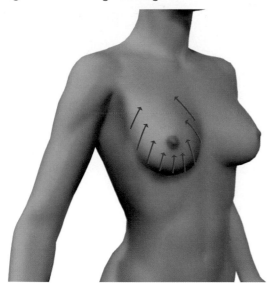

Firm pressure. Hold one probe fixed under the collar bone (flat). The other probe should be lifted up towards it over the whole area of the breast. (If the breasts are large, you may require the client to lift her arm). Hold movements for 8 seconds.

Programme 4: Firming

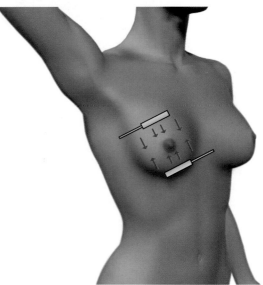

Very firm pressure. The arm behind the head, elbow bent. The client supplies active contraction by trying to move the elbow against a resisting force (RES). The probes are placed at each end of the pectoralis major muscle, pressure is exerted and held, pushing the two as if together but without sliding. Hold movements for 8 seconds.

Buttocks

Programme 1: Circulation

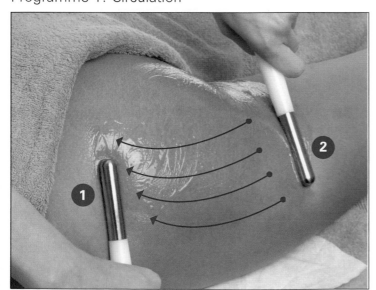

Firm pressure. Place one fixed probe ❶ at the top of the gluteal muscles. Move the other probe ❷ from below the cheek up to meet the fixed probe. Cover the entire cheek.

Programme 2: Tightening

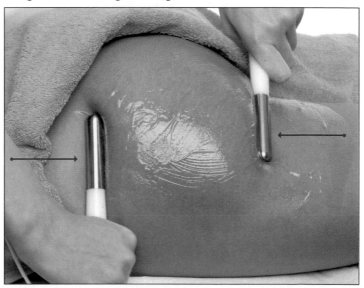

Very firm pressure. Hold the two probes approximately 12.5 cm apart. Slowly push them together to meet. Split the buttocks up into sections depending on the size. Hold movements for 8 seconds.

Programme 3: Tightening

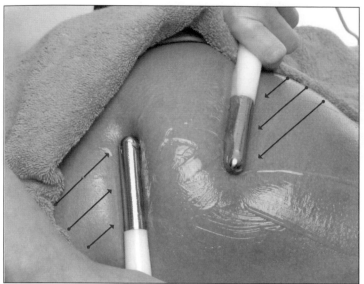

Very firm pressure. Repeat programme 2 but in diagonal sections.

Programme 4: Firming

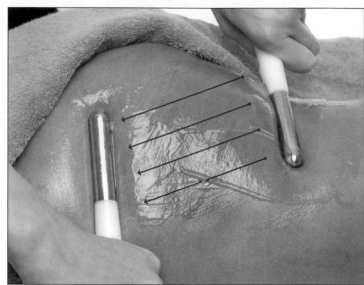

Firm pressure. Repeat programme 1 but in diagonal sections.

Abdomen lifting

Programme 1: Circulation

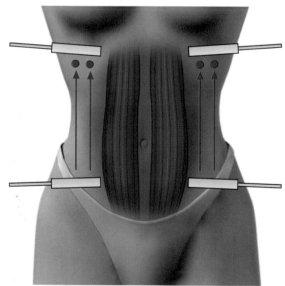

Firm pressure. Hold one probe fixed just below the ribs. Lift the other electrode up from the pubis over the whole surface of the abdomen. Move across in three or four sections.

Programme 2: Tightening

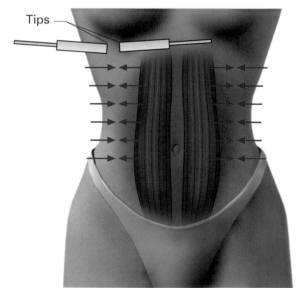

Very firm pressure. With the muscles stretched (arms lifted), move from the pubis to under the ribs. Pinch the lateral edges of the muscle with the tips of the probes. Move across the abdomen in sections. Hold movements for 8 seconds.

Programme 3: Tightening

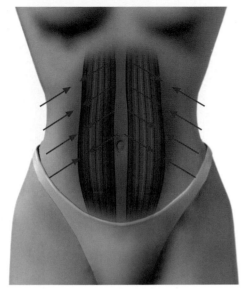

Very firm pressure. Repeat programme 2 but in diagonal sections.

Programme 4: Firming

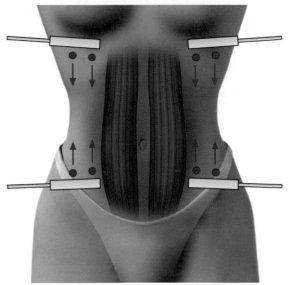

Firm pressure. Abdominal muscles stretched with active contraction (client must raise head and chin towards the sternum). Probes placed at both ends of the abdominal muscles and pressed as if together but without slipping. Hold movement for 8 seconds.

Gyratory vibration

This is the most widely used mechanical massager in salons, health spas and cruise ships. The gyratory machine is often called a 'G5'. G stands for gyratory and 5 is the number of detachable heads which offer a variety of depth, pressure and sensation.

Why 'gyratory'?

A rotary electric motor inside the unit causes the crank and peg to fit into the massage head of the machine creating a gyratory movement.

Popularity of the G5

The G5 is popular because:

* it is labour-saving for the therapist
* it is ideal for large muscular areas, so is suitable for male clients
* it is economical to run
* it is collapsible, so ideal for the mobile therapist
* it offers a deeper massage and can therefore be extremely beneficial.

Vibratory treatments

There are three forms of vibratory treatment for the body:

* percussion
* vibration
* directional stroking.

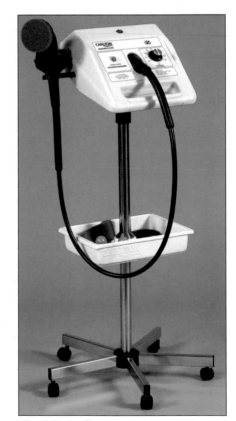

The G5 machine

These treatments may be applied by two types of machines – the more generally used large gyratory vibrators, or for localised effects, the smaller percussion or audio-sonic vibrators.

Gyratory vibrators for general body work are normally floor standing, with the weight of the motor supported by the main shaft or pedestal of the apparatus. This makes for greater safety as well as permitting long periods of use without undue fatigue.

Hand-held versions of these heavy-duty machines are also available. They produce similar effects for a lower cost but are more tiring to use. They look a little like an iron, and are quite heavy for the therapist. As they give quite a deep massage, they are really only suitable for dense muscle and clients with enough body tissue to take the pressure – a contra indication would be a slight figure, or bony areas.

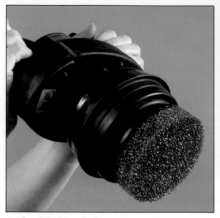

A double-handed gyratory vibrator

> ## Keys to good practice
>
> - If vibratory treatments are used simply to complement and reinforce manual massage, rather than as treatments in their own right, a hand-held gyratory unit may well be adequate.
> - Whatever physical form the vibrator may take, it must be adequate for the task required and should have an air-cooled, heavy-duty motor capable of running for long periods without overheating.
> - The smaller vibrators normally used within facial therapy can be used on the body but are suitable only for localised areas.
> - Gyratory vibrators operate on a vertical and horizontal plane, creating a circular movement while vibrating up and down, thus achieving effects similar in action to manual massage. By altering both the applicator heads and the method of use, effects similar to effleurage, petrissage and tapotement can be achieved. This will help you to decide which applications are suitable and which contra-indicated.

> ## Remember
>
> It is important to tell the client that the sensation felt during vibratory treatment is totally different from the feeling of manual massage movements. In practice, most vibratory treatments are applied in a combined form. In this way, the client gains both the personal touch of massage, and the power and depth of the vibratory unit. It can also be used as a quick method of heating the area prior to other electrical treatments.

Effects of gyrators

- Increases blood circulation.
- Aids desquamation.
- Increases metabolism.
- Promotes relaxation through warming of the tissues.
- Helps break down nodules of tension and relieves tightness in the muscles.
- Helps improve the texture of dehydrated and dry skins.
- Helps well-being if used alongside a diet and exercise programme.

Advantages of vibratory treatments

- They add variety to the treatment routines.
- They save time and prevent fatigue.
- They are less personal, so are useful in treating male clients.
- A deeply effective result can be achieved without the therapist using up a lot of energy, so helping her to conserve energy for other work.
- The time saving can help vibratory work to be more profitable.
- Clients enjoy vibratory massage and feel it is helping them in their fight against figure problems. They see value for money and have a sense that something is actually being achieved.

Contra-indications to gyratory massage

- Skin disorders/diseases.
- Infected acne conditions.

- Bruised areas.
- Cuts and abrasions.
- Recent scar tissue.
- Sunburn.
- Sensitive and fine skin.
- Loose crepey skin.
- Oedema.
- Glandular swellings.
- Highly vascular conditions.
- Over bony areas.
- Varicose veins, thrombosis or phlebitis.
- Very hairy areas.
- Over the abdomen during menstruation or pregnancy.
- Clients with epilepsy or diabetes – a doctor's approval should be obtained.
- Failure of the sensitivity testing on any area.

Effects and benefits of vibratory treatments

- Vibratory treatments act as enormous encouragement to clients in their figure improvement plans, helping them to achieve results more swiftly and maintaining interest in their reduction programmes.
- As the effects of vibration are general stimulation of the circulatory system, the pattern of application can be varied to meet personal needs. The method of application follows body contours and works with the venous return towards the heart. Its effects are on the subcutaneous tissues of the body, bringing about an increase in circulation, without any chemical or muscular contraction.
- The muscular system is improved by fresh interchange of blood through the tissue, but vibrations do not excite the muscle fibres to bring about a contraction.
- It produces a skin toning effect, both by improved nutrition to the skin's dermal layer and by increasing desquamation.
- Tense muscle fibres are relaxed and muscular pain relieved.
- Established fatty deposits are made more available to the general circulation and lymphatic systems, to be used up by the body when on a reduced food intake.
- Vibratory treatment can be extremely relaxing if combined with heat therapy and the more active stimulatory elements are excluded.
- Gyratory vibrators penetrate into the subcutaneous and cutaneous layers of the tissues, having their greatest effect on the skin's surface. Bony areas should be avoided to prevent resonance.

Method of use

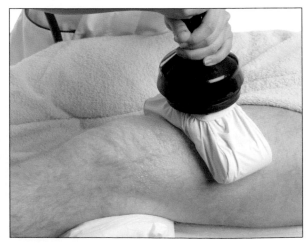

G5 application to the front of the legs using saddlehead with protective cover

The client is prepared for normal body treatments and may have had some form of pre-heating to aid relaxation of muscle tissues. Always explain the treatment to the client and test on yourself. Work as you would for a manual massage procedure, going towards the lymph nodes.

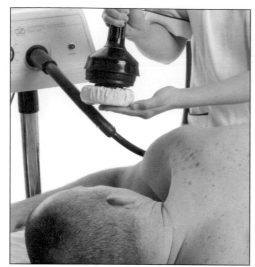

Test on self

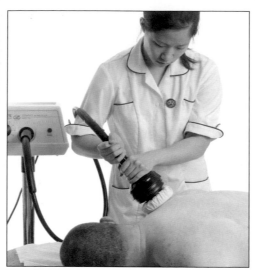

Depth of pressure will be dictated by size of client

If the effect desired is relaxation only, then the application should concentrate on the soothing strokes and gentle vibratory effects of the treatment. If stimulation and figure reduction elements are needed, then a full range of applicators and a varied pattern of strokes should be used. The concentration then is local rather than general, working on areas of established adipose tissue and heavy muscle groups.

A smooth-surfaced applicator – sponge or soft rubber – starts the treatment. This is used with a light application of a talc medium, applied via the therapist's hands with effleurage strokes.

The treatment is applied with long sweeping strokes in an upward direction, towards the heart, as in a normal manual massage treatment. The strokes follow the natural contours of the body and can break contact gently or return with superficial strokes.

Different applicators may be used for variety – both simple round forms and those pre-shaped to mould around an area such as the leg.

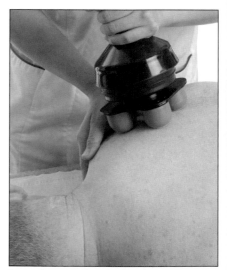

Use alternate heads for massage variation and depths of pressure

Both legs may be treated superficially, one at a time, interlinking vibratory and manual strokes, and then using the ball-studded applicator deeply on the thighs. The deeper movements are performed in a kneading, compression manner, with the therapist's hand providing support and resistance to the strokes, and interlinking them with effleurage. More superficial circular movements can then be performed using the brush type applicator on areas of adequate subcutaneous fat. Poorly textured skin and bad circulation will also benefit from the instant erythema produced by this method of treatment.

The legs should then be covered and the abdomen treated. The application starts with the sponge applicator, following the body contours, and is followed by kneading along the ascending, transverse and descending colon, using the ball-shaped applicator. Manual movements interlink and re-establish relaxation, and then the routine can proceed to stimulating movements on the sides of the waist if indicated.

The studded or short-brush type rubber applicator is used to produce erythema and increase circulation in the area.

The abdominal area is then covered and the arms and chest are treated. It starts with stroking and progresses using the short spiky applicator on the upper arms. Softening of skin over the biceps and triceps muscles indicates the stimulating, abrasive effects of this application.

The arms only may be treated, or the strokes can be extended to include the chest on either side. Choice will depend on the amount of tissue covering the sternum area.

Turn the client over and treat the back of the leg and buttocks, remembering to keep the back and leg not being treated wrapped in towels to keep in the heat and keep the client comfortable.

The G5 is particularly effective on the back, and the ball-shaped applicator, the ball-studded applicator and the short brush can be used on top of the gluteals, just below the waist. When treating the top of the buttocks, be careful not to separate the gluteals fold, as this is very near the sciatic nerve and pressure should be avoided on the area, just as it should be on the vertebral column and borders of the scapula.

Types of applicator

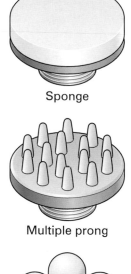

Sponge

Multiple prong

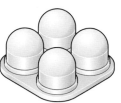

Four-ball firm rubber

Half-ball firm rubber

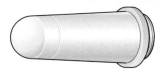

Blunt tipped firm rubber

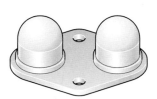

Two-ball firm rubber

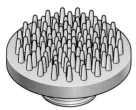

Scalp and skin surface

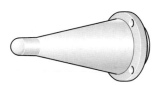

Pointed tip firm rubber

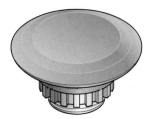

Hollow hot-cold use

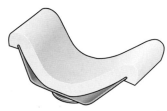

Curved flexible sponge and rubber

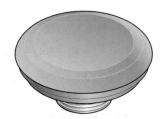

Large firm rubber

G5 applicators

Keys to good practice

Good technique depends on the smooth making and breaking of contact between the applicator head and the client's skin. Control of the heavy equipment comes only with practice and strength in the arms and wrists, and relies on working in the correct postural position.

Remember

The skin will be quite pink and hot in the area after the treatment if the full effects of vascular interchange and improved skin texture are to be effective.

Aftercare

Keep the client warm – to keep the heat in the muscles – while you prepare the equipment for the next part of the treatment.

If G5 is the finishing treatment, allow the client time to become aware of his or her surroundings, put the client into the semi-reclining position and offer a glass of water.

Follow aftercare and home care as for manual body massage (see Unit BT17, Provide head and body massage treatments, page 378).

Keys to good practice

The size of the client will dictate the most suitable applicator head. Changing heads unnecessarily should be avoided as it breaks the continuity of the treatment and can be irritating to the client.

Knowledge check

1   What are the three methods of body consultation you can use during a consultation?

2   Why is it essential to record the height of your client as well as the weight?

3   Give three examples of factors that contribute to poor posture.

4   How would you recognise the condition Lordosis?

5   Why do you take the blood pressure?

6   Why does the skin have to be clean and grease-free prior to a body electrical treatment?

7   List two ways of warming the area prior to treatment.

8   Why is it important to carry out a thermal and sensitivity test prior to electrical treatments?

9   What are the effects and benefits to the skin of a direct high-frequency treatment?

10   When would you give an indirect high-frequency treatment?

11   Does an anti-cellulite treatment require a desincrustation or an iontophoresis galvanic current?

12   Give five important safety points to check prior to giving a body faradic treatment.

13   What is a microcurrent used for?

14   List five effects on the body of a vibratory treatment.

15   What are the aftercare recommendations for a G5 treatment?

other practical
UNITS

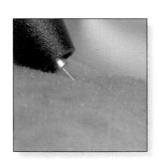
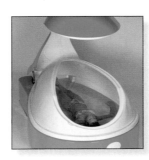
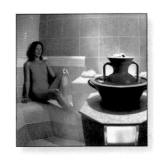

Epilate the hair follicle using diathermy, galvanic and blend techniques

Unit BT16

Galvanic or direct current was the first method of electrical epilation. As a means of permanent hair removal, it was first used in the late nineteenth century in the USA. By the 1940s, diathermy had become the main method. Since then, electrolysis has become increasingly popular, with more than 300 colleges in the UK offering electrolysis courses.

Within this unit you will cover the following outcomes:

BT16.1 Consult with the client
BT16.2 Plan the treatment
BT16.3 Prepare for the treatment
BT16.4 Treat hair follicles using diathermy, galvanic and blend epilation techniques
BT16.5 Complete the treatment.

As you work through this unit, you will need to refer closely to the **Professional basics** and **Related anatomy and physiology** sections.

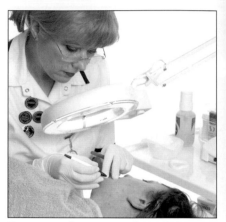

Permanent hair removal can help people feel more confident about their appearance

Consult with the client

BT16.1

In this outcome you will learn about

- hair growth definitions
- the electrolysis consultation
- pain sensitivity
- demonstrating progress.

To support your work on this outcome, you should refer to the structure and function of the skin, the endocrine system, and blood and lymph systems in **Related anatomy and physiology**.

Hair growth definitions

Your hair performs three functions – it protects you, regulates your temperature and acts as adornment.

Superfluous hair growth

Superfluous (excess) hair growth is a general term. Females with low levels of female hormones (oestrogen and progesterone) and higher levels of the male hormones (androgens) can develop superfluous hair growth. Superfluous hair is, however, a matter of opinion and cultural preferences, and only the client can judge what is excessive for him or her.

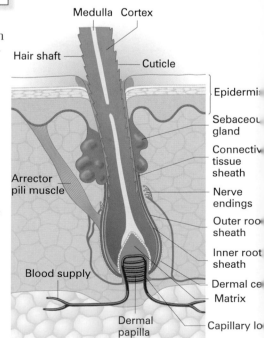

The structure of the hair and its follicle

Hirsutism and hypertrichosis

Hirsutism and hypertrichosis describe excessive hair growth. Some men may have excessive hair growth on the bridge of the nose, ears, cheekbone area, neck, back, chest, arms and hands, and may also have unusual amounts of hair on the legs.

The electrolysis consultation

This provides an opportunity:

- to discuss client expectations and agree on the treatment
- to advise the client on the achievable outcomes of the treatment
- to aid client understanding of the treatment
- to discuss suitability of the client for treatment
- to allow the client to ask questions about the treatment
- to explain all possible reactions to the treatment
- to discuss the probable causes of hair growth
- to examine the client's skin and hair type
- to discuss any previous methods of hair removal
- to plan the course of treatments
- to discuss costs
- for the client to experience the treatment
- to record in detail client hair growth and, if possible, take a photograph as visual evidence.

With electrolysis, the consultation and record-keeping are of utmost importance and new levels of empathy and consultative skills will need to be developed. A balance must be found so that the client feels confident about the therapist's professionalism and skills but also relaxed and able to communicate on the subject of unwanted personal hair growth.

It is one of the most difficult and awkward subject matters for some clients to talk about. Clients will often feel apprehensive, emotional and intimidated. A good therapist is one who can make the client feel relaxed and special, but most importantly feel a normal human being and not some freak of nature! A polite and reassuring manner should be shown to the client at all times, throughout the preparation process, the treatment itself, through aftercare and home care advice to the end of the treatment.

No two clients are the same, even when the underlying cause of the problem may be the same. All clients vary in their response and commitment to treatment. Each treatment and each course of treatments must be tailored to suit the needs of each individual client.

The first electrolysis consultation should last at least 30 minutes, with 20 minutes allocated to the consultation and 10 minutes for a patch test treatment. It is advisable to encourage clients to start the course of treatments straight away if possible; otherwise they may get 'cold feet'.

Pain sensitivity

Most individuals describe electrolysis as uncomfortable – a warm, burning or stinging sensation – rather than painful.

> ### Key term
>
> **Hirsutism** –usually reserved for females. It refers to the growth of hair on the face and body, which is usually characteristic of masculinity. Caused by an over-abundance of the hormone androgen in the blood. The dormant follicles are stimulated to grow hair, and existing vellus and terminal hairs grow larger in diameter.

> ### Key term
>
> **Hypertrichosis** – used for both men and women. It describes a general overgrowth of terminal hair affecting the entire body surface. It is not hormone dependent, and results from ethnic or genetic predisposition.

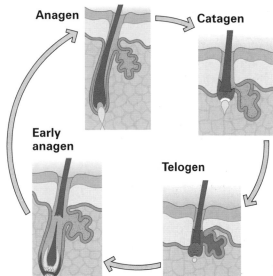

The hair growth cycle

> ### Remember
>
> Pain thresholds and sensitivity vary from client to client and appointment to appointment.

Factors which increase discomfort
Poorly motivated clients
Age – young clients are less motivated
Sensitive body areas, e.g. upper lip
Too long a treatment, too soon
Too high a current, for too long
Poor insertions
Defective needles
Defective equipment
Inflamed skin (reworking over the same area)
Failure to adjust settings
Too small a needle
Individual sensitivity changes, e.g. tiredness, headache, nervousness, menstruation
Hairs requiring high current
Dry, sensitive skin type

Factors which relieve discomfort
Motivated client
Relaxed and comfortable atmosphere
Using the minimum effective current
Varying intensity/duration and techniques with blend
Topical anaesthetics
Acclimatising client – start with less sensitive areas
Concentrated treatments rather than jumping areas
Ice packs to cool and help numb the area
Aftercare products to reduce oedema and erythema
Therapist showing a confident and professional manner
Ensuring an efficient and effective treatment
Upgrading and improving skills with further training
Finger pressure as a distraction
Distraction for the client, e.g. music, aromatherapy scent
Choice of modality to suit client
Treatment planning to avoid times of menstruation, etc.

Factors which increase or relieve discomfort

Demonstrating progress

Where possible and with the client's agreement, it is a good idea to photograph the client before and after a course of treatment to demonstrate to the client the progress made. With a slow process such as epilation, it is sometimes difficult for the client to 'remember' how significant the original problem may have been. These pictures are best used only for an area, not for a whole headshot where the client can be easily identified. The pictures must remain private and confidential and never be shown to anyone without the written permission of the client. These photographs can also be included in an in-depth treatment plan to demonstrate improvement over time as a result of treatment.

Plan the treatment   BT16.2

In this outcome you will learn about

- agreeing treatment outcomes
- present and past hair management
- causes of hair growth
- the epilation record card

Agreeing treatment outcomes

With any new client, you will need to discuss causes of hair growth, contra-indications, medical history and emotional condition before beginning treatment.

It should be explained to the client from the outset that although the results of epilation are permanent, it is a progressive treatment. Each hair has to be treated separately and a number of times. The hairs will become finer, lighter in colour, less dense and eventually will disappear, but this may take considerable time. Do not give an estimation of the expected duration of the treatments required to destroy the hair. This is a difficult estimation, even with experience, as every client is different.

Explaining the treatment

You will need to explain the treatment fully to the client. If possible, show step-by-step visual graphics or photographs with a 'summary' under the pictures. Ensure that you cover the following points.

- A tiny probe (some clients have a fear of needles) the same diameter as the hair is inserted into the follicle opening – an opening that is already in the skin, so no discomfort should be felt as the skin is not pierced.
- The probe is charged with a small amount of electrical current and the client will feel a sensation very similar to a slight sting. This sensation will feel more noticeable in some areas than others, where there are more nerve endings in the skin. The hair is then gently lifted from the skin with tweezers and the client should feel no plucking or pulling of the hair. Each hair must be treated individually with enough current and correct insertion to provide a solution that is eventually permanent.
- Explain to the client the stages of hair growth – anagen, catagen and telogen.
- The client will need to tell the therapist the areas that he or she would like treated. This should be clearly stated on the consultation card.
- All elements of the treatment should be recorded in great detail before treatment.
- Realistic outcomes of treatment must be explained to the client, who should be made aware of the commitment required.

A treatment plan should be completed with the client. If the unwanted hair problem is severe, it may be necessary to 'clear' one area at a time, which means the client will need to continue to use his or her own personal 'hair management' system (see page 401).

The various methods of epilation could be used on a client, for example blend and diathermy. Diathermy on the majority of the area will ensure that the client leaves the salon hair-free, as a greater number of hairs can be removed at any given time, but blend concentrated in a small area will ensure the quickest results. Once the blend area is permanently cleared, an additional blend area could be started.

Keys to good practice

Demonstrating to the client the quicker results achieved with blend is a tried and tested way of successfully changing diathermy clients onto blend.

In the salon

A question clients will ask during consultation:

What happens during the treatment?

Answer: 'The skin is cleansed with an antiseptic lotion, a new sterile disposable probe is used on each visit and this will be opened in front of you. This probe is inserted into the hair follicle, a natural opening in the skin, and as this does not involve any piercing of the skin it will be painless. When the probe is in the correct position, the current is discharged, treating the part of the follicle that produces the new hair. The treated hair is then gently released from the follicle with a pair of tweezers. Over time, the treatment gradually makes the hairs finer and finer until they no longer grow.'

Remember

Actively encourage clients to ask questions and clarify any points of which they are unsure, especially during the consultation and at any time during and after the treatment. The more informed a client is, the more effective the treatment is likely to be.

Unrealistic aims	Realistic aims
Hair will never grow back again after one treatment	Each individual hair will need to be treated a number of times
It's quick and easy	It is a slow but permanent treatment requiring great skill from the therapist
It doesn't hurt at all	A level of discomfort is involved – some areas are more sensitive than others. A sting will be felt with diathermy, and this will last a second or two. With blend, a more gentle build-up of warmth will be felt for about 3 seconds. Galvanic feels similar, with a build-up of warmth, and can feel painless for a number of clients. With experience, the therapist can use local topical anaesthetics
It works well on large areas	Large areas can be treated, but electrolysis works best on small areas because of the treatment time required
It won't matter if I don't keep appointments	Regular appointments and a good deal of commitment are required from the client in order to achieve satisfactory outcomes
The hairs grow back with a sharp, spiky feel	The hair is removed from the root, therefore the hair grows back with its natural tapered end, feeling smooth to the touch
All the hairs grow back at the same time	Hairs grow back spasmodically, as the hair growth cycle varies for each follicle and area

Realistic and unrealistic aims of electrolysis

Epilation clients

Epilation clients are very varied, and may include both men and women. Areas requiring treatment may include the face and neck, underarm, bikini-line, chest (male and female), and for experienced therapists, the most intimate areas – pre-operative or post-operative transsexuals' genitalia. (See **You and the skin**, page 188, for male skin behaviour, structure and product use; see also the section on ingrowing hair, page 422.)

Present and past hair management

Hair management techniques

Epilation currently offers the only permanent method of hair removal. However, there are many different ways to remove unwanted hair temporarily and the client may well have used some of these, including waxing, plucking, depilatory creams, shaving and laser. The use of any other method will have a bearing on future epilation treatments and can affect the client both psychologically and physiologically. It is important for the therapist to establish how the client has been managing the hair problem and to suggest the best way forward.

If the client has been using temporary methods of hair removal, you will need to establish whether he or she was under the false impression that these methods were permanent. Then, with this knowledge, you will need to carefully consider the treatment programme and decide whether it should be revised as the hair growth, skin, and the client's sensitivity may well have been altered in some way.

Another factor that might affect treatment will be the client's own need to 'manage' hair growth between treatments to make it acceptable to him or her. Only cutting is recommended, although occasional shaving is acceptable. Cutting does not damage the hair follicle in any way. With the popular blend method of epilation, however, distorted follicles can be successfully treated.

Remember

Client confidentiality is vital at all times. Of all beauty therapy practices, epilation in particular deals with the client's hormones and self-image, sometimes resulting in very emotional clients who may unburden some of their most intimate secrets to you. Never comment on or discuss a client's treatment with anyone but the client, ensure record cards are stored in a secure place and always comply with the Data Protection Act (see **Professional basics**).

Remember

If you suspect that the client might have an underlying medical condition which is exacerbating the hair growth problem, refer the client to his or her doctor for advice.

Method	Effect
Facial discs/abrasives	Gently abrasive, rather like an ultra-fine sandpaper. Only really suitable for very fine hair and not suitable for epilation as it makes it difficult to follow the line of the hair into the follicle
Hair removal creams	Establish how long these have been used for. Were there any allergies, soreness, etc.? Is the skin sensitised? Any sign of infection? When was the last treatment? If very recent, it may be necessary to wait for the skin to desensitise before electrolysis. Depilation creams can also result in brittle hair, making hair difficult to release from the follicle without breakage during electrolysis
Bleaching	Clients may bleach their hair to disguise it, using a number of specialised colourants. While this minimises the appearance of unwanted hair, it can result in the hair becoming brittle and liable to break, as well as sensitising the skin, both factors causing difficulties for the therapist

(continued on next page)

Method	Effect
Plucking/threading	Plucking can sensitise the skin. Has the client caused skin damage from over-enthusiastic plucking? If so, this must be brought to the client's notice, recorded on the record card and if new scarring (less than one year old) is apparent, this would be a contra-indication to treatment and the immediate area would have to be avoided. Has incorrect plucking been carried out, e.g. causing breakage of the hair or performed in the opposite direction to the hair growth? When the hair is plucked out in the opposite direction to the natural fall of the hair growth, the follicle is likely to have been distorted. Therefore, blend or galvanic epilation should be the preferred choice of treatment. It is widely believed that plucking may cause topical stimulation to the area and encourage the growth of more hair, although the evidence does not always support this theory
Electrical appliances/shaving	Shaving can sensitise the area and products used, e.g. aftershave, may contain alcohol that can further sensitise the skin. Therefore, special consideration must be given to the condition of the skin. Also, any nicks or cuts that may have resulted from shaving would be a contra-indication to treatment. Shaving cuts the hair, leaving it feeling blunt to touch and thicker and can also result in ingrowing hairs. As with plucking, it is claimed that shaving results in topical stimulation (massage of the area stimulates the blood supply that 'feeds' the hair), so exacerbating the problem. However, some experts claim that encouraging the client to shave a few days prior to treatment can show the therapist exactly which hairs are in anagen by the longer appearance of those hairs. This then ensures that the hairs treated are the active growing ones, thereby resulting in the most effective treatment. Electrical plucking or threading (see above) rips the hair out from the root. However, this is not always successful and hairs often break. Electrical plucking can result in distorted follicles and sensitised skin as well as ingrowing hairs and hairs which have been dislodged from the dermal papilla, sometimes resulting in infected follicles and affecting an electrolysis treatment
Waxing/sugaring	Waxing is also said to cause topical stimulation, although the evidence does not always support this. Waxing rips out hairs in the opposite direction to growth, which in turn causes distortion of the hair follicle, and this will have a bearing on the method of epilation used. Blend or galvanic methods which both allow the treatment of distorted follicles should be chosen
Laser/IPL	Laser is the most recent newcomer to hair removal. Legally, laser manufacturers can claim permanent hair reduction but not (to date) removal, and it is said to be an effective method of hair management. Currently, laser cannot successfully treat light blonde or white hair and indeed can strip the colour from some hairs, often leaving white hair remaining which can be removed with electrolysis

Types of hair removal and how they may affect epilation

Visual aids

During the consultation, illustrations, pictures or graphs can be used to assist your presentation to the client. You can draw your own or obtain them from manufacturers, who supply skin and hair charts and even three-dimensional models of the skin. A good therapist understands that it is his or her job to give the client as much relevant information regarding the treatment as possible. Certainly visual aids can help clients to 'see' rather than 'hear' explanations and will greatly assist in demonstrating that the skin is not pierced in epilation but rather the needle or probe travels down an already existing cavity (the hair follicle).

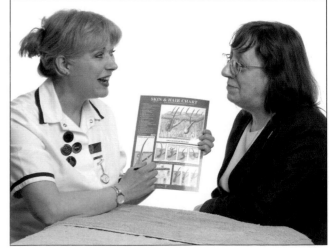

A graphic can be used to explain to the client exactly what is involved

Causes of hair growth

Causes of abnormal hair growth range from illness to hormonal reasons. What is considered excessive hair growth in one country can be considered normal in another, and what is considered ugly by some can be attractive to others. Some clients may feel they are 'freaks' and all clients must be taken seriously. If a client feels that he or she does not fit into the 'norm' in a society, it can seriously affect his or her general well-being.

The human body is covered with hair follicles that can be dormant or active and can grow no hair, fine vellus hair or thick terminal hair. All hair growth – normal or abnormal – is controlled by hormones and it is the over-secretion of male hormones that causes excessive hair growth. Hormones are chemical messengers that are circulated by the bloodstream. Research has shown that most excess hair is due to a combination of over-abundant androgen (the male hormone) secretion and an enzyme in the follicle that is sensitive to androgen increase.

Classification of hair growth

Causes of hair growth are classified as:

- congenital
- topical
- systemic.

Congenital

This is hair growth that is present from birth. Some people are born with greater amounts of facial and body hair that is both normal and hereditary, for example eyebrows, eyelashes, nostrils, scalp and body hair. People vary considerably in their skin sensitivity to androgens and females who have low levels of the female hormones (oestrogen and progesterone) and higher levels of androgens can develop superfluous hair.

Topical

Friction or stimulation to an area of skin can cause excess hair growth. Topical causes include plaster casts, plucking and waxing. This hair, formed as a protective mechanism of the body, grows deeper and coarser because of stimulation of the blood supply to the skin in that area. Moles and birthmarks often have excessive hair growth because of the multiple and unusual development of capillaries near the surface of the skin.

Systemic

These are normal and abnormal hormonal changes that can stimulate hair growth – see the table opposite.

Normal systemic causes of hair growth

At puberty, hormone levels start to rise. The process starts when the hypothalamus stimulates the anterior pituitary gland to secrete gonadotrophic hormones which activate the sex glands. Hormones secreted by the anterior pituitary gland at this time are:

Normal	Abnormal
Puberty	Cushing's syndrome
Pregnancy	Adrenogenital syndrome
Menopause	Archard-Thiers syndrome
	Polycystic ovary syndrome
Stress	Anorexia nervosa
Medication	Acromegaly

Systemic causes of hair growth

- adrenocorticotrophic hormone (ACTH) – this stimulates the adrenal cortex to produce oestrogen and progesterone in the female, testosterone and a little oestrogen in the male and androgens in both sexes

- follicle stimulating hormone (FSH) – stimulates the development and ripening of ovarian follicles and produces oestrogen
- luteinising hormone (LH) – stimulates the formation and secretion of the corpus luteum, which in turn secretes progesterone.

During pregnancy, women can have increased hair growth which may be temporary and will disappear without treatment after the birth. However, often the fine vellus hair appearing throughout pregnancy can develop into terminal hair and electrolysis is required. The many hormonal changes and often temporary imbalances result in the androgen level being raised, resulting in superfluous hair growth.

During menopause, the ovaries begin to degenerate as their reproductive function is no longer required and a reduction in the levels of oestrogen, progesterone and androgens occurs. However, the adrenal cortex continues to produce androgens and this can lead to the production of superfluous hair in the male growth pattern. A premature menopause can be brought about by surgical removal of the ovaries and womb (total hysterectomy).

Long-term stress causes secretion of hormones from the adrenal cortex and these androgens will stimulate superfluous hair growth in the male pattern.

Many types of medication can encourage superfluous hair growth, including anabolic steroids and some makes of the contraceptive pill. It is estimated that there are over 500 different drugs that can affect hair growth.

Anorexia nervosa is a psychological disorder, mostly affecting adolescent girls, and involves the nervous, endocrine and digestive systems. A strong conviction that the sufferer is overweight and a general lack of self-esteem cause the sufferer to become malnourished and severely underweight, and can even be fatal. Lanugo hair (baby hair) develops all over the body, while there is a thinning of hair on the head.

Endocrine disorders affecting hair growth

To learn more about the endocrine system, see **Related anatomy and physiology**, page 175.

Endocrine disorders include the following:

- Cushing's syndrome. Increased levels of ACTH lead to an excess of androgens, which possibly lead to hirsutism. Symptoms include osteoporosis, muscular weakness and wasting of the limbs, thinning skin, rounding of the face, high blood pressure, oedema, and obesity of the trunk.
- Adrenogenital syndrome is very rare. It is present from birth and is a genetic defect causing overproduction of androgens by the adrenal cortex. Symptoms include enlargement of the genitals, dehydration, weight loss, low blood pressure and hypoglycaemia.
- Archard-Thiers syndrome is a very rare condition with symptoms similar to Cushing's syndrome. Women with diabetes can suffer from this where the adrenal glands and ovaries produce too much androgen.
- Polycystic ovary syndrome produces symptoms including enlarged ovaries with numerous follicular cysts, irregular or absent menstrual cycle, and weight gain. Polycystic ovaries are capable of secreting large quantities of androgens, causing the development of excess hair.
- Acromegaly is caused by the hypersecretion of growth hormone. Symptoms can include large hands and feet, coarse facial features and the secretion of excess androgens that stimulate excessive hair growth in the male pattern.

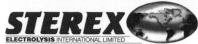

Client's name:

ELECTROLYSIS CONSULTATION RECORD

Date of Consultation:

Address:

Postcode:

Home Tel no:

D.O.B.:

Recommended/referred by:

Occupation:

Work/Mobile Tel no:

No of children: Ages:

Medical Information

Doctor's name:

Address:

Medical History:

Under medical care?   yes / no

Medication (topical and/or oral):

Allergies:

Contra-indications

Contra-indications for G.P. Referral: (circle where applicable)

Diabetes	Epilepsy	Heart Condition
History of Cancer	High Blood Pressure	Circulatory Problems

Date G.P. letter sent: G.P. letter received:
                                          (to be attached)

Contra-indications - not to be treated: (circle where applicable)

Haemophilia Pacemaker	Hepatitis/Aids/HIV	Pregnancy (Blend below neck)

If in treatment area: Metal pins/plates   Skin disorder   Bruising/Swelling

Recent scar tissue   Loss of tactile sensation   Varicose veins

Previous Treatment History

Areas to be treated: First noticed growth:

Previous hair removal methods:

Waxing ☐   Tweezing ☐   Depilatory creams ☐   Shaving ☐   Cutting ☐   Other ☐

Previous electrolysis treatment?   yes / no   Previous laser treatment?   yes / no

For how long: How often:

Healing rate/skin reaction to previous methods?

Reasons for discontinuing treatment:

Skin/Hair Observations

Area to be treated:

Skin type and condition:

Any scarring present and location:

Hair type and density:

An epilation record card

The epilation record card

In addition to the standard information, the epilation record card should include:

- previous hair removal treatments
- hair type
- skin type
- method of epilation
- intensity of current
- needle size and type
- date and timing of sessions
- treatment remarks and details, length, etc.
- machine settings
- reaction to treatment
- aftercare advice
- products purchased.

During consultation and throughout a course of treatments, the condition of the client's skin is vital to the success, effectiveness and comfort of the treatment. A full skin diagnosis should be carried out and details noted on the client's record card. As well as general skin type, great care must be taken to record, in great detail, the condition of the skin in the direct working area. Any changes in the skin (good or bad) throughout the treatment should be recorded.

After a full consultation, the content of the record card should be clarified with the client to ensure that the correct information is recorded and that no misunderstandings have arisen.

Keys to good practice

Clients should carefully check, sign and date the record card at the end of the consultation, stating that all the information is true to the best of their knowledge. It is also a good idea to ask clients to sign and date a statement that they have been given aftercare advice and that they will follow the advice, e.g. 'I agree to follow the written and verbal aftercare advice which has been given'.

Remember

A skin in good condition ensures for the client:

- more comfortable treatments
- more effective treatments
- quicker healing time
- less erythema.

A good skin condition ensures for the therapist:

- easier treatments
- satisfied clients.

The information on the client's record card should be checked every time he or she visits the salon to ensure that there are no changes; for example, has the client started HRT and not informed you? This could affect her hormonal balance and therefore her hair growth, skin and general well-being.

Contra-indications

Electrolysis guidelines about restricting treatments or requiring medical referral are given below. This is not necessarily a comprehensive list. For any condition you are uncertain of, a doctor's permission must be sought.

The following contra-indications will either prevent or restrict treatments.

- Electronic implants, e.g. pacemakers.
- Haemophilia.
- HIV or hepatitis.
- Epilepsy.
- Skin cancer (treatment area).
- Pre-malignant/malignant lesions.

Remember

Failure to keep up-to-date, accurate records could result in unsafe treatment and possibly to legal action being taken against you and/or the salon.

- Recent scar tissue (treatment area – advisable to wait 12 months).
- Cuts and abrasions (treatment area).
- Warts and moles.
- Heart valve disorders.
- Viral infections e.g. herpes simplex.
- Bacterial infections e.g. impetigo.
- Fungal infections e.g. ringworm.
- Infestations e.g. scabies.
- Any contagious or infectious disease or disorder.
- Severe psoriasis/eczema/acne/dermatitis (treatment area).
- Severe stress or anxiety.
- Loss of tactile sensation.
- Varicose veins (treatment area).
- Hyperpigmentation and hypopigmentation.
- Keloid scarring.
- Metal plates or pins (treatment area) – this is especially important with blend or galvanic currents.
- First three months of pregnancy.
- Below neck area during pregnancy with blend or galvanic currents.
- Avoid breasts or abdomen in pregnancy particularly during the last three months.

Always seek medical approval if your client has:

- insulin-controlled diabetes
- lupus
- emphysema
- asthma
- hiatus hernia (affects positioning of client)
- endocrine disorders/hormone imbalance
- moles and pigmented naevi
- heart problems
- pregnancy.

Clients aged under 16 will also need a doctor's permission before treatment can be carried out.

In addition to these contra-indications, skin sensitivity can be affected by other skin care treatments which may inhibit or prevent epilation, for example glyconic peels, microdermabrasion and laser.

Prepare for the treatment   BT16.3

In this outcome you will learn about	
• planning a treatment	• the correct working position
• equipment and materials	• hygiene and safety.

Planning a treatment

It is vital to discuss with clients a treatment plan to cover the course of their treatment. This will ensure that they are aware of the commitment that they must make and that appointments need to be regular and, in some cases, for a period of months, if not years. Advise on the best possible skin care and products to ensure the skin is in the best possible condition – this will make the treatment more comfortable, easier and more effective. Facials, particularly exfoliation treatments, can assist epilation treatment ensuring ease of operation, and when aftercare is discussed, products to calm, soothe and assist with healing should be recommended and sold to the client. It is imperative that clients follow the therapist's advice, as the use of incorrect products could be detrimental to their skin and health.

It is important to organise treatment time carefully – clients will want value for money and not to be rushed. Always start the treatment with the darkest and most noticeable hairs first. Ask clients which hairs bother them the most (the answer may not necessarily match your opinion). With a dense growth it is advisable to treat every other hair to prevent over-treatment of the area and cause either the build-up of heat (diathermy) or sodium hydroxide (blend or galvanic) as this can cause tissue damage, oedema and/or erthyema and sensitisation of the skin. Treat all hairs of the same type, texture and diameter. When these have been treated, it may be necessary to reduce the needle size to complete the treatment. It is important to work in a systematic manner so that you are not jumping from area to area, both for client comfort and to prevent touching areas that have been treated.

The treatment plan

The treatment plan should include:

- area to be cleared and a consistent, organised visual aid showing how to attain the final desired result
- date
- time and timing of treatment
- area worked
- size and type of needle
- hair removed (clients should be told how many hairs are removed and with the 'treat and leave' technique, it is easy to count them).

All hair management techniques should be discussed as part of the treatment plan to manage the client's hair growth between treatments and while the course of epilation is continuing (see the section on hair management techniques on page 401).

Working cost-effectively

It is important to complete services in the given time so that you are cost-effective. It is not advisable to over-treat or go over time and you must ensure the client pays for work carried out and is not overcharged.

The costs of individual epilation treatment and courses of treatment vary considerably around the UK and depend not only on region but location, standard of premises, experience of therapists and client base. In addition, single treatments vary in time to suit a variety of clients and their own personal hair growth problems. Appointments can range from 5 minutes to 2 hours. Prices usually get less expensive the longer the session and a course usually offers a reduction of some type. On the other hand, many therapists offer a free aftercare product if a course is booked. This way you can ensure the client receives an excellent product, which will ensure good aftercare.

Remember

A skin in good condition will yield the hair on removal, preventing breakage and will ensure smoother insertion, making the treatment more comfortable.

Check it out

Research the competition! Find out what the rates for epilation treatments are in your area.

Regular treatments

Regular treatments are essential to achieve permanent hair removal. The following factors will affect the regularity of treatments and the speed of results:

- the scale of the hair growth problem
- the financial considerations
- the area to be treated
- regrowth time
- the size of the area to be treated
- the type and strength of hair
- the type of skin
- any underlying medical problem
- the healing rate of the client
- the client's pain threshold.

Hair growth rates

The growth pattern of the hair will influence present and future treatments. All hair goes though a life cycle that is timed by genes. This cycle can vary from a few months for an eyebrow hair to up to six years or even longer for a scalp hair – see the table below.

Type of hair	F = Female; M = Male	Regrowth time
Upper lip (vellus hair)	F	8–9 weeks
Upper lip (terminal)	F/M	4–6 weeks
Chin (vellus)	F	6–7 weeks
Chin (terminal)	F/M	5–6 weeks
Bikini line (terminal)	F	5–6 weeks
Eyebrows	F/M	5–6 weeks
Underarms (terminal)	F/M	7–8 weeks
Neck/nape (terminal)	F/M	5–6 weeks
Breast (terminal)	F	7–8 weeks
Chest (terminal)	M	6–7 weeks
Abdomen (terminal)	F	8–9 weeks
Fingers, toes (terminal)	F/M	6–8 weeks

Guideline estimates for regrowth of hair

It is advisable to be aware of the estimated rate at which hair grows on different parts of the body so that you can prepare an effective treatment plan and to understand that hairs that grow in treated areas before the normal regrowth time are hairs growing from untreated follicles. The client must understand that latent early anagen hairs account for the largest percentage of the 'regrowth problem'. If you feel at any time that progress is not being made or that the hair growth problem is getting worse, then it may be advisable to refer the client to his or her doctor for investigation into any possible underlying medical problem.

Each area of the body has a set number of hair follicles from birth. Most hair follicles are dormant or grow hair invisible to the human eye. New hair results only if a dormant follicle becomes active. There can be approximately 5,000–10,000 hair follicles per square inch depending on the part of the body.

Equipment and materials

Trolley layout

On a clean and sterile trolley, lay out the items shown below. The tiers of the trolley may be lined with couch roll. However, always read manufacturers' instructions as some epilation units must be placed on a clear surface as they are designed for continuous use and have a cooling fan which can get blocked with tiny tissue particles.

A suggested trolley layout

First tier:

Epilation unit and accessories
Bowl with cotton wool pads
Client record card/treatment plan
Alcohol steriliser (e.g. Steritane)
Aftercare creams/gels (small selection)
Kidney bowl with a sterilised pair
  of tweezers
Timer

Second tier:
Sharps box
Box of tissues
Boxes of needles – a good selection
Aftercare leaflets
After creams/gels (further selection)
Skin and hair graphics

Third tier:
Bowl for the client's jewellery
Box of disposable gloves
Mirror
Fresh towels
Space for the client's belongings, e.g. handbag

- covered container with sterilised chuck cap and tweezers
- sterilising fluid container
- covered container for used tweezers and chuck caps

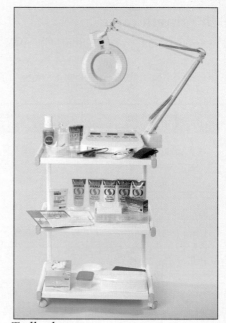

Trolley layout

The working area

- The trolley and magnification lamp should be within easy reach of treatment.
- Ensure the treatment room is not too hot. Otherwise the client may perspire, which will make epilation more difficult as the skin will become moist. This can cause the therapist to 'slip' and be unable to stretch the skin properly. Remember that an electrical current can be intensified when the skin is moist, and that perspiration forming on the skin would make the hair difficult to grip. The skin will have to be blotted with tissue frequently.
- Lighting is of major importance with epilation. Not only is good basic lighting required but also lighting from the magnification unit.

Magnification lamps

There are many different types of magnification lamps available including fixed or free standing, with attachments for the wall or attachments for trolleys. Some offer individually operated lights on both sides of a square-shaped glass (these allow shadows to be cast to assist removal of very fine blonde hair), others offer natural light or a high level of flexibility and are lightweight. If you opt for a flexible, lightweight round lamp without the individually controlled lights that the square lamps offer, then a tip is to have a snake wall light near to the areas worked in order to enable you to use this to cast shadow.

Keys to good practice

Use of magnification lamps is strongly recommended. For good clear vision, safety, hygiene and sometimes discretion, they are essential. The positioning of the lamp is vital in order not to distort the hairs or limit probing. Look through the centre of the magnification lamp and not at the edge – this can distort the image – and position it so that it is equidistant between the client and you.

With advanced epilation, it is possible to have a minute splatter of bodily fluids and the magnification lamp will protect you from this. It will also protect both your eyes and your back from strain, because you will not have to crouch so close to the client to see. When working on intimate areas such as the bikini line, a lamp will offer the client some discretion.

The correct working position

Great care must be taken with your own posture and positioning to ensure that back and shoulder fatigue or repetitive strain injury (RSI) do not occur. Correct positioning of the magnification lamp helps ensure the back and neck are kept straight, and a correct height for the stool also helps to prevent leaning over the client, which can cause back and neck strain or possible injury. Below are some tips for good posture:

- Keep your back as straight as possible.
- Have both feet firmly planted on the ground.
- Do not cross your legs.
- Ensure your neck and shoulders feel relaxed.
- Ensure your stool is the correct height.
- Change positions when working on different areas of the body.
- Ensure the couch is in a central position so you can move around it.
- Do not be afraid to move the client into a position that is comfortable and effective.
- To aid with accurate insertions, position yourself so that the wrist and elbow are aligned with the direction of hair when possible.
- Occasionally, you may need to lean on the client – use body weight lightly.
- Ensure equipment is easily accessible.
- Ensure correct positioning of the magnification lamp – the lens should be parallel to the treatment area, with enough space left to move the hands freely without touching the lens and with similar distance from the therapist's face.
- Ensure a clear view of the epilation unit for adjustment of the dials at all times.
- If right-handed, the therapist should sit on the right side of the client as he or she is lying down and vice-versa for left-handed therapists.

Remember

Always release each section of a magnification lamp by turning the nut to slacken and then move the section into position. Once positioned, tighten nut. This will ensure the magnification lamp remains stable. Failure to do this will result in a 'floppy' or unusable lamp.

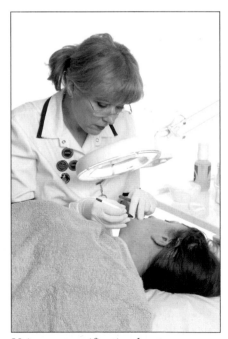

Using a magnification lamp

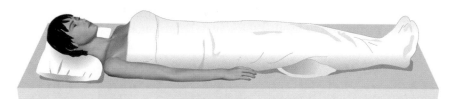

Standard supine position.

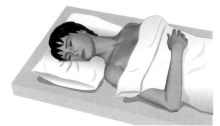

Side face – left

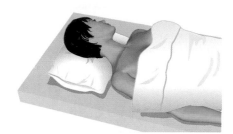

Side face – right

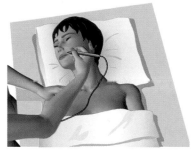

Lip, upper and lower

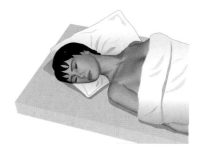

Chin – left

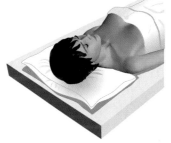

Chin – right

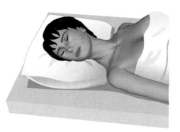

Under chin and throat – left

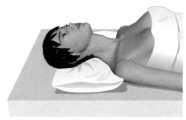

Under chin and throat – right

Facial working positions

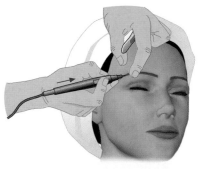

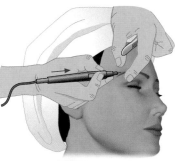

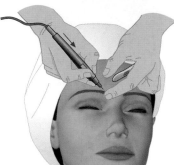

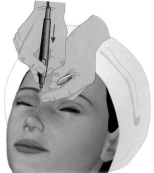

Positioning for eyebrows

> ### Remember
> These sequences are written for right-handed practitioners, so it is vice versa for left-handed practitioners.

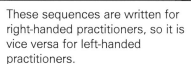

> ### Remember
> If right-handed, position yourself on the right side of the client as he or she is lying down. Vice versa for left-handed therapists. The therapist can also position herself behind the client for eyebrows or other areas when the direction of hair growth demands it.

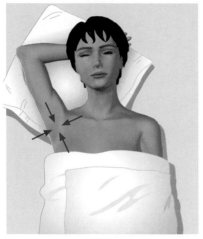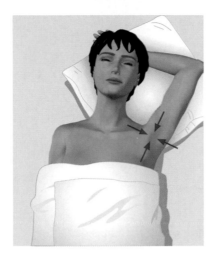

Positioning for underarms

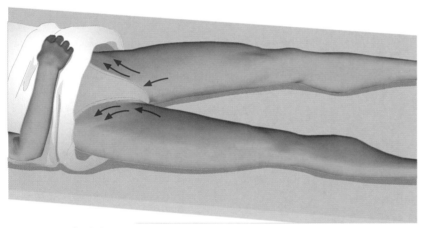

Positioning for bikini

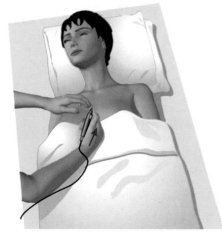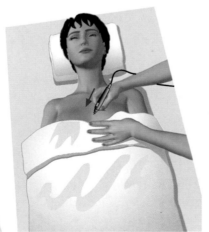

Positioning for breast

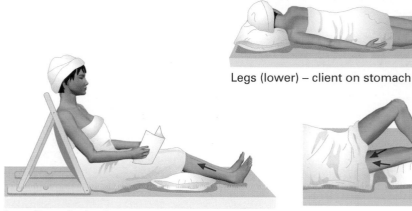

Legs (lower) – client on stomach

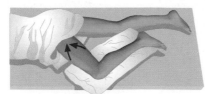

Legs – upper left outside

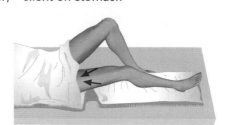

Legs – upper right outside

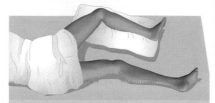

Legs – upper left inside

Legs (lower) – back rest

Positioning for legs

Hygiene and safety

As a therapist treating hair follicles using diathermy, galvanic and blend epilation techniques, you have responsibilities as laid down by:

- the Health and Safety at Work Act
- the Control of Substances Hazardous to Health Regulations
- the Electricity at Work Act
- local bye-laws relating to electrical epilation
- registration and approval from the local environmental health office. It is your responsibility to contact the local environmental health office to register with them. An environmental health officer will visit the salon and check on a number of criteria including sterilisation and disinfection methods used.

(For more information on hygiene and safety legislation, see **Professional basics**, page 50.)

Throughout the treatment, safety and hygiene are of vital importance for both the client and therapist's health and safety. For example, any waste products such as cotton pads or tissues used for wiping the skin must be disposed of immediately into a covered waste bin.

At the end of each treatment (or day at the salon), used chuck caps and tweezers should be gently scrubbed in hot water using a mild antiseptic wash and a special brush (e.g. baby's toothbrush) kept specifically for the purpose. This will ensure that any contaminated material present will be removed, and should be performed by the therapist with gloved hands for protection. The items should then be rinsed, dried and put in either an autoclave or liquid sterilant. This will ensure that any contaminated waste is not baked onto instruments used and that the sterilant is not contaminated or diluted, thereby allowing it to work effectively. (For information on the autoclave, see **Professional basics**, page 48.)

When ready to begin the treatment, wash your hands with an antibacterial hand wash, then dry with tissue, hot air or a clean towel. It is strongly recommended that you wear gloves for the treatment. It is advisable to have everything ready and prepared prior to treatment as it is pointless once gloved to perform other tasks such as placing the client's belongings on the trolley, positioning the bin nearer you, blowing your nose or coughing as the gloves will have picked up bacteria prior to treatment.

Keys to good practice

RSI can also be caused by incorrect tweezer technique. There are a number of different tweezer methods – try them to find out the one that suits you.

Keys to good practice

Each treatment requires a new needle, a new sterile chuck cap and a new sterile pair of tweezers!

Keys to good practice

Always protect your hands with rubber gloves when dealing with blood, chemicals or body fluids.

Remember

The sequences on page 415 are written for right-handed practitioners, vice versa for left-handed practitioners.

tep-by-step

Tweezer method – technique 1

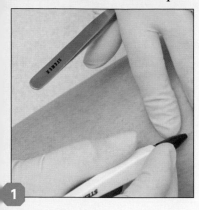

1 Hold needle holder in your right hand and tweezers in your left hand. Rest the tip of the tweezers between your thumb and the palm of your hand

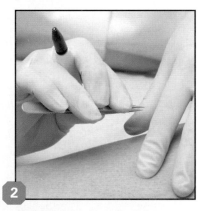

2 Slide the needle holder between your 2nd and 3rd fingers, using your thumb to push into place

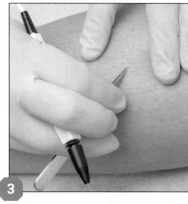

3 Take the tweezers from your left hand, with the thumb and forefinger of your right hand, and gently release epilated hair

Tweezer method – technique 2

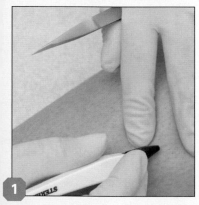

1 Hold needle holder in your right hand and tweezers in your left, with tip facing away from your client

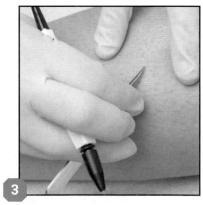

2 Slide the needle holder between your 2nd and 3rd fingers, using your thumb to push it into place

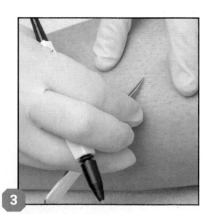

3 Take the tweezers from your left hand, with the thumb and forefinger of your right hand, and gently release epilated hair

Tweezer method – technique 3

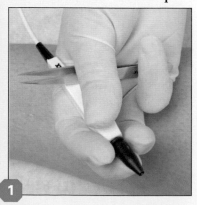

1 Hold tweezers and needle holder in the right hand and approach hair for epilating as in techniques 1 and 2

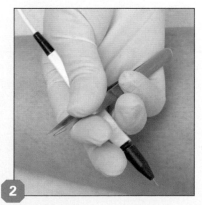

2 After treating, slide the needle holder between your 2nd and 3rd fingers, using your thumb to push it into place

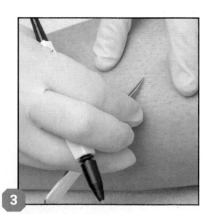

3 Manoeuvre the tweezers into position between your thumb and forefinger, and gently release the epilated hair

415

	Hazard (What can go wrong?)	Who could be harmed?
Hygiene	Cross-infection, contamination of equipment	You, the client, other therapists and colleagues and visitors to the salon
Equipment	Ineffective treatment Damage associated with faulty equipment, possible burns, skin blemishes. See contra-actions on page 436	The client; the salon owner and/or therapist because of possible litigation
Magnification lamp	If a lamp is left uncovered by a window on a sunny day, it will generate enough heat to burn or set fire to fabrics close by Injury to the client due to a loose-fitting joint connecting the lamp and its support	If a fire starts, everyone is at risk
Needles/tweezers	Needle stick injuries	Client/therapist
Allergies (see You and the skin)	Skin reaction caused by allergy to nickel/cotton wool fibres/product ingredients/latex and powder used in gloves	Client/therapist

Risk assessment for epilation

Prevention (How can I prevent this?)	Monitoring (How can I check?)	Corrective action (What do I do if things are not right?)
Use the most up-to-date effective methods of sterilisation Use sterilisation equipment and products in accordance with the manufacturers' recommendations Ensure your inoculation certification is valid Ensure regular maintenance of autoclave and other methods of sterilisation, scrupulous personal and salon hygiene Work to HASWA recommendations	Regularly test equipment Maintain inoculation records correctly Ensure regular inspection visits from professional bodies for insurance validation	Replace and regularly update equipment Follow the correct procedures for reporting infectious diseases and disorders (RIDDOR) (see **You, your client and the law**, page 74)
Ensure regular testing and maintenance of equipment Hold a valid certificate of insurance Ensure regular training and updating of skills	Maintain equipment correctly Machinery should have a sticker noting last service date	Ensure manufacturers' recommendations are followed Ensure spare accessories are available
Cover the lamp – follow manufacturer's instructions Avoid keeping lamp near to a window Use correctly following manufacturer's instructions Loosen nuts to move and tighten when positioned	Be aware of possible dangers Ensure regular maintenance of equipment	Maintain fire extinguishers and hold fire drills – all staff should be aware of evacuation procedures (see **Professional basics**, page 61) Withdraw from service if faulty
Follow manufacturer's instructions when loading and unloading needles Ensure correct treatment procedure is followed	Follow manufacturer's instructions	Injury to therapist – stop treatment immediately and follow first aid procedures Injury to client – immediately apply pressure to assist clotting and help prevent bruising
Hold a full consultation with client Use alternative products and specialised needles designed for allergies Use gloves without powder, and latex free	Monitor client reaction during treatment Hold a consultation update each visit/specifically check for delayed reactions Follow manufacturers' instructions for products and gloves	For client – immediately stop treatment, remove product if necessary and apply cool compress For therapist – wash hands and change gloves

You will also need to take preventative measures against cross-infection – see the risk assessment below (page 419). Viruses such as HIV and hepatitis B and C are transmitted by blood and blood-stained body fluids. Prevention of cross-infection can be achieved through:

- attention to personal hygiene
- thorough cleaning of treatment rooms
- cleaning and sterilisation of all equipment, tweezers and using disposable needles
- keeping cuts and abrasions covered
- hand washing before and after all client contact
- gloves worn at all times – a fresh pair for each client and for different areas worked
- correct disposal of clinical waste – an approved refuse collector must remove sharps boxes and contaminated waste. Contact your local council refuse department, which will arrange regular collection. The health and safety officer will provide information on contaminated waste removal, and sometimes local pharmacists or hospitals will dispose of your sharps boxes.

(Refer also to Unit G1, Ensure your actions reduce risks to health and safety.)

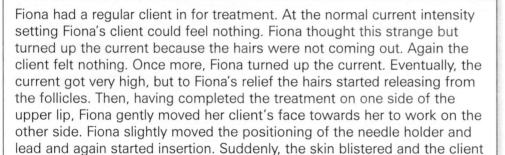

In the salon

Fiona had a regular client in for treatment. At the normal current intensity setting Fiona's client could feel nothing. Fiona thought this strange but turned up the current because the hairs were not coming out. Again the client felt nothing. Once more, Fiona turned up the current. Eventually, the current got very high, but to Fiona's relief the hairs started releasing from the follicles. Then, having completed the treatment on one side of the upper lip, Fiona gently moved her client's face towards her to work on the other side. Fiona slightly moved the positioning of the needle holder and lead and again started insertion. Suddenly, the skin blistered and the client jumped in pain.

- What did Fiona forget to do?
- What should she do now?

Remember

Always check that the electrical machinery you are about to use shows its electrical maintenance check date and that it is current. Ensure that the wires and leads are not frayed or loose and follow the manufacturer's recommended test to ensure that the leads are in good working order. Leads are made of very fine copper fibres, which if coiled too tightly can break. This can cause the current to become intermittent and unpredictable.

Treat hair follicles using diathermy, galvanic and blend epilation techniques

BT16.4

In this outcome you will learn about

- aseptic procedures
- skin and hair types
- sizes and types of needles
- carrying out the treatment
- possible faults
- contra-actions
- aftercare and home care.

Aseptic procedures

Loading and unloading the needle holder

A new sterile needle is required for each client. You must avoid contaminating the needle by ensuring fingers, tweezers, etc. do not come into contact with it.

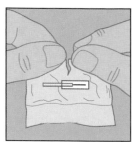

1. Slacken chuck cap ready to accept the needle but do not remove it. Tear open the packet and withdraw the sterile needle by the protective sleeve (some needle holders have removeable chucks; if yours is one of these remove the chuck first.

INSTRUCTIONS: Follow these simple instructions and you will be able to load your needle quickly and easily without contamination.

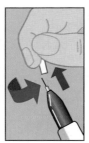 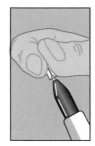 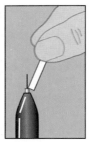

2. The needle, complete with protective sleeve, should be inserted fully into the chuck and the cap tightened.

3. Now remove the protective sleeve with a twist and pull. Your needle is now ready to use.

4. If you wish to alter the position of the needle, slacken the chuck slightly and use the plastic sleeve

Needle loading instructions

It is important to load the needle into the needle holder correctly. Manufacturers have produced many different needle holders and needles which all load differently, so whichever needle holder you use, follow the manufacturer's instructions to ensure aseptic loading. If the needle is contaminated in any way, cross-infection could take place and infections or diseases could be passed on. If the needle is damaged, for example upon removal of the plastic sleeve or knocking the magnification lamp, then it should be disposed of and a new one loaded. Not only could cross-infection occur but also once a needle is bent, the metal is weakened and current could build up or be discharged at the weakened section, resulting in skin damage.

To load the needle into the needle holder:

*   Wear gloves.
*   Unscrew the chuck cap so that it is loose but do not remove.
*   Open the needle sachet without touching the needle.
*   Holding the plastic cap, position the needle into the needle holder.
*   Screw the chuck cap back on until the needle is held tightly.
*   With gloved fingers, twist and pull the plastic covering off.

To unload the needle from the needle holder:

*   Wear gloves.
*   Unscrew the chuck cap.
*   Position the needle holder facing downwards, over the sharps box, holding the loosened chuck cap. Gently tap the holder to allow the needle to fall into the box.
*   If the needle does not move, slacken the chuck cap a little more and repeat the procedure.
*   If the needle still does not move, gently grip and pull out the needle with tweezers while positioned facing downwards over the sharps box.

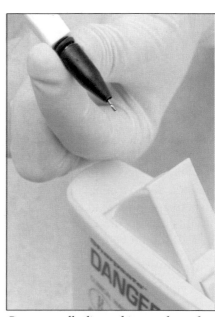

Correct needle disposal into a sharps box

If the needle cannot be removed easily, check that the clamps supporting the needle underneath the chuck cap are of the correct grip. If loosening is required, gently press on these grips to pull them apart fractionally. However, if they are too loose, apply gentle pressure with a small pair of pliers to tighten them. This should then ensure the correct disposal of the needle.

Skin and hair types

The outer appearance of the skin and hair both act as a guide for different strategies when giving an effective electrolysis treatment.

The thickness of the epidermis affects the treatment. For example, a thin epidermis will react with almost immediate erythema because the epidermis is nearly transparent and the blood can be seen through it, whereas a thicker epidermal region with a deeper hair follicle may not react so quickly and may require deeper than normal insertions with a regular needle rather than a short one. The length of the needle depends on the average depth of the hair follicles in the area to be treated. In general, dark terminal hairs lie deeper than fine dark and vellus hairs.

A firm or soft skin can also affect an epilation treatment because of the ease or otherwise of needle insertion:

- the chin is an example of a firm area
- the breast an example of a soft area where a greater stretch will be required with difficult insertions because of the skin's resilience in this area
- the abdomen is surprisingly sensitive with the hair proving very strong, therefore a firm stretch is required due to the resilient nature of the skin and lack of underlying bone support
- fingers and toes are sensitive and hair can be difficult to remove. The depth of insertion generally is superficial, so a low intensity for a longer time is recommended.

Type of hair growth

The type of hair growth – vellus, coarse/terminal, fine, curly, straight or compound – will affect the choice of method of epilation, intensity and timing. Fine hair is often accelerated lanugo or vellus hair and although the hair is fine, it will be anchored into the follicle very firmly and will require more time on a lower intensity. Fine vellus hair may have no papilla and may be located in and feed off the sebaceous gland. Darker and thicker hairs require higher intensity than finer, less dense hairs. Curly hairs may have distorted hair follicles and probing accuracy can prove difficult with no obvious or clear insertion, with the blend method offering most success. Insertions too close to each other result in over-treatment of the area (often performed on dark deep terminal hairs with a close proximity to each other) and can cause hyperpigmentation to occur and possible pitting. If the hairs are too long to treat, cut them, allowing the angle of growth to be seen more easily. The darkest and heaviest growth should be removed first so that the client can see immediate progress.

Curvy follicle growth
- The hair replacement cycle of curly hair is just the same as straight hair.
- Curved follicles can be found on white as well as black skin, but are predominantly found in black skin.
- The amount of follicle curvature is related to the flatness of the hair shaft.
- In most curved superfluous hair, the lower quarter of the follicle turns at an obtuse angle from the follicle proper and this angle causes the flattening of the hair structure. It is the flattened shape which gives rise to the curling of the hair shaft.

> **Remember**
>
> To analyse follicle depth, grasp the hair with the tweezers at the surface of the skin and gently tweezer it out following the direction of growth. The distance from the tweezer to the root of the hair is the depth of the hair follicle. Select a needle that is slightly longer than the measured depth and ensure the depth of insertion is accurate.

- The curl of the hair above skin level is greater than the follicle curvature in the skin. This is because the part of the root encased in the root sheaths is still in a newly formed, moist condition – the hair does not begin to curl until it has left the sheaths and it begins to dry.
- Treatment for curved follicle growth must be given special consideration. Insert the needle on the underside of the hair. It may be necessary to push past a tissue obstruction and continue down about half as far again and release the current. When the hair releases, check the depth and use this depth as your guide.

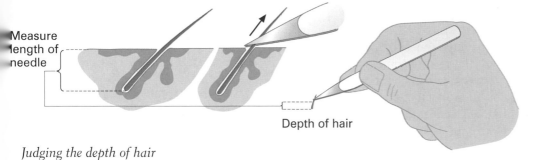

Judging the depth of hair

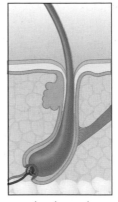
J - shaped

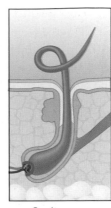
Corkscrew

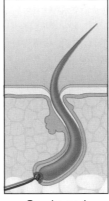
S - shaped

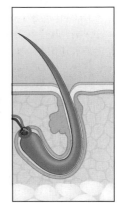
U - shaped

Distorted hair follicles

Corkscrew hair

This is a distorted hair follicle and is produced by the remains of an almost destroyed pilosebaceous unit, which has become disorientated and has not re-formed properly. To treat, see curly follicle growth above.

Single hair

A single hair grows from a single follicle and is treated by lining up the needle with the hair and inserting gently into the follicle. Adequate current is used and the needle is removed. The hair is then gently released from the follicle by the use of tweezers.

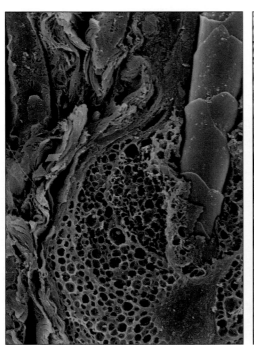
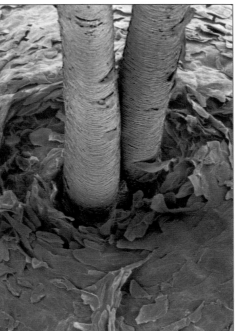

Different types of follicle – single and compound

Compound hairs

These are also known as pili multigemini. The follicle has two or more dermal papilla, which results in two or more hairs growing from the same follicle. Treat the larger hair with the current. This may well affect both hairs. Gently release the treated hair and then try to remove the second hair; if it has been successful, the hair will epilate easily. If using the blend method wait to see if the hair releases after some time has passed. If not, the hair can be treated as a single hair when deemed appropriate and not overtreated. If the hairs are 'blasted' separately, then too much current may be unnecessarily used and could cause skin damage.

Ingrowing hair

An ingrowing hair is one that grows abnormally under the skin having been covered by an overgrowth of skin. There are several reasons for this: some people are genetically disposed towards them; waxing or tweezing hairs often cause them, when the hair breaks at the weakest point just below the surface of the skin. Waxing, in particular, can distort the hair, especially if pulled against the direction of growth. The hair then tends to grow under the surface of the skin rather than up and out of the hair follicle.

Men with heavy hair growth can have this problem. When they shave closely, the hair pulls back into the hair follicle and sometimes its direction of growth is altered, causing ingrowing hairs. The hairs can continue to grow just beneath the skin's surface and may become infected. If not infected, the trapped end should be freed from the skin to release it either using a one-piece needle, a microlance or a professional sterilised pair of sharp-tipped tweezers. Once released, if not infected, the hair can be treated with epilation or allowed to heal as required. If infected, antiseptic cream should be applied and if necessary antibiotics prescribed by a GP. Ingrowing hairs often resolve soon after electrolysis is started.

Embedded hair

These can be recognised by the appearance of bumps on the skin, irritation, erythema and hair being seen under the skin. There are many causes including friction, irritation and dry skin. To treat this condition, see ingrowing hair above.

Unshed telogen hair

Telogen hair that fails to shed appears in the form of a shaved or clipped stump and can become infected. It is usually colourless and occurs when a telogen hair that is quite wide reaches the skin's surface. Telogen hair is difficult to see and does not usually grow in length. It lacks pigmentation because the hair has lost contact with the source of pigmentation after separating from the dermal papilla. Treat these hairs as normal in telogen stage.

Tombstone hair

This is a small hair that has been epilated in the anagen stage of hair growth, but remains in the skin. The therapist will probably have removed a hair from a follicle in the telogen stage, without realising a new anagen hair was forming underneath. Such hair is thick, very dark, brittle and looks like a 'foreign body' or 'rotting stump' at the surface of the skin. It does not usually need to be epilated – cleansing and exfoliating the skin or tweezing it out is usually sufficient.

Lanugo comedones

These are a tiny bundle of lanugo hairs protruding from a follicle or follicles. They may appear as a short, thick brown hair, resembling a comedone. When examined closely, this is made up of a number of very fine lanugo hairs held together by sebum, as they can arise from the sebaceous gland. There is a tendency for them to be found on oily, seborrohoeic skin. These comedones can be tweezed out without traction.

Skin types

Refresh your memory about skin types and the skin's structure and functions by referring to **You and the skin** and **Related anatomy and physiology**.

The following skin type information applies mainly to white skin, although it is possible to have several aspects relating to ethnic skins. Clients must be treated as individuals based on the information obtained at consultation, especially clients who may have a combination of the differing skin categories.

Oily/combination skin

Sebum is found in abundance in this skin type. It is the insulating properties of sebum that are of benefit during a short wave diathermy treatment. Provided there is correct probing technique and intensity of current, as it reaches the surface of the skin the sebum will protect the epidermis from the effects of the current. However, any surface oil should be completely removed. The moisture content of this skin type is usually good, which plays an important part in conduction of the current. Insertion of the needle will usually be relatively easy because of dilated pores common in this skin type. Care must be taken when working near any papules or pustules as the pH balance of the skin may also be affected, which could cause infection in the area. The skin texture is often thicker than that of normal or dry skin.

Dry or dehydrated skin

Dry skin is usually lacking in sebum and moisture content and will take longer to heal, so additional space should be left between probes as well as a longer time between treatments to ensure a safe and effective outcome. Dry or dehydrated skin can present difficulties because both short wave diathermy and direct current require moisture to work effectively. Dead skin cells may also block the follicle opening, causing difficulty with needle insertion. It is important to also consider the skin's reaction.

Moist skin

This skin type has a high moisture content in both the epidermis and dermis. When there are varying degrees of moisture found on the facial area, there may be changes to the intensity, timing and skin reaction in the various areas, and these must all be noted. Blend is the more suitable current because of the lower intensity of short wave diathermy current. The use of short wave diathermy current on this skin type is not recommended as the current may rise too quickly to the surface of the skin before effective treatment of the lower follicle.

Sensitive/mature skin

This skin type will react quickly to epilation with a pronounced erythema and the client's pain threshold may also be affected, so the current intensity should be as low as possible. Length of treatment, spacing of insertions and treatments will also have to be taken into consideration, to ensure no unfavourable reactions occur. The blend method may prove more suitable for this skin type because of the lower intensity of the short wave diathermy current. Skin sensitivity can appear, with allergy to products or treatment.

Global origins

Clients' ethnic origins will directly affect the type of treatment chosen. Their follicle shape and depth will impact on all aspects of the treatment including the treatment plan and needle choice.

There are a number of differences between the structures of white, black, Asian and Chinese-type skins, so each skin type should be treated differently when epilation is being carried out. People of different ethnic origins have differing amounts of hair. Northern Europeans (including people from Britain and Scandinavia) have less hair than people from Asia. Black people have relatively little hair, while people with Chinese-type skin have the least body hair.

Black skin

- The stratum corneum of the epidermis is much thicker and skin desquamates more easily.
- Collagen fibres are more numerous, making it stronger.
- The ageing process is slower because the elasticity in the skin lasts longer.
- Sebaceous glands are more numerous and larger.
- A greater number of sebaceous glands open onto the skin's surface instead of into a hair follicle.
- Suderiferous glands are more numerous and larger.
- The suderiferous duct opens onto the surface of the skin – it is longer and more obvious.

Advice on epilation

- Curly and distorted hair follicles are a consideration.
- Black skin tends to hyperpigmentate more than white skin (although this can rectify itself).
- When a hair regrows in a hair follicle that has been treated previously, it grows straight and very shallow. This hair can then be treated as for hair on white skin.
- It is difficult to detect erythema, so there is a risk of over-treating.
- The area can be prone to heat retention and swelling as the skin is extremely sensitive to heat.
- The skin is prone to keloid scarring – ensure a full and accurate consultation.
- Complete a short test treatment to assess healing rate.
- The preferred method of treatment should be blend so that the sodium hydroxide (lye) produced reaches the curved hair follicles effectively. Consider a gold needle for less skin reaction. If using short wave diathermy, use an insulated needle so that the current is concentrated at the tip of the needle to reduce surface reaction, and ensure current is of a low intensity.
- Difficulty probing a curved hair follicle can be experienced as the hair shaft is usually flattened. Ensure firm but light stretch is used and positioning of body is correct.
- Use the correct diameter of needle, matching the diameter of hair treated.
- Space out the treatments and the probing area – one in five to prevent overheating of the skin tissue.
- Ensure aftercare is applied immediately – use a compress of witch hazel or aloe vera gel.
- Discuss home care advice and give the client an aftercare leaflet.
- Book the next treatment after sufficient healing time has occurred.

Key terms

Keloids – elevated fibrous enlargements of the skin, most commonly found at the site of a scar. A skin reaction to injury, they are usually raised, smooth and firm. They are most frequently found on black skin and the person usually has a congenital disposition to keloid scarring.

Asian skin

- Normally a finer texture than black skin.
- The skin colour can vary from dark brown to light brown.
- The hair growth tends to be fine, dark and dense, although dark and coarse hairs may be found among the finer hairs.
- The fine hairs usually grow from follicles that are small, straight and superficial to the skin's surface.
- This skin type is prone to sensitivity and increased pigmentation.
- The pigmentation may not be evident for several days or weeks and can take many months to fade.

Advice on epilation

- The blend method is recommended, teamed with a gold needle to combat sensitivity and problematic reaction.
- If the short wave diathermy method is used, ensure a low intensity and use an insulated needle to keep the intensity in the lower half of the follicle.
- Space out the treatments and the probing area.
- Avoid over-treating the area and allow sufficient healing time.

Chinese-type skin

Chinese-type skin is prone to pigmentation, sensitivity, discoloration and pit marks due to over-exposure to heat.

Advice on epilation

- See the advice for Asian skin above.
- The pores will usually be small and tight, so a size 2 or 3 short needle may be required.

Sizes and types of needles

There are many manufacturers of needles, including Sterex, which developed the world's first sterile disposable needle. Types of needles include two-piece, one-piece, gold and insulated needles. Needles are made from the highest quality materials, with a polished tip for perfect insertion comfort. They are most commonly sterilised using gamma irradiation and are guaranteed for five years with a visible date mark.

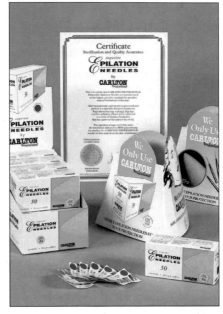

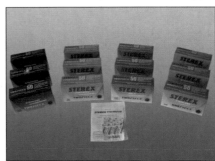

A selection of needles

> *Needle types*
> - Two-piece needles: available in stainless steel, gold and insulated.
> - Stainless steel: available in sizes 2, 3, 4, 5, 6 and 10 (size 10 for advanced techniques).
> - Gold: available in sizes 2, 3, 4 and 5.
> - Insulated: available in sizes 2, 3, 4 and 5.
> - One-piece needles: available in sizes 2, 3, 4 and 5.

Remember

The electrolysis needle fulfils two roles:

- to position the needle
- to conduct the current.

The smaller the size number, the thinner the needle. Therefore, when treating fine hair, a 2 or 3 needle which is 0.02 or 0.03 of a millimetre would be selected. To work on very coarse hair, a size 6 might be chosen; 4 and 5 are used for hairs of in-between thickness.

The choice of diameter of needle is essential to the effectiveness of the treatment. A smaller needle is easier to insert into a larger follicle. It is wrongly believed that by using a smaller needle than is suitable, less discomfort is caused. In reality, a greater discomfort is caused because the same current is released from a smaller surface area, thus causing a more concentrated expulsion of current.

Importance of using the correct diameter of needle

It is important to use the correct diameter of the needle:

*   to ensure that the destructive agent (heat or chemical) is adequate to be effective
*   to help prevent (diathermy) heat rising to the surface and damaging the surface of the skin
*   to prevent skin damage and over-treatment if too large a needle is used
*   to prevent needle movement within the follicle if the needle used is too small
*   because the smaller the size of the needle, the smaller the surface area and the sharper it is, causing a more intense sensation for the client.

Two-piece needles are also available in different shaft lengths (the part that goes in the follicle) – short is 3/16th of an inch long; regular is $\frac{1}{4}$ of an inch long. Short is recommended for the face and regular for the body, but all clients are different and it really is a matter of the therapist's personal preference and client requirements.

There are also different shank sizes (the part that fits into the needle holder) – F and K. F is the standard size for the UK. They are both the same length, but F has a larger diameter than K, which is much thinner.

The difference between two-piece and one-piece needles

A two-piece needle is a strong yet flexible needle offering the therapist essential flexibility and 'feel'. This type of needle flexes when it meets resistance, indicating to the therapist whether the insertion is correct or incorrect.

The one-piece needle is more rigid, and is ideal for advanced techniques and for the experienced therapist.

Gold needles

The benefits of using gold needles include the following.

*   Smoother insertion. Gold is a very smooth metal and glides into the follicle more easily than other needles, proving more comfortable for the client, with less erythema.
*   Gold ensures a more comfortable treatment. It is an excellent conductor of electricity, which sometimes allows the current to be reduced resulting in a more comfortable treatment for the client and less erythema.
*   Gold is hypoallergenic and is suitable for those with allergic reactions to metal and for sensitive skins.

Insulated needles

These are coated with a medical-grade insulation material and are used in hospitals in the lining of catheters, heart bypass tubing and endoscopes. They are recommended for the client who has sensitive skin and are suitable for the flash technique.

They offer the therapist more choice and freedom to treat even the most difficult skins. By insulating the needle all the way down its surface leaving only the very tip exposed, they help prevent heat (diathermy) rising to the surface of the skin, concentrate the current at the hair root and offer a smooth insertion. Insulated

> **Remember**
>
> Always follow the manufacturer's instructions when using needles.

> **Remember**
>
> The client may be allergic to nickel, in which case gold needles should be used, or if allergic to gold, insulated needles may be used.

> **In the salon**
>
> The flash technique uses a very high current for a very short period of time. This method is popular in the US but is not widely used in the UK. The heating pattern is very different with a narrower field of current spread. Specialised equipment is required for this technique.

needles are recommended for diathermy only as there is evidence to suggest that the insulation material can be distorted by the chemical sodium hydroxide produced when using blend or galvanic.

Carrying out the treatment

There are many different types of epilator available, including:

- computerised units costing many thousands of pounds that will calculate the amount of hair that is removed and allow you to program in the client's details
- units that will allow you to operate DC and AC separately (or together)
- modern digitalised units which offer three-in-one modalities
- simple straightforward diathermy or galvanic only units.

Methods of epilation

To refresh your memory about the types of electrical current, see **Facial treatments – theory and consultation**, page 225.

There are three different methods of epilation:

- galvanic (meaning 'direct current')
- high frequency
- blend.

Galvanic electrolysis

This is the first form of electrical epilation and uses a direct current (a current that flows in one direction only) through a circuit consisting of one negative and one positive electrode. When a direct current passes through an electrolyte containing ions, the ions move in opposite directions.

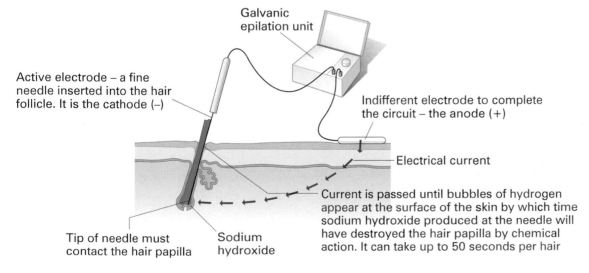

Galvanic epilation unit

Active electrode – a fine needle inserted into the hair follicle. It is the cathode (–)

Indifferent electrode to complete the circuit – the anode (+)

Electrical current

Current is passed until bubbles of hydrogen appear at the surface of the skin by which time sodium hydroxide produced at the needle will have destroyed the hair papilla by chemical action. It can take up to 50 seconds per hair

Tip of needle must contact the hair papilla

Sodium hydroxide

Destruction of the hair follicle by galvanic electrolysis

The ions carry the current. When this is applied to tissue salts and moisture or a salt/water solution, 'electrolysis' takes place. The salt and water split into their chemical elements, which then rearrange themselves to form entirely new substances. In galvanic electrolysis, the client holds the anode connected to the positive outlet on the epilation machine and the needle holder electrode is connected to the negative outlet and therefore negatively charged. A needle is inserted into the hair follicle which contains water (H_2O) and salt (NaCl) which together act as a natural electrolyte. This increases the conductivity of the skin and allows the current to flow freely through the skin. The direct current causes a chemical reaction resulting in the atoms of the salt and water breaking down.

The atoms split into negatively and positively charged ions called cations and anions which rearrange themselves to form completely different chemical substances – sodium hydroxide (NaOH), a strong caustic alkali, provides the destructive force in galvanic electrolysis, and hydrogen gas (H_2) at the cathode and chlorine gas at the anode, which in turn change into hydrochloric acid.

Galvanic electrolysis is a very effective method of permanent hair removal and offers a wide field of tissue destruction which is useful for curved and distorted follicles. However, a minimum of ten seconds is required for each hair, making it an effective but slow treatment.

Formulation of lye

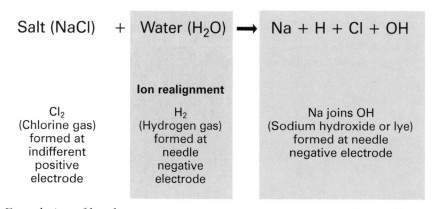

Formulation of lye chart

Source: Sterex

Benefits of galvanic

- Generally less discomfort than other methods
- Chemical reaction has a wider field of destruction
- More effective (but much slower) method
- Can treat distorted follicles
- Current is attracted to the area of greatest moisture (the dermal papilla), therefore less risk of surface over-treatment as the moisture gradient of the skin ensures the action is kept below the skin's surface.

High frequency treatment

High frequency, radio frequency, thermolysis or short wave diathermy is an alternating (oscillating) current of very high frequency and low voltage ranging from 2–30 MHz or 3–30 million cycles per second. This method directs the radio frequency to the moist tissue at the base of the hair. The moisture in the cells resists the radiant energy and heats up only to be dehydrated and destroyed. These light waves heat the moist living tissue and the dry keratinised tissue of the epidermal wall of the surrounding hair follicle is left unaffected. This is similar to placing meat in a paper bag into the microwave – the meat will be heated enough to be cooked, yet the bag will be unaffected.

By the 1930s, short wave diathermy began to replace the galvanic method because of its ability to destroy tissue in milliseconds rather than minutes. However, the disadvantage of short wave diathermy was its high percentage of regrowth coupled with its inability to treat curly or distorted follicles.

In short wave diathermy treatment, the molecules within the tissues are altered. The rapid agitation of atoms causes them to vibrate against each other resulting in friction which, in turn, causes heat to concentrate close to the needle tip, known as the high frequency field. Therefore, the friction that is produced by these oscillations (cycles) produces heat that builds up in the hair follicle and destroys tissue by either cauterisation or coagulation. Therapists aim at coagulation (where the cellular structure in the tissue breaks down and protein is congealed) of the lower hair follicle in order to destroy it without damaging the surrounding tissue

Benefits of diathermy

- Quick treatment time.
- Many hairs removed in one sitting.
  a
- Flash can be used.
- Some clients prefer the sensation of short sharp sting.

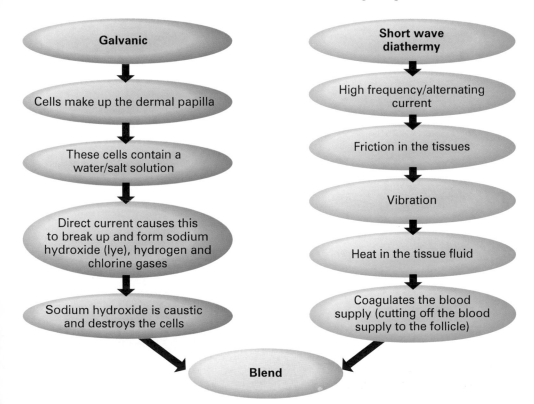

The three currents used in epilation – galvanic, short wave diathermy and blend

Blend

The thoroughness of galvanic electrolysis and the speed of short wave diathermy have been combined to produce a method of permanent hair removal known as the blend. It was introduced to the UK in 1987 and has been steadily growing in popularity because of its effectiveness. The principle of the blend is to enhance the chemical action of galvanic electrolysis with the application of high frequency simultaneously. Both currents retain their own individuality and work together to provide the most effective method in a versatile, efficient and comfortable treatment. It is suitable in treating any type of hair follicle including curly or distorted hairs because of its wide and deep field of destruction, and the regrowth experienced with shortwave diathermy is reduced.

Blend is primarily a galvanic treatment with minimal use of the short wave diathermy current. Short wave diathermy's only function (in blend treatments) is to produce warmth to speed up the chemical reaction brought about by the galvanic current. This warmth heats the sodium hydroxide (lye) as it is produced within the follicle by the galvanic current and makes it a more effective destructive pattern as well as creating more receptive skin tissues.

Step-by-step

Blend epilation application

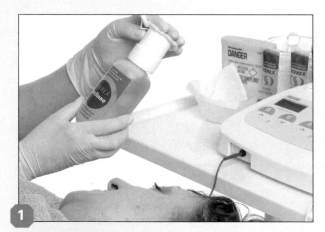

1

Prior to treatment the skin must be cleansed

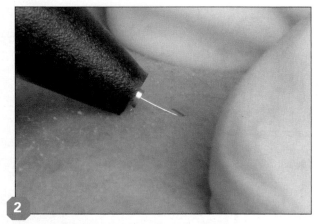

2

The needle is 'lined up' with a chosen hair

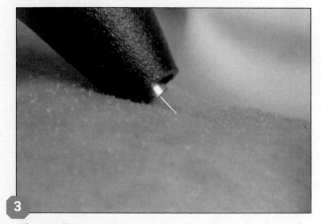

3

The needle is gently inserted to the correct depth

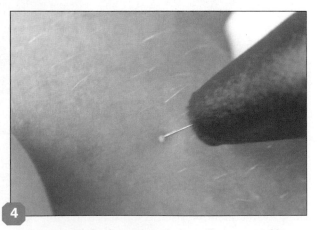

4

The current is discharged and a small amount of lye appears at the follicle opening

Benefits of blend

- Quicker treatment time than galvanic alone.
- Less regrowth than with short wave diathermy.
- Chemical reaction when mixed with warmth proving the most effective destruction pattern and results.
- Less discomfort than short wave diathermy.
- Effective on curved and distorted follicles.
- Current is attracted to the area of greatest moisture (the dermal papilla), therefore there is less risk of surface over-treatment as the moisture gradient of the skin ensures the action is kept below the skin's surface.
- When blended the lye becomes more turbulent, enabling it to invade all parts of the follicle.
- The warmth of the diathermy affects the tissues surrounding the dermal papilla, causing them to become more porous and allowing the caustic lye to diffuse into them, making the treatment more thorough.
- Research indicates that the wide field of effectiveness destroys any hair germ cells which may develop at a later date.
- Effectiveness is ensured as research indicates the lye remains in the follicle for a period of time after treatment.

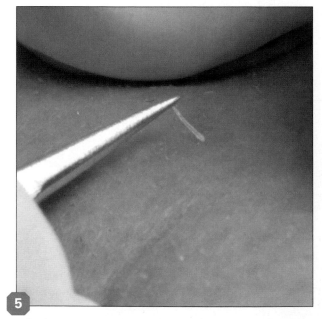

5 The hair is removed. In this instance the hair is removed complete with sheath

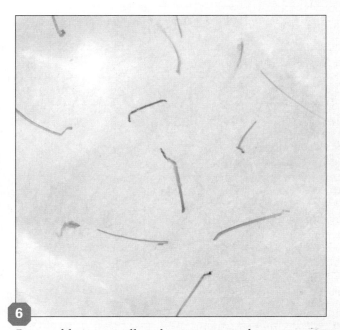

6 Removed hairs are collected on a cotton pad

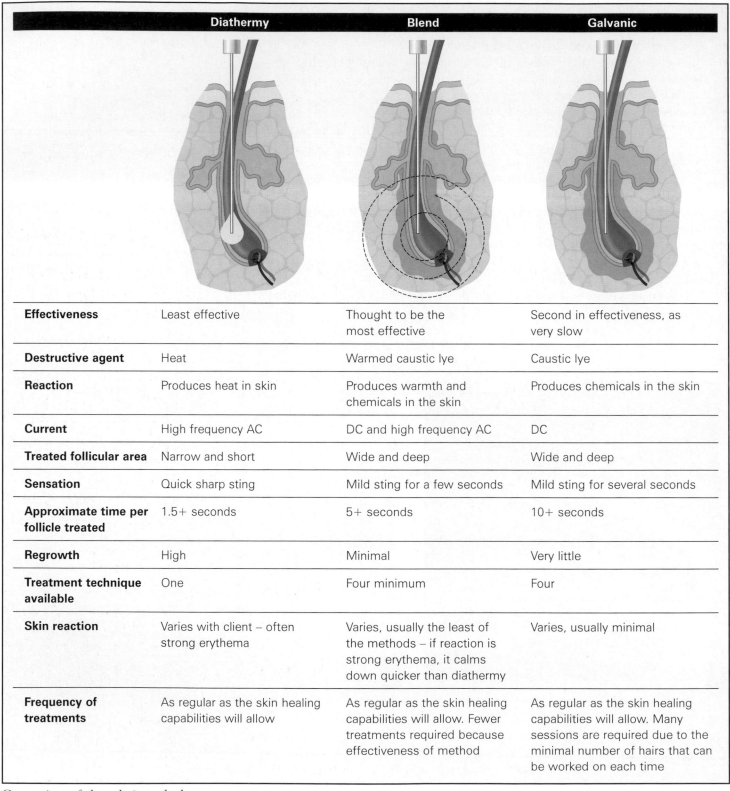

	Diathermy	Blend	Galvanic
Effectiveness	Least effective	Thought to be the most effective	Second in effectiveness, as very slow
Destructive agent	Heat	Warmed caustic lye	Caustic lye
Reaction	Produces heat in skin	Produces warmth and chemicals in the skin	Produces chemicals in the skin
Current	High frequency AC	DC and high frequency AC	DC
Treated follicular area	Narrow and short	Wide and deep	Wide and deep
Sensation	Quick sharp sting	Mild sting for a few seconds	Mild sting for several seconds
Approximate time per follicle treated	1.5+ seconds	5+ seconds	10+ seconds
Regrowth	High	Minimal	Very little
Treatment technique available	One	Four minimum	Four
Skin reaction	Varies with client – often strong erythema	Varies, usually the least of the methods – if reaction is strong erythema, it calms down quicker than diathermy	Varies, usually minimal
Frequency of treatments	As regular as the skin healing capabilities will allow	As regular as the skin healing capabilities will allow. Fewer treatments required because effectiveness of method	As regular as the skin healing capabilities will allow. Many sessions are required due to the minimal number of hairs that can be worked on each time

Comparison of electrolysis methods

Mixing methods

The method chosen should be jointly agreed between the therapist and the client. The severity of the hair growth will influence that decision. If the client has a large amount of superfluous hair, then short wave diathermy taking only one second or so per hair will clear the area in salon treatment time, allowing the psychological benefits this can bring. It may be that a section, for example just the upper lip, can be treated with blend. Once the blend area has been cleared, a further section can be set aside for blend treatments.

With this method of working, the client gains the benefit of the most effective method teamed with the greatest number of hairs removed. For example, with an area of dense and scattered hair growth, it is important to work systematically and methodically. Use short wave diathermy in order to clear the area quickly with treatment duration of up to one hour per week, which will, over a period of time, change to treating a specific area (e.g. upper lip) with blend. Then as the hair weakens and starts to disappear, move to fortnightly sessions with blend on upper lip and chin. Eventually, blend treatments only will be used for the remaining hair. The length and frequency of treatments will be determined by the appearance of regrowth, and the needle size will reduce as treatment continues.

Treatment techniques: blend

With the Sterex SX-B blend epilator, there are four main treatment techniques available. A combination of the four will enable you to tailor the treatment to suit the client.

Treatment technique number 1

Technique number 1 is the main technique and used first, but if the client feels uncomfortable, one of the other three techniques (see page 434) can be used. Ask the client after each increase if he or she is happy with the sensation, but do not inform the client that you have just increased the current, rather that you are adjusting the current. Discuss the sensations felt by the client, as you can offer other techniques and combinations of techniques to suit each client to ensure acceptable comfort levels at all times.

1 Prepare the client.
2 Give the client the indifferent electrode to hold – you may wrap a damp tissue around it if the client's hands are dry. It is recommended to remove the client's jewellery.
3 Seat yourself comfortably, and ensure you have easy access to the footswitch.
4 Use needles appropriate to the size and length of the follicle.
5 Attach all accessories.
6 Switch on the SX-B at the back of the epilator ensuring there is nothing blocking the fan situated beneath the unit, e.g. towels/couch roll.
7 Switch on the diathermy, galvanic and timer sections – the digital readouts will Register 01 or 00.
8 Using the slow up button, increase the timer to 5.0 seconds.
9 To alter the diathermy intensity, depress the foot pedal and using the slow up button increase to 3 or 4. Do not be concerned if the numbers fluctuate up or down a number as this is normal with digital readouts and does not mean the current is fluctuating.
10 To alter the galvanic intensity, depress the foot pedal and using the slow up button increase to .10 – do not be concerned if the numbers fluctuate up or down one.
11 When you remove your foot from the foot pedal, the digital readouts on the currents will go back to 00 or 01.
12 Insert the needle into a typical follicle in the area you wish to treat and depress the foot pedal. When you hear the 'beep' after 5 seconds, remove your foot from the foot pedal.
13 Test the hair to see if it will remove. If not, check the client's level of sensation and increase the galvanic current. If the client feels nothing, increase by 10 digits; if the client can feel something, increase by only 5 digits.

Remember

Diathermy, galvanic and blend epilation units are very different in their use. Follow the manufacturer's instructions or attend a training course before operating. Settings vary with different machines.

Technique number 1

Prepare the client as for diathermy.

Choose the size of needle as for diathermy.

Switch the diathermy on to 3/4.

Switch the timer on to 5.0 seconds.

Switch the galvanic on to .10.

Insert the needle and depress the footswitch.

Wait for the 'beep' and then remove your foot.

Try the hair to see if it will release.

If not, increase the galvanic intensity by 5–10 digits.

Insert into another follicle and depress the footswitch.

Increase galvanic intensity 5–10 digits at a time until you reach the working point.

14 Increase the galvanic in this manner, one follicle at a time, until you have reached the working point, then record these data on the client's record card.

15 The level of galvanic current will vary on every client. Check to ensure the client is comfortable and no adverse skin reaction is apparent.

16 The level of galvanic current may vary dramatically between clients, whereas the level of diathermy will vary less. (It may be necessary to increase the diathermy a little but remember the diathermy is there not to epilate with but as a catalyst to increase the action of the more effective galvanic.)

17 There may be more erythema and even oedema than associated with diathermy – this is a normal galvanic reaction that calms down very quickly.

Treatment technique number 2

This is known as the 'lower for longer' technique as the galvanic intensity is lowered but the time is lengthened. This technique is used if the client feels uncomfortable with the higher current and shorter time of technique number 1.

If when using technique number 1, the client says he or she is finding it too uncomfortable, then reduce the galvanic current by 5 digits and increase the time by 1 second, or reduce by 10 digits and increase by 2 seconds.

Technique number 2 will not treat as many hairs as the main technique, as you will be in the follicle for longer, but the sensitive client may prefer it. If the treatment area is the face, however, the client may decide to have the main technique, as it will remove more hairs even though she may prefer the sensation of the second.

Treatment technique number 3

This is known as the 'treat and leave' technique as you treat a group of hairs, but do not remove them immediately. If the client is sensitive but anxious to have as many hairs removed as possible, this technique is a useful and popular one to offer.

If the client says he or she is finding technique number 2 too uncomfortable, then reduce the time back to 5 seconds. Treat a group of at least ten hairs, then treat a further group of at least ten hairs. After treating the second group, go back to the first group with your tweezers and remove the hairs, then go back to the second group and remove those hairs.

The action of the lye continues for a brief period of time, even though the current is switched off and the needle is withdrawn. In this technique the therapist specifically uses the 'carry-on effect' of the lye.

The benefits of this technique are lower levels of current but with a quick treatment time, and the fact that many hairs are removed saves time, too.

Treatment technique number 4

Galvanic only is a technique that is rarely used as it takes so long. Some clients prefer the sensation of the galvanic-only technique but few are happy with the longer treatment time of 10 seconds, minimum, per follicle. It is an option, though, for the very sensitive client or those with just a few hairs. If the client finds all the blend techniques too uncomfortable, then turn off the diathermy and increase the time to 10 seconds.

With the fourth technique, if the client is not comfortable you can decrease the current and increase the time, thereby having a 'lower for longer' method, or offer 'treat and leave' as a method of increasing the number of follicles treated.

Technique number 2

Turn the galvanic intensity down 5 digits.

Increase the time by 1 second (to 6 seconds).

Technique number 3

Decrease the time to 5 seconds; leave the galvanic intensity alone.

Treat a group of approximately ten follicles.

Do not remove the hairs.

Treat another similar sized group of hairs.

Do not remove the hairs.

Remove the hairs from the first group of follicles with tweezers.

Remove hairs from the second group of follicles.

Technique number 4

Increase the timer to 10 seconds.

Switch off the diathermy.

Leave the galvanic intensity where it is.

Treat the follicle and remove hair or Lower the intensity and lengthen the time or Treat and leave.

NVQ 2 BEAUTY THERAPY: **Epilate the hair follicle using diathermy, galvanic and blend techniques**

Treatment technique using a Sterex SXT Diathermy only unit

1 Attach the switched needle holder.
2 *Or* attach a Sterex unswitched needle holder and footswitch.
3 Plug in and switch on the epilator.
4 The mains light will come on and you will hear the internal fan.
5 Switch on the on/off button.
6 Using the up and down buttons set the thermolysis/diathermy intensity to the level required. (If using a footswitch and unswitched needle holder, you will need to depress the footswitch when altering the current intensity.)
7 If working on a new client, start at 10 and increase 5 digits at a time, working on a different follicle each time, until you reach the working point. (The working point is reached when the hairs remove without traction.)
8 All clients have different tolerance levels and current intensity requirements, but as a rough guide the average working points are 20–40. Some clients will need lower levels, some higher.

Possible faults

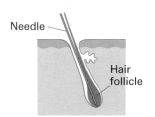

(a) Correct probing angle

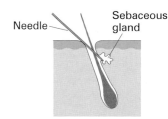

(b) Incorrect probing angle – sebaceous gland pierced

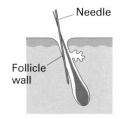

(c) Probing angle too steep – follicle wall pierced

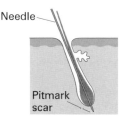

(d) Probe is too deep – base of follicle pierced. Tissue below follicle destroyed causing pitmark scar

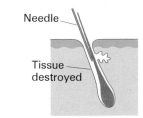

(e) Probe is too shallow – current application too close to surface. Tissue close to skin's surface destroyed

The effects of incorrect needle insertion

Accurate probing is essential for a successful epilation treatment:

- The needle should enter the follicle easily with no 'bending' of the needle.
- The needle should gently slide into the follicle with no depression of the skin.
- A steady, supportive three-way stretch helps ensure an accurate insertion by clearly 'presenting' the hair and direction and angle of growth to the therapist. When performed correctly, that is firmly but gently, it also assists with client comfort and confidence.

Remember

- Technique number 1 = higher for shorter
- Technique number 2 = lower for longer
- Technique number 3 = treat and leave
- Technique number 4 = galvanic only.

Remember

Which treatment technique is chosen is ultimately the client's choice.

Keys to good practice

With all techniques, if the occasional hair does not want to release, do not attempt to treat it again or force it, let the carry-on effect work, return and remove the hair at the end of the treatment.

- The action should be smooth, rhythmic and unhurried with no sign of traction when removing the hair from the follicle.
- Contact with the client at all times is most important. The 'supportive stretching hold' should never be removed from the client when passing over the tweezers to the needle holder hand to release the hair.
- A smooth, rhythmic change-over of tweezer to release the hair should be achieved.
- Slight resistance will be felt when the needle tip reaches the base of the follicle.
- The needle should remain stationary in the follicle, not be shaken or moved.
- The finger switch or footswitch should be depressed gently and smoothly.
- Double shots of current either by finger switch or foot pedal are not recommended. This can cause the needle to shake inside the follicle when the current is released, causing tissue damage and discomfort.
- The angle of insertion should mimic the direction of hair growth.
- The needle should not lean on the surface of the skin.
- Too deep an insertion may pierce through the follicle wall and cause discomfort, tissue damage and ineffective treatment. Repeated insertions of this type will cause pitting on the surface of the skin.
- Too shallow an insertion may cause surface skin damage, discomfort and ineffective treatment.
- A needle holder held lightly without tension ensures therapist achieves sensitivity during probing.

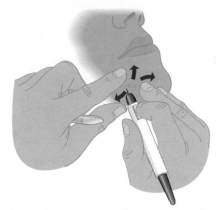

A steady, supportive three-way stretch helps ensure accurate insertion

Contra-actions

Possible contra-actions are shown in the table below.

Contra-action	Action required
Bending the needle	If the needle is bent in any way it should not be straightened as distortion of the metal in the area will have taken place. This may cause a build-up of current in that section of the needle and therefore a possible burn to the client. Remove the needle safely, replace and continue treatment. (This is not to be confused with angling of the needle, when the needle is deliberately angled from the base in order to assist difficult insertions.)
Whitening	Whitening around the follicle during insertion and treatment may be the inappropriate use of short wave diathermy on a black or Asian skin or could indicate too high a current or too superficial an insertion. Treatment should immediately stop in the area and a cold compress should be applied. The reason for the whitening should be pinpointed and rectified. Hypopigmentation marks may fade over time and exfoliation of the area and a good skin regime will help; however, sometimes pigmentation can be permanent. A build-up of whiteness under the skin surrounding the follicle during blend or galvanic treatment can be the result of sodium hydroxide (lye) building up under the skin's surface during treatment – this is not to be confused with blanching and is not an uncommon phenomenon.
Blood spot	If an incorrect insertion is made, a blood spot could appear on the surface of the skin. Immediately stem the blood with a fresh piece of cotton wool and depress gently but firmly for several seconds. This action is twofold – bruising is prevented by the pressure stopping the blood spreading under the surface of the skin; blood is prevented from spreading on to other items, e.g. gloves. The pressure and cotton wool can remain in place while the therapist continues her work on other hairs in a nearby area.

(continued on next page)

Palpitations	If the client suffers palpitations, it could be because he or she is nervous or it could indicate that the individual's breathing is restricted by being in a supine position, that is flat on the couch. Stop the treatment, loosen the client's clothing, and gently reassure the client. Fetch a glass of water to help the client calm down and raise him or her into a more seated position. Adjust your working angle to suit. It may be that the client is unsuitable for treatment.
Profuse sweating	The client may be nervous or ill, or have recently performed aerobic exercise, or it may be very hot. It is important to check the cause in order to know how to continue. Profuse sweating makes a treatment very difficult to perform. Because of the excess moisture in the skin, accuracy of insertion can be affected and also the moisture in the skin will exacerbate the current, so the current needs to be very low. Stop treatment and try to cool and calm the client as much as possible. Allow time for composure, and offer a cool glass of water. If the sweating can be calmed, continue the treatment.
Erythema and oedema	A certain amount of erythema and oedema (swelling) of the area are to be expected and is normal. Every client is different in his or her reactions to treatment. With sensitive skin, the area often becomes very red and swollen. Spacing of insertions can help, working to strict time limits and short treatments, covering perhaps two areas rather than one intensive area, and ensuring the skin has plenty of time to heal between treatments should all assist the problem. Cool water can be applied via a fresh cotton wool pad. Witch hazel is very cooling and this can be used on a fresh cotton wool pad. Some therapists use ice (ensure this is not put directly on the skin) to take the heat out of the skin and to assist with the prevention of swelling. Good camouflage products are recommended.
Bruising	A blue or black bruise appearing during or after treatment could indicate inaccurate and too deep probing which pierces or damages the capillaries. It could also indicate too firm a stretch and handhold and too large a probe. Immediate pressure should be applied with dry sterile cotton wool or a cold compress.
Weeping follicles	These could indicate that too much galvanic current has been used, resulting in excessive chemical decomposition of the tissues of the skin. A cold compress and good aftercare are recommended if over-treatment has occurred.

Contra-actions to epilation

Aftercare and home care

Immediately after treatment show the client the hair removed and discuss the progress to date. Allow the client to view the area by giving the client a mirror and checking back to the treatment plan. Follow this with full aftercare and home care advice, product sales (if required) and confirm the next treatment booking in the salon's diary and with the client.

In the salon

Lucy's client listened carefully to all her aftercare advice, including how to use the aloe vera gel Lucy recommended – it contained 95 per cent aloe whereas other similar products may contain only 2 per cent. However, the client chose not to purchase the gel. Later that night, the client cleansed her face with a product which contained a high alcohol content. This stung a little, so in the absence of a specialised aftercare product, the client spread some Vaseline over the still slightly sore and raised treatment area, thinking that this would help calm it. The next morning the area was moist, sore and swollen. The Vaseline had occluded the area (keeping the heat in by acting like cling film) and encouraged bacterial growth.

- What should Lucy have done?

There are many different aftercare products on the market specially designed for epilation. It must be impressed on the client that a good programme of hygienic home care will avoid any spots or minor infections occurring. It is important for the client to know that extra care of the treated area must be taken, especially within the first 36 hours, giving the skin a chance to settle and return to 'normal'.

Aftercare advice

- Aftercare products such as aloe vera or witch hazel gel are designed to assist in the healing process of the area. They are specifically formulated to soothe the skin and help prevent any infection of the treated follicles, which will be more prone to infection after the hairs have been removed.
- Once the skin has absorbed aftercare products, a specialised coloured cream to camouflage erythema can be used. The client's normal foundation may not be suitable as it may contain perfume or chemicals that could irritate the treated area.
- Any aftercare product should always be applied with fresh cotton wool and gloved hands, and the manufacturer's instructions should always be followed.
- Advise the client not to touch the treated area for 12–24 hours to avoid contamination. After this time, gently cleanse with perfume/alcohol-free products, otherwise the skin may be sensitised. At home, the aftercare product should be applied using clean cotton wool. Rich creams will occlude the heat (see 'In the salon' on page 437).
- Advise the client to avoid wearing tight restrictive garments on the area as this may cause further irritation.
- Advise the client to avoid heat treatments such as sunbathing, sun beds and saunas following epilation. This is because there is still heat remaining in the skin and it must be allowed to cool down and recover. Swimming is not recommended for a minimum of 24 hours as the skin is healing itself and must be given time to recover. Client participation in any of these may result in irritation, oedema, erythema, soreness or even infection.
- Advise the client on how to deal with regrowth between treatments (see the section on hair management techniques on page 401).
- An appointment should be made for the next treatment.

Remember

Aftercare leaflets are available from the manufacturers and it is advisable to give clients one after each treatment to encourage them to maintain 'best practice'.

Keys to good practice

Write the date and time of the client's next appointment on the back of the aftercare leaflet.

It is essential that the skin is allowed to heal completely between treatments. Some clients take longer than others because of individuals' different healing speeds and capabilities. General well-being and self care have a direct effect on the speed of healing. For example, vitamin C assists the body's healing process, with smokers requiring double the amount of vitamin C. Taking all these points into account, allow a healing period of one to two weeks for the majority of clients for each area of the face or body.

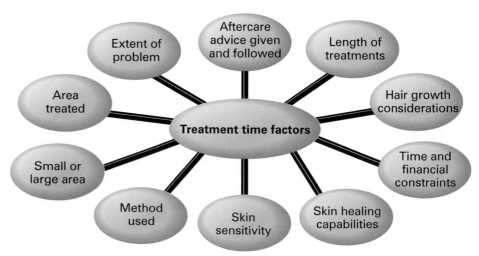

Factors affecting treatment time

Set up, monitor and shut down water, temperature and spa facilities
Provide specialist spa treatments

Unit BT28
Unit BT29

A spa is not a new experience – throughout history, communal bathing and 'taking of the waters' have been seen as both a social activity and a cure for all manner of ailments, from skin problems to kidney stones and liver complaints. Roman soldiers were said to bathe in the village of Spa, Belgium, and that is one possible source of the name we associate with water treatments. The other is the Latin phrase *Sanus Per Aqua*, meaning 'health through water'. Today, a spa experience has become synonymous with water treatments, which encompass not only the physical treatment of the body but a whole philosophy of treating the mind and spirit, too.

Spa towns were so called because of the natural mineral springs flowing through them. Bath, Buxton and Leamington Spa are all famous for their drinking and bathing waters. In the eighteenth century, the spa visit was an annual ritual. Today, the spa industry is enjoying a revival. Luxury hotels and health farms are offering extensive water treatments, and spa design has evolved from the basic and clinical to the luxurious. While treatments such as sauna, steam and spa or flotation treatments are beyond the capabilities of the smaller salon, both in terms of space and setting-up costs, the spa experience is an essential part of deluxe hotel operation.

The industry has begun to specialise in a number of areas offering a total package to the client:

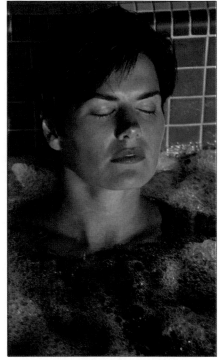

Spa treatments are a very relaxing treat

- **Wellness** – this was often perceived as simply fitness of the body, but now incorporates many alternative therapies. Some spas have Ayurvedic doctors who can diagnose clients, and offer naturopaths, homeopaths, acupuncture and Bach flower remedies – all the alternative approaches to preventative health care.
- **Medical** – onsite medical teams can carry out Botox and collagen injections, plastic surgery, electrical treatments, colonic irrigation and some screening procedures for preventative health care
- **Weight loss and health care** – this includes nutritional advice, exercise planning, toning and firming treatments, body wrapping, gyms and personal training, Pilates and meditation.
- **The spa experience** – this includes saunas, steam treatments, wet and dry flotation, spa pools, shower treatments, massage, hot and cold stone therapy, aromatherapy and marine therapy.

Within this unit you will cover the following outcomes:

BT28.2/BT29.1 Consult with, and prepare, the client for treatment
BT29.2 Provide body wrapping treatments
BT29.3 Provide flotation treatments
BT29.4 Provide hydrotherapy treatments
BT28.1 Prepare, clean and maintain the spa environment
BT28.3/BT29.5 Monitor water, temperature and spa treatments and environment
BT28.4/BT29.6 Provide aftercare advice
BT28.5 Complete shut down of treatment areas and spa environment

As you work through this unit, you will need to refer closely to the **Professional basics** section and **Body treatments – theory and consultation**. Many of the topics covered have been discussed in earlier units.

Consult with, and prepare, the client for treatment

BT28.2
BT29.1

In this outcome you will learn about

- hygiene in the wet area
- the spa treatments consultation
- blood shunting
- contra-actions to heat treatment
- general effects of heat treatment.

Hygiene in the wet area

The wet area offers germs and bacteria the perfect breeding environment, namely heat and moisture. By its very nature, the wet area has to be a suitable ambient temperature for clients, and although some of the plunge pools and showers may be a cold treatment, the atmosphere has to be warm and inviting, otherwise no one would ever want to removing their clothing and take part in the treatments. The same is true of the moisture content – air humidity is high because of the water treatments.

Hygiene is the prime consideration for any wet area manager, and the safest way to prevent bacteria and germs being bought into the treatment areas is to complete a full consultation with the client. A full contra-indication check should detect any infectious diseases present or conditions which could spread and contaminate very quickly, for example athlete's foot or impetigo. Preventing and containing the infection plays an important part in protecting other clients and staff. (For further information on bacterial, viral and fungal infections, see **Professional basics**, page 40.)

The spa treatments consultation

- Check the client fully for any contra-indications.
- The body temperature should be between 36.5°C and 37°C – anything higher could indicate the client has a fever. In this case, the client must not have any heat treatment – you should not increase the body temperature further.
- The pulse rate should be approximately 72 beats per minute. Palpitations and a high pulse rate may also cause erratic blood flow to the brain, causing the client to lose conciousness. Always seek medical approval for readings which are outside the normal.
- If the client is an existing customer, then a new record card will not be required, but you will need to re-check contra-indications. It is also professional to ask about previous treatments: what the client liked/disliked or had preferences about, including time of treatment and the products used, or if there were any contra-actions which developed after the client left the salon.
- For a new client you should take your time over the consultation, as you will need to explain the treatment process, the physical and physiological effects and the benefits and effects of products used. This will help the client make an informed decision about treatment choices.

Remember

Remember to take the client's blood pressure as high or low blood pressure would be a contra-indication. The possibility of the client fainting is higher when the body temperature is raised if he or she has this condition.

Remember

For how to take the client's blood pressure, see **Body treatments – theory and consultation**, page 307.

Remember

For how to take the client's pulse, see **Body treatments – theory and consultation**, page 308.

- Always provide a full tour of the treatment area, equipment to be used and other facilities, that is the toilets, rest area and refreshment bar. This should not include treatment rooms in use, for example a client in a flotation tank should not be disturbed, but it is important that the new client be familiar with the rooms, and general layout, in order to feel comfortable and able to relax.
- Find out the client's reasons for treatment, for example cleansing of the skin, general relaxation and de-stressing, muscular tension or as part of a slimming programme. This will also help the treatment planning for both the wet area and related electrical treatments.
- For sauna and steam treatments, the client should be told that any weight loss is only temporary, due to fluid loss, and will be replaced naturally within the next 24–48 hours.
- You should be prepared to answer fully any queries or questions the client may have. Indeed, you should actively encourage questions as clients should feel fully confident about the treatment procedure.

General contra-indications to the wet area

See individual equipment below for other contra-indications.

- Viral, bacterial and fungal infections.
- Skin diseases or disorders, e.g. scabies, eczema.
- Severe bruising, recent hemorrhage or undiagnosed swelling.
- Breathing difficulties, colds, asthma (not as vital in a steam cabinet, as the head is not involved).
- Within 90 minutes of a heavy meal (see blood shunting below).
- Clients under the influence of alcohol.
- Clients on strong medication.
- Heart conditions.
- A high or low blood pressure condition.
- Pyrexia (raised body temperature) and high pulse rate. Either may indicate illness or disease within the system.
- Headache; migraine sufferers (applies more to a sauna).
- Clients prone to claustrophobia.

For women:

- Menstruation – first two days, depending upon how it affects the client. Some clients will prefer not to wear a swimming costume, and are also more sensitive generally.
- Pregnancy or lactation (the heat could inhibit milk flow).

Always seek medical approval if the client has:

- diabetes/pancreatic disorders
- epilepsy
- fluid retention associated with kidney problems
- medication – check with the doctor
- any severe circulatory disorders, e.g. Reynaud's disease
- history of thrombosis
- dysfunction of the nervous system, e.g. Parkinson's disease
- recent operations
- severe exhaustion
- hepatitis – due to the body's inability to release toxins and maintain fluid balance.

Remember

Take into account:
- the client's skin type (see **You and the skin**, page 188, for skin characteristics)
- the client's cultural background. For example, some religious communities do not permit women to show their body to any man other than their husband. One solution is to offer women-only treatment days.

Keys to good practice

Advise the client to remove contact lenses before entering a sauna or steam room.

Blood shunting

In most spa treatments, the body temperature rises, the circulation is stimulated, and as part of the body's natural cooling process, blood is drawn towards the skin's surface – seen as a marked erythema. Because of this, the organs and brain may be slightly depleted of their normal blood supply, especially if the digestive system also requires blood to aid the digestive process. It is, therefore, a contra-indication to go in the sauna after having eaten.

The process of blood being shunted to several areas of the body at the same time may cause symptoms such as nausea, dizziness, cramp, headaches, abdominal pain and general discomfort. It may even result in the client fainting, which is the body's defence mechanism, forcing the client to lie flat, so lowering the brain to the level of the heart to enable blood to reach it.

Contra-actions to heat treatment

- Erythema.
- Fainting.
- Nosebleeds.
- Vomiting.
- Excessive sweating.
- Breathing difficulties.
- Allergic reactions (prickly heat).

If any of the above occurs, you should be nearby to assist the client. Treatment should be discontinued immediately and you may need to summon help, if required.

Contra-actions may occur if incorrect information was given by the client at the consultation, for example about consumption of alcohol, a heavy meal, or inaccurate medical information.

It is important that you supervise treatment to ensure correct timing of treatments and to watch out for heat exhaustion, burns or scalds.

General effects of heat treatment

- Rise in body temperature.
- Increase in metabolic processes in all cells.
- The heart rate increases.
- Erythema comes to the skin's surface.
- Perspiration is induced, cleaning the skin.
- Glandular activity is stimulated.
- Muscle fibres are relaxed by the heat.
- Sensory nerve endings are soothed by the heat.
- Mental relaxation is induced.

Keys to good practice

You will need to keep clients informed of the type of heat treatment most suitable for them as some generate more heat than others. For the client who does not like a lot of heat opt for a more gentle heat, or perhaps a bubble bath, rather than a hot sauna.

Provide body wrapping treatments

BT29.2

In this outcome you will learn about

- dry body wrapping
- wet body wrapping
- wraps with bandages/linen strips.

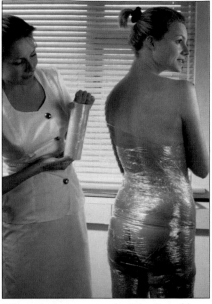

Client being wrapped with cling film

Body wrapping was discovered at an arthritis clinic in Switzerland. As a by-product of a health care treatment, patients found they were slimming down as they were de-toxifying. This was thought to help rid the joints of accumulation or build-up of salts and alleviate pain. As a result, the treatment was taken up by the beauty industry.

There are many body wraps and body masks on the beauty market, and most salons offer some form of treatment, depending upon their facilities and the client demands within the area.

Body wraps vary. They can be:

- dry – using electric blankets
- wet – using various body masks
- with bandages/linen strips/cling film/foil (depending upon the product manufacturer's recommendations)
- with heat from a dry flotation bath (see BT29.3, Provide dry flotation treatments).

Dry body wrapping

This is one treatment which the smaller salon can easily offer clients as it involves only a fairly small purchase of a heated insulating high grade PVC blanket (compared with a spa or sauna), which can be used either alone or with a preferred wrap system. This electric blanket acts as a cocoon and warms the clients' body, so helping the client maximise the treatment over a shorter period of time.

The electric blanket is coated with anti-microbic and anti-fungal agents to prevent a build up of contamination, which reduces the risk of infection. The blanket is used with inner disposable plastic sheeting to avoid the product coming into contact with the blanket. It has individual heating zones, for the neck to the abdomen, abdomen to knees, and knees to ankles, so that the separate areas get just the right amount of heat. The heating zones are fully adjustable, so that if the client prefers not to have legs heated that zone can be switched off (ideal if the client has varicose veins).

The blanket operates on a very small voltage, making it safe to use, and it folds up for easy storage. The controls are simple to use, and may be wall mounted for ease of visibility. The blanket offers up to two hours of heat treatment.

Remember

These blankets are often used with a body wrap, which gives excellent results with the heat. However, if the client wants a general warming treatment before massage, there is a single electric blanket available which heats up under the body, rather like a domestic electric blanket.

Wet body wrapping

Body masks are a good treatment to offer the client in the smaller salon, providing it has the shower facilities to rinse off the product. These moist masks can be either setting or non-setting, and they offer an all-over skin treatment, designed to aid circulation, firm and tone, and detoxify the body depending upon the ingredients used.

Body mask ingredients

Seaweed/algae
Seaweed ingredients are very popular. They contain over 104 trace elements and minerals and the composition of these elements indicates the best way to use them.

Below are some examples, and their function within body masks.

Seaweed type	Function
Focus	Increases circulation and aids slimming
Spiruline	Restructures and firms
Himanthalia elogata	Revitalises and re-mineralises
Laminaria digitata	Stimulates the lymphatic system and has diuretic properties
Focus seretus	Decomposes toxic accumulation, making the urine darker
Focus vesiculosus	Firms, tones and detoxifies

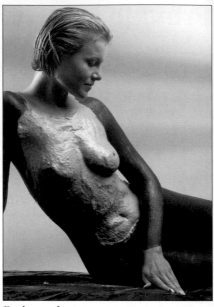

Body mask

Aromatherapy oils
These are another popular active ingredient within body masks, and can be used with seaweed.

They not only work well but are also pleasantly scented. For example:

- seaweed and peppermint oil cleanse, tone, moisturise and tighten the skin
- juniper and lemon detoxify, decongest and stimulate the lymphatic drainage system
- cinnamon, zedoary and ginger can be blended into a contour gel to stimulate lymph drainage, circulation and detoxification of problem areas.

Using different blends of oils, manufacturers provide products intended to tackle individual problems such as loose skin, fatty areas, or water retention.

Mud
Like seaweed, mud and clay from the seabed are packed with active minerals, although often, the drawback is the natural odour that they have, especially if the clay has sulphur in it! However, that can be overcome with additives of aromatherapy oils.

- Sodium regulates osmotic pressure in the cells, while potassium acts on the cell membranes' permeability to regulate cellular exchange and rehydration of the cells.
- Magnesium increases the cells' defences and has anti-inflammatory properties, which are very relaxing and soothing on the tissues.
- Dead sea mud is very popular and can be easily infused with essential oils to relax and ease muscle pain.

Alpine hay

The healing effect of Alpine hay has been known for centuries and provides a totally natural treatment with no odour, dried herbs or synthetic additives. The whole body is enveloped in soaked hay, and the even heat produced releases the valuable elements in the hay, for their healing effects. The hay bath stimulates the blood circulation, purges the body and has a relaxing effect. The temperature rises to 40–42°C, and in the moist environment the immune system is stimulated. The treatment time is 20–25 minutes, and this works very well when the body is also immersed in a dry flotation tank, or with a heated wrap or blanket.

Application of wet body wrapping

The masks can be applied by hand or with a large brush – a paint brush or wallpaper paste-size brush is ideal. Application is just like applying a face mask, but as it is on the body, try to get an even application, without the product being too thin or patchy. Ideally, the client will have the minimum of clothes on – paper or disposable pants – although some clients may be happy to wear nothing in order to get a thorough coverage of the mask.

Body masks work well, either left to set on the body or, in the case of non-setting masks, wrapping the body in a thermal cling film, or foil, which keeps in the heat which the body has generated. Non-setting masks leave less mess on the couch. Most masks can be showered off, along with the accumulated dead skin cells, toxins and perspiration.

The male client

Men are a little more shy about having firming and toning treatments, but the benefits of body packs often appeal because of the muscle relaxant aspect of the treatment, especially for sportsmen who often regard body masks as a therapeutic muscle treatment.

As with most male grooming products, smell is very important and so is the marketing of the treatment. Any treatment which is flowery or highly perfumed will not be a success with a man. Men are more likely to prefer the smell of sandalwood or a muscle balm or an embrocating type of fragrance such as camphor.

If a salon markets a male treatment day, with a separate treatment description using language like 'eases post-sport muscular pain', 'improves muscle tone, so muscle performance is enhanced', then the treatment will have much more appeal.

Males tend to accumulate fatty deposits from the abdomen up through the face and throat, rather than on the hips and thighs, as women do. This means that they tend to respond well to an inch-loss treatment such as a fabric wrap, and the de-toxifying effects of a body wrap will often help disperse the beginnings of a 'beer belly'.

A salon associated with a gym or health club is likely to have great success offering treatments which appeal to the male market – this is a little less threatening than entering a salon which may be seen very much as a female domain.

Wraps with bandages/linen strips

The body wrap is a quick and effective body treatment to help lose unwanted inches, disperse cellulite and achieve a general toning and firming effect. The treatment can be used in conjunction with a healthy lifestyle as part of a slimming and weight-loss programme, but body wrapping is also ideal as an individual appointment before a special occasion.

> ## Remember
>
> The clients' dignity. Avoid pasting the mask over the genital area, although the breast and buttock skin will benefit from treatment. A small hand towel will preserve the client's modesty, and the room should be warm enough to allow the client to be uncovered if he or she wishes.
>
> If the client would like to be wrapped up in towels, then have some at hand. The product will easily wash off them.

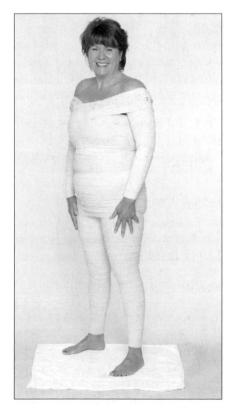

Body wraps with bandages/linen strips

Body wraps:

- will balance the figure
- will detoxify and firm
- are quick and effective
- use safe, natural ingredients.

Contra-indications to body wraps

While this is a safe treatment to carry out, you will need to check the client for the following contra-indications:

- high or low blood pressure
- heart disease
- kidney disease
- slipped disc
- skin ailments (e.g. eczema)
- pregnancy
- breast-feeding mothers
- epilepsy
- varicose veins.

Always seek medical approval if your client:

- has recently had an operation
- has a serious illness
- is post natal (within six months of the birth).

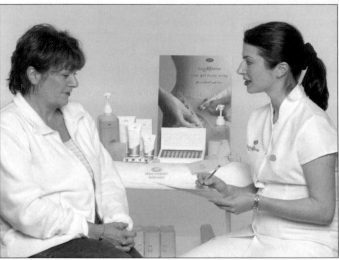
A body wrap consultation

Benefits of body wraps

The active gels used in the treatment are formulated to achieve inch loss through the intra-cellular drainage of the lymphatic system. This is achieved by the combination of compression bandages, which allows the stimulation of the deep and superficial veins, and the active ingredients in the Slim Gel that detoxify the body. The gels are concentrated and contain essential oils, seaweed extract, herbs, distilled witch hazel, aloe vera and mineral salts, horse chestnut and sweet fennel. The ingredients in most gels are diuretic, purifying and tightening.

This treatment is suitable for all skin types. The body wrap is beneficial to anyone who wants to lose inches or to detoxify. To maintain results, the treatment should be taken in conjunction with a healthy diet and regular exercise programme.

Body wrap preparation

Half an hour before the client arrives, place a sufficient quantity of the chosen active gel (see box on next page for suggested amounts) in a container and stand it in warm water or on a radiator. This will ensure that the gel will be applied to the client at a comfortable temperature.

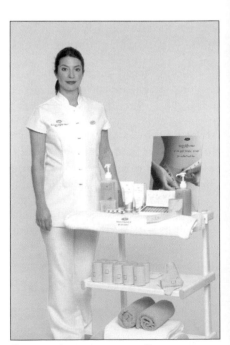
Prepare the treatment trolley

Taking measurements

Having discussed the treatment with the client, use a tape measure to measure the areas where the inch loss is required.

With a water-soluble pen or crayon, gently mark the skin in two places above and below the tape measure at each measurement position.

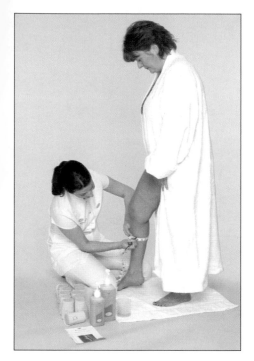

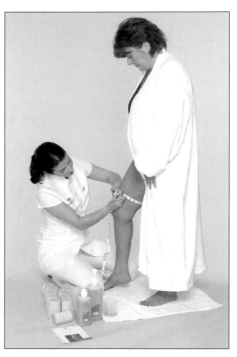

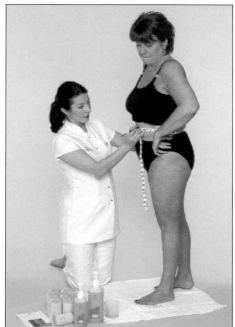

Measuring the client

Remember

Never warm the active gel in a microwave.

Approximate amount of gel required

20 ml for mini-lift facial
60ml for a partial wrap
100 ml for a full wrap
120ml for a full wrap including mini-lift facial
These amounts will depend on the size of the client.

Keys to good practice

Apply the active gel to a clean skin free of any oils and creams. Do not apply after waxing.

These guide marks will enable you to locate the exact measurement positions after the treatment.

Record the first set of measurements in the 'Before' column on the Slim Gel leaflet.

MEASUREMENT RECORD CHART

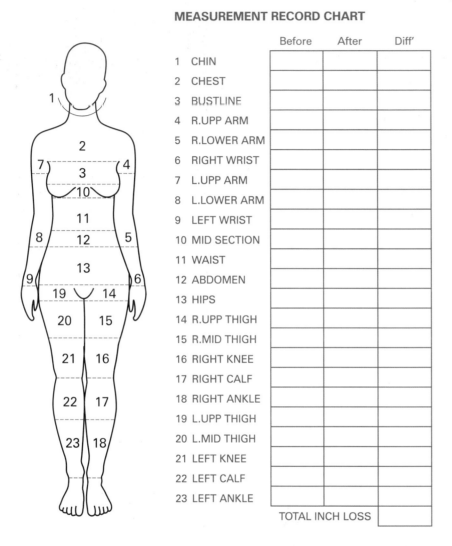

		Before	After	Diff'
1	CHIN			
2	CHEST			
3	BUSTLINE			
4	R.UPP ARM			
5	R.LOWER ARM			
6	RIGHT WRIST			
7	L.UPP ARM			
8	L.LOWER ARM			
9	LEFT WRIST			
10	MID SECTION			
11	WAIST			
12	ABDOMEN			
13	HIPS			
14	R.UPP THIGH			
15	R.MID THIGH			
16	RIGHT KNEE			
17	RIGHT CALF			
18	RIGHT ANKLE			
19	L.UPP THIGH			
20	L.MID THIGH			
21	LEFT KNEE			
22	LEFT CALF			
23	LEFT ANKLE			
	TOTAL INCH LOSS			

Recording measurements on the Slim Gel leaflet

Also record the date and if your client is having this treatment as part of a slimming programme. You may also record the client's weight.

Step-by-step

Body wrapping technique

1 For best results, the client should shower before treatment using body scrub as this will remove dead skin cells and help absorption of the product. Advise the client not to wear any body oil or lotion as this will stop the gel absorbing effectively.

2 Apply the active gel liberally to the areas being treated, stage by stage, making sure that the gel does not dry out before wrapping.

3 Each pass of the bandages should overlap by at least 5 cm. Pull the bandages firmly using the squares on the bandages to judge compression, while supporting the client with one hand and maintaining an even tension (see 'Tips to ensure correct application of bandages', page 451). Secure each bandage with a clip.

4 Legs. Commence wrapping, from above the ankle joint towards the knee. Bandage loosely over knee area. With legs apart, wrap upwards towards the groin. Pull the bandages firmly and maintain an even tension. Repeat this process on the other leg using the squares for guidance.

5 Hips and buttocks. With legs at hip width apart, secure the bandage at the top of the thigh. Continue bandaging firmly around the buttocks, shaping and lifting as you work.

6 Waist contour. Take an unrolled bandage, approximately 1 m in length, and pass around the back of the waist with about equal length on each side. With the client holding one end at hip height, smooth the bandage over the waist, passing across the abdomen. Pull the end down towards the hips, taking it around under the buttocks, securing with a clip to the bandage at the top of the thigh. Repeat the for other end.

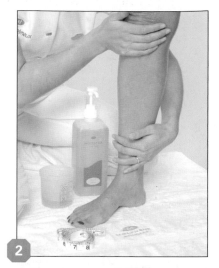
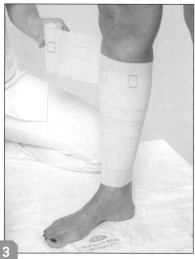

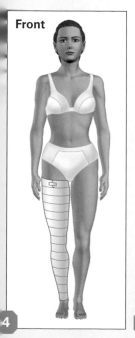
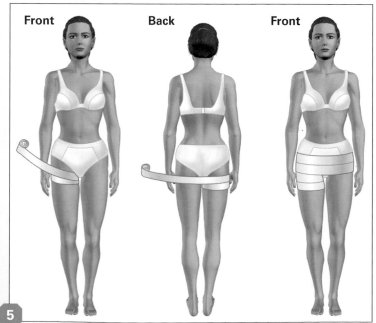
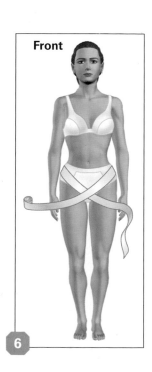

7 Stomach. Attach a bandage to the hip area. Continue wrapping upwards as firmly as is comfortable for the client, overlapping the bandages and covering the waist contour. Continue over the rib cage without restricting breathing. Finish under the bust. If the client has a hollow back or small waist, do not bandage too tightly or the bandages will roll into the waist and become uncomfortable.

8 Arms. Using gentle pressure, commence wrapping upwards from above the wrist stopping just below the shoulder joint. Repeat for the other arm.

9 Bust (optional). Clip a bandage to the back of the left arm and take the bandage under the right arm, bringing it around to the front. Using light pressure lift and mould the bust, bring the bandage up between the cleavage and over the opposite shoulder. Repeat this action overlapping the first crossover. Attach the bandage to the back at shoulder level with a clip. Repeat for the other breast.

10 Cover any remaining areas of skin that are showing.

11 Assist the client to lie down on the couch and keep him or her warm and comfortable. Cover the client with sufficient blankets to maintain warmth for a period of 60 minutes. It is important to check that the bandages are not too tight around the joints and are not causing a restriction to the circulation. If necessary, ease the bandages at the relevant joint using the method taught on the training day. While the client is resting, a further treatment may be offered, e.g. a facial, lash tint, make-up or manicure.

12 Never leave the client unattended.

Front

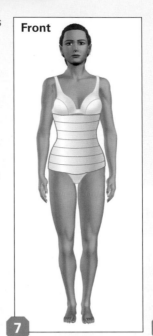

7

Back

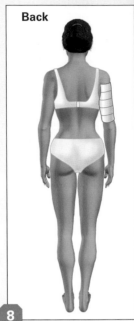

8

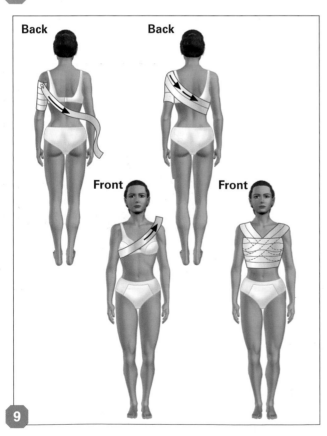

9

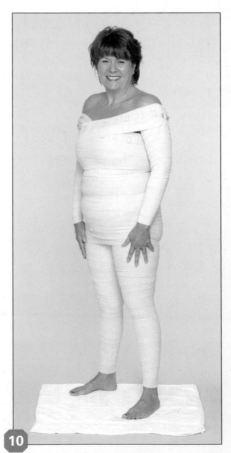

10

Remember

The bandages should overlap by 50 per cent covering the squares marked on the bandage (see 'Tips to ensure correct application of bandages', page 469 below).

Remember

Use the bandage technique as taught on the training day.

Mini-lift facial

1 Measure from under the chin to the top of the head and note the measurements on the leaflet. Apply Slim Gel to the face and neck. Place sterile gauze over the area and smooth upwards with a mask brush.
2 Apply a headband below the chin and pull gently to secure the gauze and fasten with a clip on top of the head. Leave on for 20 minutes.
3 Remove headband and using sponges and warm water, thoroughly dampen the gauze. Gently roll gauze downwards to remove. Massage the neck and face with the appropriate pre-mixed facial oil for 10 minutes.
4 Blot, tone and moisturise with appropriate skin care preparations. Re-measure the chin area.

High or moderate compression?

If a client is not used to compression therapy or is of slim build, moderate compression should be used.

Tips to ensure correct application of bandages
- A simple visual guide is indelibly printed (will not wash out) on both sides of the bandage. The visual guide consists of coloured rectangles which become squares when the correct extension is reached.
- On one side of the bandage are *brown* rectangles, which will give *high* compression, and on the other side, *green* rectangles which will give *moderate* compression.

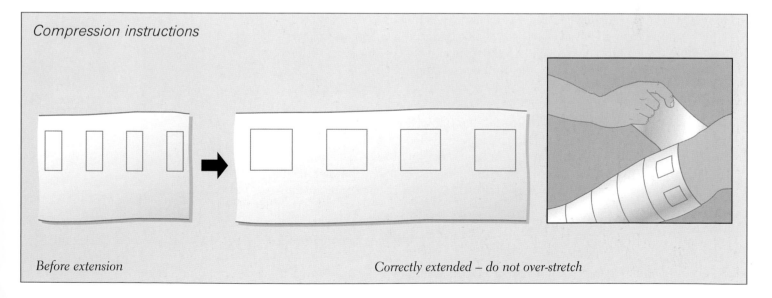
Compression instructions
Before extension — *Correctly extended – do not over-stretch*

Re-measuring

1 After 60 minutes, help the client off the couch and unwrap the bandages. Re-measure the client using the guide marks you made earlier to ensure that measurements are taken in the same position.
2 Enter the new measurements on the Slim Gel leaflet and calculate the difference.

451

After the treatment

Stress to the client the importance of a healthy diet and exercise programme. The client needs to drink eight glasses of water daily to help flush the toxins through the body.

Give the client the Slim Gel leaflet which contains the before and after measurements and aftercare notes. Also recommend the appropriate skin care preparations for home care.

Laundering bandages

Wash at 40°C, using a non-biological washing powder and allow to dry naturally. Do not bleach, iron, dry clean or tumble dry. Bandages may start to lose elasticity after 20 applications, but this should not affect the treatment significantly. Further bandages can be purchased separately.

Aftercare

A body wrap detoxifies the system and helps the appearance of cellulite. Unwanted inches are lost during treatment and the body appears firmer and more toned.

To further aid the detoxification process and to help maintain the inch loss that has been achieved during the treatment, you should advise the client of the following simple procedures:

1 Do not shower off any residue of active gel from the skin – keep it on for approximately 8 hours.
2 If cellulite is a problem, then a body therapy gel should be used morning and night as part of a home care routine.
3 Avoid consuming the following for at least one week: tea, coffee, salt, fried food, sugar, carbonated drinks, low-calorie drinks, alcohol and junk foods. For long lasting results, a calorie-controlled diet and an exercise programme should be followed.
4 Drink at least eight glasses of water a day between meals. Herbal teas are also helpful and a healthy alternative to drinking tea and coffee. (For more dietary advice, see **Body treatments – theory and consultation**, page 316.)

Points to consider

- The body wrap method works on intro-cellular transaction through the lymphatic system as a result of compression therapy. There is a reduction of cellular fluids in the fat tissues. It does not involve fluid loss by perspiration and the inches do not return after a drink. Lost inches stay off for around 3–6 days, but if a healthy lifestyle is adopted, the inches may not return, giving the client a great incentive and morale boost.
- The main lymphatic nodes must be covered during the treatment for it to work properly. Therefore, calves cannot be treated without covering the nodes in the groin and the same is true for the waist, that is the whole area must be treated.
- The most popular treatment is the partial wrap – from under the knees to just under the bust including the upper arms. Other areas which may be treated are the bust and chin. It is important to bandage upwards to encourage lymphatic drainage and to bandage loosely over joints such as knees and elbows so as not to impair circulation. If the client complains of tingling in the toes or fingers, loosen the bottom bandage by pulling sharply down. Then rub the limb to encourage circulation.
- Do not apply over body oil or creams or after waxing. Check for contra-indications.

Remember

Use the right bandages for the gel. You should purchase the product and bandages from the same supplier. If you mix the product and bandages, the results cannot be guaranteed.

- To reduce the chin, apply the active gel to the neck and chin only. Apply surgical gauze to the area, brushing upwards. Now apply either a headband or bandage to the area under chin, pulling gently. Secure with a clip on top of the head and leave for 20 minutes. Remove bandage or headband; moisten gauze with plenty of warm water and sponges. Gently roll the gauze downwards to remove.
- If the client is having a steam cabinet or sunbed treatment also, this should be taken before the body wrap treatment or the gel will be sweated out of the pores. Clients should not shower after the treatment as the gel will go on working for around 8 hours after the treatment. Toning tables or an exercise bike can be used for part of the treatment while the client is bandaged.
- The treatment can be repeated after one week and then again after about 3 weeks, depending on the client's concerns and body shape. Try to sell a course of three treatments initially. Thereafter the client can have a treatment once a month.
- Soft fat and cellulite respond best to the treatment. In the case of cellulite, give the client follow-up advice. Changes in diet and amount of exercise are important. With cellulite, remind the client to drink eight glasses of water a day between meals.
- Complementary treatments to follow up the body wrap include anti-cellulite treatment and bust-firming treatments such as faradic, G5 and vacuum suction (see Unit BT18, Improve body condition using electro-therapy).
- It is important not to guess how many inches will be lost during treatment as the client may lose less than you suggest and so be disappointed. Individual clients will respond differently to the treatment.

Treatment timings

The average body wrap takes around 90 minutes in total. This allows 30 minutes to measure and wrap and 60 minutes for the client to rest.

Provide flotation treatments   BT29.3

In this outcome you will learn about

- benefits of flotation therapy
- ailments which flotation can help alleviate
- wet flotation
- dry flotation.

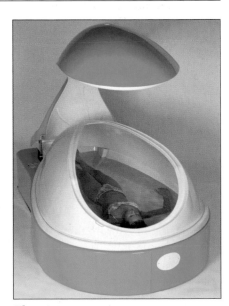

Flotation treatment

Flotation therapy involves placing the body into a state of total relaxation. Flotation can take place in:

- a bath
- a pool
- a tank
- a bed.

Flotation therapy is based on a single important principle. While we are active in the ordinary world, we experience stress and conflict that is incorporated into our daily routines and habitual patterns of activity. These habitual patterns often become locked into neurotic and energy-depriving actions. Some people smoke, or drink to cope with this 'normal' situation of anxiety and stress. The flotation treatment is a therapeutic one which breaks these habitual responses and reactions, and allows the mind and body to regenerate their natural energy without interference from the patterns of the outside world.

There are two types of flotation treatment:

- wet flotation
- dry flotation.

The wet therapy utilises flotation in salt water, while in the dry therapy a modified restricted environmental stimulation therapy (REST) environment is created (see below). The latter therapy separates the floater from the water with a 15 mm polymer membrane.

Benefits of flotation therapy

- Warms the tissues and softens them.
- Eases aches and pains in the joints and muscles.
- Produces a sleep-inducing and relaxed mental state.
- Eases pressure points through water buoyancy.
- Produces a calm and relaxed client.
- Ideal as a warming pre-treatment prior to massage.

Ailments which flotation can help alleviate

- Pre-menstrual tension.
- Arthritis.
- Asthma.
- Back pain.
- Jet lag.
- Irritable bowel syndrome.
- Muscle and skeletal conditions.
- Anxiety.
- Panic attacks.
- Lack of concentration.

Wet flotation

This usually occurs in a specially constructed bath or tank, or small pool. The water has salts and minerals dissolved into it to enable the body to float. There are close similarities between this form of therapy and eastern techniques of meditation.

The flotation tank experience isolates the client from all external stimuli, enabling him or her to forget the body and concentrate on the mind. It is based upon a scientific approach to deep relaxation called restricted environmental stimulation therapy (REST). Dr John Lilly, who is considered to be the father of flotation therapy, believed that if the brain's workload is reduced by up to 90 per cent, the body conserves energy and has a chance to heal and rejuvenate itself. During his training at the National Institute of Mental Health, Dr Lilly experimented with physical isolation in an effort to discover what keeps the brain going and what its energy sources were. One answer was that the energy sources are biological and internal and do not depend upon the outside environment. The theory was that if you cut off all stimuli to the brain, then it would go to sleep. Dr Lilly decided to test this theory using a flotation tank.

Gravity

Due to the high salt levels in the water, the flotation tank or pool creates a zero gravity environment. Zero gravity allows you to relax every single muscle, your neck, arms, back and even ears. The tank enables you to find those areas you are holding tense, so you can let go. Finding where gravity is and in which direction, then computing how you can move and not fall over, takes about 90 per cent of the brain's activity on a daily basis. When you start to float, you are free from all the gravity computations and the physical world, which leaves the brain free to relax.

Temperature and touch

One of the major sources of stimulation in humans is the temperature gradient change on the surface of the body, through the nerve endings within the skin. Temperature inside the flotation tank is isothermal over the surface of the body, so that nerve endings no longer perceive a separation between the skin and the solution inside the tank. This means that the nerve endings in the skin also have a chance to relax and stop working so hard.

Sound

The flotation tank is sound proof and so is the treatment room in many health clubs. During treatment the client wears earplugs and the ears are below the surface of the solution, which cuts out external sounds. Many people find that gentle music, from the underwater speakers in the tank, helps them to relax.

Light

Floating in darkness allows areas of the brain which are always in use when awake to be freed from their work. Tests have shown that there is a drop in electrical activity of the brain and the darkness during floating also induces a balance between the left and right sides of the brain. There is a shift from the normally dominant left side of the brain (logical, analytical, and rational) to the right side (intuition, mental clarity and creativity), so both sides of the brain are in harmony and the balance restores full brain function. The visual cortex for light reaction within the brain is allowed to rest.

Benefits of wet flotation to the body

The client lies in a tank for up to two hours without any physical stimulation. The body has nothing to react to, therefore the levels of stress hormones, like epinephrine or adrenaline, as well as cortisol in the blood, are reduced. This therapy also has another effect in that the endorphins or natural painkiller hormones increase, providing a state of deep relaxation. Stress disorders are reduced and are unlikely to manifest themselves under flotation therapy. Chronic pain can also be controlled through the release of the endorphins that this therapy produces.

The process works in the following way in the case of muscle pain. Because the endorphins released through deep relaxation stop the pain from a chronic ailment reaching the brain, the muscles relax and healing takes place much more rapidly. This therapy can aid patients suffering from ailments like arthritis. Psychological ailments can also be assisted and even cured through flotation therapy. This is especially the case when treating obsessive and addictive behaviour. This is due to the fact that this type of behaviour is often initiated and exacerbated by stress.

Contra-indications to wet flotation

The contra-indications are the same as for the wet area.

Keys to good practice

If the client has a history of psychosis or other psychological disorders, he or she should not undergo flotation therapy. This also includes claustrophobia, as this phobia may be aggravated by the confines of the flotation tank.

The salts used in flotation therapy may have an adverse effect on some skin conditions. Advise the client to seek medical approval before embarking on a course of therapy. You must not carry out treatment without this.

The wet flotation tank

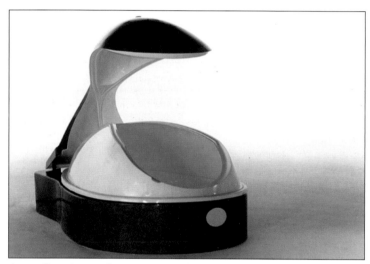

A wet flotation tank

These vary in size and shape but the principle is the same: the body must be able to float suspended in shallow salt water (25–30 cm deep), which is heated to body temperature.

The flotation tank is a fibre-glass capsule containing water with a very high concentration (up to 318 kg) of Epsom salts.

The approximate capacity of a wet tank is 600 litres of water with a saturation level of 85 per cent salts. The water is heated to 35°C. The resultant high density allows the body to float naturally and spontaneously without effort. The Dead Sea in Israel has a saturation level of 100 per cent, which means that as you stand up, the water evaporates and the salt immediately crystallises on the body. This does not happen with wet tanks – the water just feels like a silky solution and you are not aware of the salt. Even the head floats – the centre of buoyancy and the centre of gravity of the head are in about the same place, so the client can tilt the head back comfortably without fear of sinking.

As the water is salty, any broken skin will need to be covered with some form of waterproof, protective barrier cream such as petroleum jelly, although infected areas of skin would be contra-indicated.

Remember

The client who is unable to swim should feel perfectly safe in the shallow water.

Keys to good practice

With any heat treatment which raises the body temperature even a little, the body needs to replace the moisture lost, so always offer the client a drink after treatment.

Tank maintenance

- The tank should be checked and filtered regularly for any loose hairs, scum lines or oily film on the water. These can be avoided by asking the client not to apply body lotion or moisturiser on the skin prior to the treatment.
- The inside of the tank, above the water line, must be cleaned once a week or as necessary, although a daily check is advisable.
- The temperature should be monitored and the water re-heated between clients if required – a floating thermometer can be used, but remember to remove it before the client enters the tank.
- The pH of the water should be 7.6. This should be checked daily.
- The level of bromine must not be higher than 2 parts per million and must be checked a minimum of once a week.

Frequently asked client questions about wet flotation

- *How long does it take?* Each session lasts 60 minutes, but the treatment can be flexible. If clients require a longer or shorter float, they should discuss this when they book. Clients should come 10 minutes prior to their first float so that a consultation can be done and their queries answered. Clients will be offered a showering time before and after the float so they can dry their hair and have a drink.
- *Can floating really change my life?* There is a growing movement towards natural solutions that counteract the stresses of modern life. The benefits of floating are natural, long-term and cumulative. Every time the client floats, the health benefits of the relaxation response are reinforced.
- *Will I feel claustrophobic?* The client is in complete control of his or her surroundings and can float in the light or dark or even with the lid open. There is no feeling of being in a confined space.
- *Will my skin become wrinkled?* The water contains high salt levels, which leaves the skin soft but not wrinkled.
- *How is water hygiene maintained?* All flotation spas adhere to strict hygiene regulations. The water contains salt and a balance of chemicals to keep it sterile and these levels are checked daily. Between each session the water is thoroughly filtered and the inside of the tank sprayed with the solution, so maintaining hygiene.
- *What if I fall asleep?* Some people fall asleep. The salt in the water keeps the client afloat so there is no chance of turning over or sinking. If the client is concerned about running over time, advise him or her that the tank can be controlled from reception. Gentle music is played throughout the therapy which gradually gets louder towards the end of the treatment to wake the client. As a last resort, the therapist can open the tank door automatically and switch on the lights to wake the client.
- *Is it private?* The client is shown into a private room which has a shower for use before and after the session. There is a lock on the float room door so the client can maintain privacy at all times. The door to the tank does not lock – it is motorised and opens and closes when the client presses a button. However, it can be easily pushed open so the client will never get trapped inside.
- *What do I do in the flotation tank?* Nothing at all! Floating automatically induces deep relaxation. The client may day dream or drift off to sleep.

Remember

As the muscles are so relaxed, massage is extremely therapeutic after a flotation treatment, but to extend the after-effects of the treatment, the client should avoid stimulating or noisy electrical treatments.

Remember

When checking and/or cleaning flotation tanks, remember to bend at the knees and not from the spine, where possible. This will help you to avoid bad posture and muscle strain.

- *Can I float with someone else?* Flotation tanks only accommodate one person at a time. The aim of floating is to reduce environmental stimulation, and to have another individual in the tank would defeat the object.
- *How often should I float?* The natural reaction triggered in the flotation tank is reinforced each time the client floats. Regular floating benefits the body because the client learns to relax more quickly. Frequency is a matter of individual preference and lifestyle – some people float once or twice a week to keep the body and mind in perfect tune, others float when they are experiencing a demanding time in their lives and require relaxation. Clients will need to float about three to five times before they become fully acclimatised to the tank and get the maximum benefit. Most wet flotation tanks have the added safety feature of an intercom, so that the therapist outside can check that the client is comfortable.

Aftercare

Helping clients out of the tank is important, as they may be disorientated, having been in the dark and warmth for up to two hours. Rather like waking up from a deep sleep, clients may wonder where they are! Be supportive and allow them to rest and wake fully before they either move on to other treatments or leave the salon. It is particularly important to ensure clients are wide awake if they intend driving or returning to work. Ideally, the client should go home to sleep to get the full benefit of the soporific (sleep-inducing) feeling.

After treatment, the client will need to shower off the salty water.

Dry flotation

In dry floatation the body does not come into contact with the heated water – it is protected by a membrane or lining of heavy duty vinyl. Dry flotation is rather like being on a waterbed, with warm water in it, or on a very relaxing mattress. However, it does not have the same effect as wet flotation as the body is not sensory-deprived in quite the same way. It is important that the client is aware of the difference.

Unlike wet flotation, in which no body preparations should be used, the dry flotation method is often used with body packs so that the heat works with the active ingredients to help penetrate the skin, or it can be used on its own, depending upon the client's needs and personal preferences (see page 453 for ingredients and their benefits).

The dry flotation tank

The dry flotation tank can be used either as a couch or bed, and the client is massaged while on it, or it can be lowered into the water.

A dry tank is like a larger than average bath tub, and is usually a stainless steel frame containing a tank of water which can be thermostatically controlled, covered with a thick vinyl lining, and with a duckboard on which the client lies. The board can be lowered to suspend the client in water with no pressure points. The water tank is completely sealed by a flexible membrane with upholstered and padded side panels.

Some manufacturers are now producing the same wet tank format, with an inner membrane covering the water, so the client gets the best of both worlds, but does not get wet.

Remember

Flotation therapy maximises the benefits of fitness training through improved circulation and deep relaxation of muscle fibres, aiding regeneration of tissue. This would appeal to the male market, especially keen sportsmen.

Remember

Flotation helps to stimulate the body's own powers of healing and regeneration and maintains homeostasis within the body.

Dry flotation therapy

After the consultation, the client showers and has a suitable body pack applied, depending upon the treatment aims, and then lies on top of the board. The therapist covers the client and then lowers the duckboard.

The lights within the room can be dimmed or the client may wish to have the eyes covered with a sleep mask. The client can then be left to drift away into a relaxed state.

Time the treatment and then gently arouse the client into a more focused state. The board can then be lifted up to the level of the top of the bath to enable the client to climb off. The client should shower off the products.

Aftercare is the same as for wet flotation treatments.

Remember

Ensure the client removes all jewellery, spectacles and contact lenses.

Provide hydrotherapy treatments

BT29.4

Prepare, clean and maintain the spa environment

BT28.1

Monitor water, temperature and spa treatments and environment

BT28.3/BT29.5

In this outcome you will learn about

- the sauna
- steam hydrotherapy
- spa pools
- baths
- pools
- showers
- tepidarium.

Hydrotherapy comes from the Greek word *hydor* meaning water and *therpia* meaning therapy. It includes all forms of water treatment. Like spas, hydrotherapy is not new. The Romans had 'hot rooms' and their communal bathing rituals led to the use of hydrotherapy in the Middle East.

The sauna

There are three types of sauna:

- the traditional Finnish sauna, designed for communal use
- the less intense Roman laconium sauna, also designed for communal use
- the personal sauna, which can be for individual use and can have added features such as oxygen infusion or it can vibrate.

The Finnish sauna

Sauna cabins come in log or panelled versions, and are usually made of low-sap pine. Between the panels are air spaces filled with an insulating material which helps save on running costs (electricity) and prevents heat from escaping so allowing the temperature to remain constant.

Seven air changes are required each hour to keep the air healthy, and the low-sap pine wood allows this interchange. Heating is by electric stoves which heat special stones placed in a recessed tray, piled on top of the stove. Heat rises, so the top bench is hotter than the lower one.

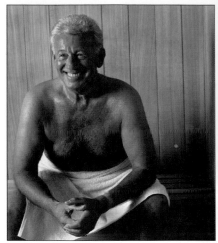

Finnish sauna

Remember

Advise new clients to stay on the lower bench until they acclimatise to the heat.

Saunas produce a very dry heat, with only 10 per cent humidity – the water evaporates on the coals very quickly and clients should be wet when they go into the sauna to induce perspiration.

Regular visits to the sauna are an ideal anti-stress programme and promote the deep cleansing of the skin. The client should be encouraged to come out of the heat and take a cool shower, or visit the plunge pool every 10 minutes. The interplay of hot and cold stimulates the body's physical functions, especially blood circulation and irrigation. In addition, the body's own resistance is promoted, the heartbeat stimulated and blood pressure positively influenced.

Finnish sauna

- Wooden cubicle.
- Electrically heated.
- Temperature: 80–100°C.
- Dry environment (stones are wetted towards end of warm-up).
- Purges the body and cleans the skin.
- Helps reduce damaging environmental influences and stress.
- Stimulates circulation; promotes the body's defences.
- Recommended time in the sauna: 15–20 minutes (heat-up), two to three times a week.
- Follow up with 20–30 minutes' rest.

Remember

Advise the client that the weight loss from a sauna treatment is temporary, due to water lost during the perspiration process – the body adjusts, the thirst mechanism is activated and the weight is put on when water is replaced.

Remember

Most sauna cabins have a window in the door, so you can observe the clients and check on their well-being without having to keep opening the door, which will cause a draught and heat loss.

The laconium

This is a relaxing, dry, aromatic environment creating a Roman sauna atmosphere, with lighting and sound effects to stimulate the senses. There is 15–20 per cent humidity in the laconium, so it is cooler than the very dry heat of a pine sauna. It has fully heated tiled walls, floor and contoured benches for communal bathing of six to eight people. A Kniepp Hose can be used to refresh and cool the body so enabling the client to enjoy a longer treatment time (see Kniepp therapy, page 479).

The body is so warmed up that after a short time it is thoroughly cleansed by intensive perspiration. The circulation is stimulated, the elimination of metabolic waste accelerated and the body's own defences are mobilised. The regular perspiration in the laconium helps to reduce stress over the long term. The heartbeat is stimulated and blood pressure regulated. The result is a feeling of freshness and deeper mental and physical relaxation. The time spent in the laconium depends on individual preference, but the purging effect starts after 15–20 minutes.

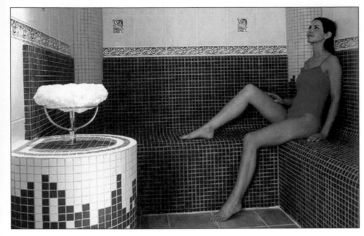

The laconium sauna

Laconium

- Mild form of Finnish sauna.
- Temperature: 55–65°C.
- Dry environment.
- Purges and decontaminates the body.
- Helps reduce damaging environmental influences and stress.
- Stimulates the heartbeat and circulation.
- Recommended time in the sauna: 15–20 minutes, two to three times a week.
- Follow up with 20–30 minutes' rest.

The personal sauna

A personal sauna is a single pod, a little smaller in size than a wet flotation tank, which offers individual treatment. It is suitable for the client who either does not want to share a sauna or who likes to be in control of the settings and have a more personal treatment. Some individual saunas also have the facility of Shirodhara – the ancient soothing Ayurvedic technique of pouring a stream of aromatherapy oil on to the centre of the forehead, which is the third eye chakra. Oxygen infusion helps the skin, and promotes good cellular activity.

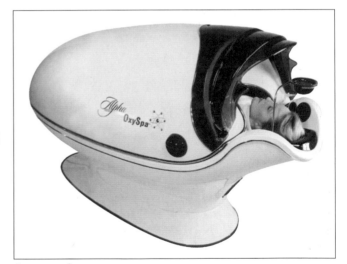

A personal sauna

It is a dry heat sauna, and inside the capsule, the body is bathed in gently heated air. The temperature is adjustable from 26°C to 82°C.

There is an adjustable pulsating vibratory surge in variable waves under the massage bed, and the rhythm can be adjusted from rapid strokes to long, deep waves that allow multiple therapies, from delicate to deep penetration of the tissues.

The aromatherapy system allows clients the choice of scents to flow over the body and fill the capsule. The blend of oils can be prescriptive, to suit the client's needs. The massage bed is ergonomically designed to fit the contours of the body and eliminates any pressure points by evenly distributing body weight.

The pod includes a sound system with CD player, so clients can listen to their own choice of music through speakers or head phones, and a fan which blows cool air across the face – ideal for the claustrophobic client or one who gets over-heated in a traditional sauna. There is also a canopy which can be pulled over the head, to infuse oxygen on to the face, which is an added facial therapy for those clients who like to be totally immersed in a sauna.

The alpha Oxyspa has 18 pre-set programmes, which can be customised to suit the individual client, and can be used with body wraps and body masks. It is also useful for the client starting a detox programme.

Personal saunas:

- helps to detoxify and cleanse the body
- increase circulation
- ease muscular tension through the heat
- aid in stress management
- burn calories and promote weight loss
- provide a private, personal sanctuary
- promote deep relaxation.

Sauna hygiene

The laconium is completely tiled and is therefore easy to wash down and keep clean. However, maintenance is required on the tiles to ensure they do not crack or chip, but they can be easily replaced, and sanitised with a cleansing solution, as recommended by the supplier.

With Finnish saunas, sebum and skin particles adhere to the wood, but it is impracticable to use soap solutions due to the need for large quantities of rinse water. Equally, disinfectant substances could cause noxious fumes. Although the air in a sauna is too hot for the active growth of bacteria, the walls and furnishings are not. The sauna must be scrubbed out daily using fresh clean water.

As clients go barefoot in the sauna, there is a risk of spreading foot infections such as verrucas and athlete's foot. It is advisable to place disposable couch roll on the floor of the wooden duckboards, to avoid this.

Personal saunas can be lined with disposable sheeting, if a body wrap is used, and the capsules can be wiped out with a recommended solution for deep cleansing after each client.

For maximum hygiene, it is advisable:

- to limit client occupancy – there should be adequate room for each individual to sit without being in body contact with another person
- for clients to wear the bottom half of a bathing suit
- for clients to sit on a paper towel
- to change the water in the sauna bucket daily and empty at the end of each day (see below).

Sauna temperature and humidity

The temperature in a sauna can range from 70°C to 110°C – higher than the boiling point of water!

However, the air does not feel as hot as it is: first, because hot air does not have as high a heat capacity as water and is soon cooled on contact with the skin and secondly, because as the body perspires, the sweat evaporates, resulting in a cooling effect on the skin.

Humidity means the dampness in the air. The rapid evaporation of sweat which occurs in a sauna is because the relative humidity of the air is very low. Humidity is measured

Remember

To ensure hygiene and client safety, always use the products recommended by individual sauna manufacturers. Otherwise, you risk causing chemical build-up, the accumulation of fumes and cross infection.

The manufacturers' instructions will guide the temperature settings:

- 70°C is a mild sauna.
- 90°C is a strong sauna heat.
- 110°C is a very hot sauna.

Remember

Small saunas with small stoves can be plugged into the normal household supply, but the larger ones need a special power cable similar to that used for electric cookers. They must be installed professionally.

by a hygrometer. It usually contains human hair which expands when it is moist and contracts when it dries. This expansion and contraction is used to turn a pointer on a dial. The hygrometer is usually found next to the thermometer in the sauna.

The sauna stove

The heat is provided by a powerful electric stove. On top is a tray of stones or 'coals' on to which clients may pour water.

Because of their power ratings, sauna stoves cannot be run from a socket. They must be wired directly from the consumer unit.

SAUNAS
A User's Guide

The potential hazards are:

❖ adverse reaction caused by excess heat or overuse, including giddiness and fainting
❖ burns caused through contact with the sauna stove and light fittings
❖ cross infection from unhygienic sauna bench surfaces
❖ shock due to sudden, extreme changes in temperature induced by use of plunge pools or cold showers
❖ allergy to chemicals used in the plunge pool disinfection process
❖ fire or fumes from towels placed on or above the sauna stove
❖ slipping injuries caused by wet flooring.

Be aware that:

❖ a sauna operates at a temperature of 85-100°C. Ensure this is comfortable for you
❖ jewellery, watches, etc. should be removed before using the sauna
❖ the warmest part of the sauna is diagonally opposite the stove. The higher benches are the warmest
❖ the sauna controls should only be adjusted by an authorised person
❖ contact lenses and glasses should not be worn in the sauna
❖ care should be taken when adding water to the stove. The sauna is intended to be a dry heat bath, it should not be so dry that it is uncomfortable to the nose and throat.

You should not use the sauna if you:

❖ suffer from heart disease or circulatory problems, high or low blood pressure or from any condition which may affect your reaction to heat
❖ are suffering from infections, skin diseases, sores or wounds
❖ are suffering from an illness causing an inability to perspire
❖ are taking anticoagulants, antihistamines, vasoconstrictors, vasodilators, stimulants, hypnotics, narcotics or tranquillisers or any other medications that makes you unsure as to the advisability of using saunas
❖ have had a heavy meal within one and a half hours
❖ have consumed alcohol within one and a half hours
❖ have recently exercised. Time should be allowed to enable body temperature to return to normal levels
❖ suffer from any condition that makes you unsure as to the advisability of using saunas.

A user's guide to the sauna

Keys to good practice

The use of essential oils in the sauna, such as sandalwood and eucalyptus, enhances the treatment and helps clear a stuffy head. However, essential oils are highly flammable. Never add them directly to the coals – there is a risk of fire. Add a few drops to the water in the bucket, which dilutes the oil, and then add to the coals.

Remember

Ask the client to read the user guides for the wet area.

Remember

The term 'bather load' refers to the number of people using a spa pool or sauna, usually in relation to a period of time, that is number per hour. However, it is not just the number of clients in the sauna – in the case of a pine sauna, it is also their combined weight. Most saunas specify six to eight people at one time, but this will depends on their size – the sauna bench seating needs to be sturdy enough to take their total weight.

Pouring water on the coals

The users of a sauna are provided with a bucket of water and ladle. They ladle water on to the coals. The water boils and the steam from the boiling water increases the humidity. This reduces the rate of evaporation of sweat, so lessening the cooling effect – the sauna feels hotter. This lessens the water loss from the body and the risk of dehydration. It also lessens the likelihood of scorching the lungs.

Steam hydrotherapy

Steam is a moist heat, with up to 90 per cent humidity. It works rather like a kettle does – water is heated in a container and the steam being made is channelled into either:

- a steam cabinet
- a steam room
- a caldarium
- a hamman.

The steam cabinet

This is an ideal individual treatment for clients who do not like the dry heat of a sauna, and who prefer their head to be out of the heat. The high humidity provides a relaxing climate. The circulation is stimulated, muscle tension relaxed and the skin becomes pliant and supple.

Steam cabinet

- Temperature: 50–55°C.
- Moist environment (warm steam is fed in).
- Cleanses the skin and respiratory tract; stimulating.
- Recommended time in the cabinet: 10–20 minutes, two to three times a week.
- Follow up with 20–30 minutes' rest.

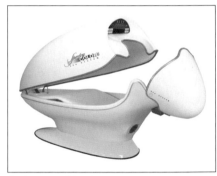

A steam cabinet

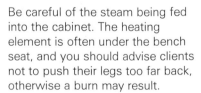

Remember

Be careful of the steam being fed into the cabinet. The heating element is often under the bench seat, and you should advise clients not to push their legs too far back, otherwise a burn may result.

Steam cabinet preparation

1 Fill the reservoir of the steam unit to within 1.25 cm of the top. The unit will heat up more quickly if hot water is used.
2 Place a towel and paper tissue on the seat. Try to arrange the towel so that the client's legs are protected from the steam, but do not block the flow.
3 Place paper tissues/couch roll over a towel on the floor treads.
4 Place a towel and paper tissue on the floor outside the cabinet, placed to the side so that the client can stand on it before entering and leaving the unit.
5 Set the thermostat dial to the required position. Refer to the manufacturer's instructions for the appropriate setting. Place a towel over the open top to prevent the steam from escaping.
6 Switch on the unit and set the timer control to 10 minutes to pre-heat.
7 When the cabinet has heated up, the client can then be brought from the shower/changing area.

Steam cabinet procedure

1 The therapist assists the client into the steam unit. (She will need to ensure that heat loss is kept to a minimum.) As the client sits down, the therapist checks the seat height is correct. The client passes his or her towel covering to the therapist who slowly closes the door.
2 The therapist places a large towel around the client's neck to prevent the steam from escaping.

3   The therapist sets the minute timer and temperature control to the appropriate settings to suit the individual. (Refer to the manufacturer's instructions, which should always be on display near the cabinet.)

4   The therapist must stay with the client during the treatment and adjust the temperature control if necessary.

5   When the treatment is complete, the therapist removes the towel placed around the client's neck. As the therapist opens the door, she passes a large fresh, clean towel to the client.

6   The therapist assists the client out of the steam cabinet.

7   The client should finish with a cool shower once the treatment is complete.

8   Following this, the client must rest at room temperature until body temperature returns to normal.

Steam cabinet hygiene

Steam cabinets are an ideal breeding ground for germs and bacteria, so you will need to ensure that:

- the cabinet is washed out thoroughly with disinfectant after every client and is scrubbed regularly with detergent to remove oils and greases
- all water is removed from the cabinet
- at end of day, the door is left open to allow the cabinet to air dry.

The glass fibre construction of a steam cabinet resists the growth of many organisms.

Precautions to take when using the steam cabinet and shower

- Female clients may wear bikini bottoms; male clients may wear swimming trunks. There are disposable panties and slippers available, which should be issued to all clients prior to a treatment.
- Long hair must be tied up, to avoid contamination.
- Paper must be used on the floor of the shower as a barrier method to prevent fungal/viral infections and should be disposed of after use.
- Individual soaps should be used to prevent cross-infection, or shower gels applied to client's own flannel. Flannels and soaps should not be communal.
- Ensure that there is a good non-slip covering on the floor in and around the changing cubicle.
- Make sure that dressing gowns and towels are only used once before being laundered.
- Towels or disposable paper should be used for drying the body and immediately placed in a plastic-lined linen basket for washing, or the paper can be disposed of.
- Take the client's pulse rate and body temperature before and after treatment; check feet for fungal infections.
- Check equipment temperatures before use and at frequent intervals to guard against thermostat failure. Do not have the thermostat controls where they are accessible to the client.
- Make sure that there is an efficient guard around the heater or steam inlet.
- Keep the client in view throughout the treatment.
- Do not treat the client for too long.
- Do not over-heat the cabinet.
- Take special care with new clients unused to the treatment.
- Give the client clear instructions as to correct usage of the equipment and display the instructions in a prominent position nearby.
- Make sure that there is adequate resting space.
- A place should be provided for clients to cool down and have a drink before leaving the premises.

Risks when using the steam cabinet

- Scalds.
- Burns.
- Fainting.
- Heat stroke and exhaustion with resulting collapse.
- Falls.
- Headaches.
- Infection.
- Fatigue.

The steam room

The steam room works on the same warm, moist air principle that a cabinet does, except it is much larger, and used for multi-occupancy, instead of one individual.

Some swimming pools and larger leisure centres have a steam room, often working on a payment system – place a pound into the timer and you are guaranteed 15 minutes of steam.

STEAM ROOM
A User's Guide

The potential hazards are:
- adverse reaction caused by excess heat or overuse, including giddiness and fainting
- scalding form direct contact with steam from the steam pipe
- shock due to sudden, extreme changes in temperature induced by use of plunge pools or cold showers
- slipping injuries caused by wet flooring.

Be aware that:
- a steam room operates at a temperature of 40-50°C. Ensure this is comfortable for you
- the steam room controls should only be adjusted by an authorised person
- jewellery, watches, etc. should be removed before using the steam room
- prolonged stays in the steam room are not recommended because the continued effects of higher levels of humidity on the body an be dangerous.

You should not use the steam room if you:
- are pregnant
- suffer from heart disease or circulatory problems, high or low blood pressure, or from any condition which may affect your reaction to heat
- are suffering from infections, skin diseases, sores or wounds
- are suffering from an illness causing an inability to perspire
- are taking anticoagulants, antihistamines, vasoconstrictors, vasodilators, stimulants, hypnotics, narcotics or tranquillisers or any other medications that make you unsure as to the advisability of using steam rooms
- have had a heavy meal within one and a half hours
- have consumed alcohol within one and a half hours
- are a child under the age of 8
- suffer from any condition that makes you unsure as to the advisability of using steam rooms.

A user's guide to the steam room

Unlike the cabinet, the client's head is in the steam, so the respiratory tract is cleansed, but it can be slightly claustrophobic for a client, and when the steam room is full of steam, it can reduce visibility, so often clients cannot see who they are sitting next to! The effects and precautions are the same as for a steam cabinet.

A caldarium

This is based upon a Roman-style steam room, with an aromatic moist atmosphere either to relax or stimulate the senses, depending upon the oils used. The oils can be added electronically by injecting them into the steam or adding them to the water. Lavender, rose, jasmine and summer meadow are most commonly used, but as the oils have to suit all the occupants of the caldarium, they cannot be prescribed for the individual client's needs.

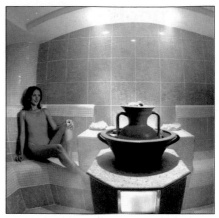

A caldarium

The caldarium operates at between 42–45°C ambient air temperatures with steam. Fully tiled heated walls, floor and lounge benches provide seats for up to 10 people. A Kniepp hose is used to refresh and cool the body, which enables the client to spend longer periods in the caldarium.

The interplay of heat and moisture stimulates the circulation and thoroughly and gently cleans the skin and respiratory tract. Muscular tension relaxes, stress is reduced, limbs and joint pains are eased. The caldarium is a mild but effective means of relieving stress and helping regeneration.

Caldarium
- Temperature: 42–45°C.
- Moist environment (steam with natural herbal essences).
- Cleanses the skin and respiratory tract; stimulating.
- Recommended time in the caldarium: 20 minutes, two to three times a week.
- Follow up with 20–30 minutes' rest.

A hamman

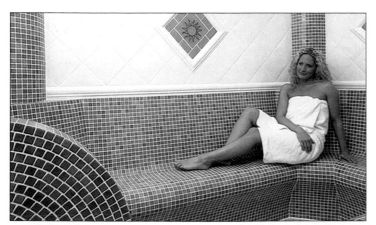

A hamman

This is a variation on the theme of steam baths. Originating in Turkey and the Middle East, it is a communal bath house. The hamman is easily identified by its the characteristic Ottoman blue and yellow tiling and motifs. The bath has a moist aromatic atmosphere – it is usually a hot steam room with a cold plunge pool used to rapidly bring down the body's temperature.

Spa pools

The spa pool is also known as a whirlpool, jacuzzi, aqua spa pool or hot tub. The term 'hot tub' originally referred to the wooden, barrel-shaped tubs first introduced in the 1960s. Early hot tubs were simple devices – they held hot water with room for two bathers. The wooden tub has evolved to include amenities such as seating, jets of water and air, and is now made of moulded acrylic or plastic shells, with seats for up to ten, depending upon the space available and the supporting structures within the spa or leisure centre.

Whatever the type of spa, the principle of the mechanics is the same – the pool holds a set amount of water, which is heated, forced around the pool system by a pump, and then filtered and re-circulated. Once the water is in the spa, it is only drained every two to four months, depending upon the individual manufacturer's instructions. Most colleges will only drain their spa at the end of every term for cleaning and maintenance.

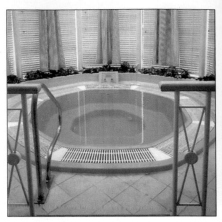

A spa pool

Spa pool hygiene

Hygiene is maintained by:

- filtering the water – the filters collect debris, hair and any foreign matter
- a chemical balance – ensuring the water is user-friendly for human skin.

Filters

These can be made of:

- sand
- graphite
- paper
- polyester micro-pore fabric.

Sand and graphite are contained in boxes and the water is forced through them – the fine grains catch any larger debris, such as hairs, fibres from swimming costumes, or grass if the spa is outside. These boxes are usually found in older spa units, and have mostly been superseded by paper or fabric filters.

Paper and polyester micro-pore fabric filters are pleated into a cone shape, with a centre core where the water passes through. They are held in place by moulded end caps and the pleats catch all the debris, so that the water can then be passed through the heater and re-circulated out through the jet holes.

Depending upon the bather load, the filters should be cleaned every two weeks and replaced every time the spa is emptied. Paper filters are very hard wearing but will need replacing before the polyester fabric ones. They clean up very well, either through soaking overnight in the recommended commercial filter cleaning compound, or by rinsing every pleat with fresh water, to dislodge all foreign matter.

Using a filter rotation method, where one is being soaked, and a new one is in the spa, means that the client should never have to wait for a treatment.

Check it out

Find out your job role for monitoring the spa, testing the water and cleaning filters. If the task is duplicated by staff through the day, then the chemicals added will be more than required, and will not only be wasted but could cause an overdose which might be harmful to clients. Check the rota to ensure the task is not duplicated, or missed altogether!

Keys to good practice

For added protection and to increase the life of the filter, some spa pool manufacturers recommend a 'scum sock', a stretchy sock which fits over the whole filter and prevents debris from clogging it. This is particularly effective for a domestic spa which may be housed outside – grass gets into the water from the feet, and bugs and flies are attracted to the water, especially if the spa does not have a cover on it. Older models may have a skimmer basket, just in front of the filter bank, which performs the same task.

Keeping the spa clean

The other method of keeping the water clean is to ensure the client knows spa etiquette. During the consultation, you will need to advise the client of the following:

- Tie up long hair, both for hygiene reasons and for the client's safety.
- Avoid using highly foaming shower gels and shampoo prior to entering the spa – the pressure action of the water and air jets will create a lot more foam, even if there is only a trace of soap gel left on the client's swimwear from the shower.
- Avoid applying body lotion or oil beforehand, as this creates scum on the water which cannot easily be got rid of by chemical means. Often the only solution is to drain the spa and clean it out!
- Remove all make-up. Eye make-up, for example, often runs down the client's face as it liquefies in the heat, and causes an oily film on the water. If hairspray is used, the client will need to wash this out before getting in the spa pool.
- Remove plasters, jewellery or bandages. These can easily be lost in the water and clog the filters.

Never leave clients unattended in the water, and when they enter the spa pool, make sure the jets of water and air are switched off so that the floor can be easily seen, and clients are sure of their footing.

Keys to good practice

Do not heat the spa over 40°C as it may cause damage to the spa and could be hazardous to the client. Most heater units have a fail-safe system, whereby the heater cuts out if the temperature rises above 44°C. The temperature can be read by a floating thermometer, which should be removed from the water during setting up, prior to the client getting into the water.

Contra-actions

Stop the treatment if the client experiences:

- nausea
- light headedness
- headache
- dryness or burning sensation in the nose/mouth
- lethargy or listlessness
- breathing difficulties
- skin irritation.

Controlling the water balance

This involves:

- balancing and maintaining total alkalinity (TA) and pH
- checking hardness levels
- adding scale and stain pre-emptors.

Remember

The pH scale is explained in **You and the skin**, page 197.

When the mineral components of spa water are in correct proportion, the result is 'balanced water', in other words the water is neither too alkaline (high pH), which causes destructive scale build-up on the equipment, nor too acidic (low pH), which may erode plumbing and cause costly damage to spa pumps, seals and heaters. Balanced water has a pleasant feel to the skin, and allows the sanitiser to work more efficiently.

Total alkalinity is important to test. It is the measure of all the alkaline material in the water and is an indicator of the ability of the water to resist changes in pH, the water's buffering capacity. Too high TA is much less of a problem than too low. Always adjust TA first, then check pH. Maintaining the proper TA will often bring the pH into line automatically. Water is balanced by adjusting its TA and pH with compounds such as Alkalinity Increaser, pH Decrease and pH Increase.

The hardness level of spa water – measured as the amount of dissolved calcium – is also important. This will depend upon the hardness of the water in your area. Insufficient calcium hardness can cause equipment to corrode and also results in water foaming problems. Although there is no practical way to reduce high hardness levels, it is easy to increase levels which are too low by adding Hardness Increase.

Chemical balance

There are several types of micro-organisms which can grow in spa water – bacteria, fungi, protozoa, and viruses. Some of these are pathogens (cause disease). The organisms come from a variety of sources including humans and animals, from the ground, from water or even airborne sources. In a poorly maintained spa they can form biofilms on surfaces, particularly in nooks and crannies. Left unchecked, they will multiply rapidly.

To ensure that delicate human skin is not irritated or infected, and to remove the possibility of cross-infection from others, regular testing of the water and adding chemicals to get the correct balance is essential.

The water should be between 7.2 and 7.6 pH and the level of bromine 2–4 mg per 1 litre. Any other readings will encourage the following.

- **Algae** – these are aquatic plant life, which can grow on spa surfaces or float in the water. Although harmless to bathers, algae discolour the water and indicate incorrect sanitisation – which will put clients off. The spa would need to be drained, and then treated with an algaecide, used to kill algae and prevent regrowth. The addition of bromine will kill bacteria and algae, either dispensed using a flotation dispenser, or a granule form added to the filter.
- **Bacteria** – microscopic organisms continually enter the water via bathers, airborne dust, etc. and the moist and hot conditions are an ideal breeding ground for bacteria, many of which carry disease or infection. (See **Professional basics**, page 40, for a list of infections and their causes.)
- **Pseudomonas** – these bacteria can cause hot tub folliculitis, a condition often seen where spa hygiene is failing. The most common symptom is an itchy rash or small reddish bumps, sometimes resembling insect bites. It can develop into more serious problems. This condition usually clears without scarring. It may recur if

the infected hot tub is not properly cleaned and disinfected. Pseudomonas can affect ears, eyes, skin and the respiratory tract. The micro-organism that causes legionnaire's disease is commonly found throughout our environment, particularly in soil. It can thrive in warm water where the sanitiser level is inadequate, and has been known to become airborne via the action of the air jets in spas. Another is mycobacterium avium, which can cause flu-like symptoms. Interestingly, researchers have found that many people who complain of 'allergic reactions' to sanitising chemicals are actually suffering from skin rashes caused by bacteria due to inadequate sanitiser levels!

Hot tub folliculitis symptoms

- History of using hot tub within last three days.
- Itchy, bumpy, red rash appearing within two days of hot tub exposure.
- Bumps may develop into dark red tender nodules.
- May develop small blisters.
- Multiple members of family or party with same rash and same hot tub exposure.

Bromine tablets

Bromine is a member of the chemical family of halogens, which also includes chlorine. Bromine kills micro-organisms and bacteria by attacking their cell walls through oxidation, and destroying the enzymes and structures inside. This makes them harmless.

When hot tubs first appeared, many people used pool chlorine (TriChlor or cal-hypo tablets) as a disinfectant. This type of chlorine is *not* well suited for hot tubs because it has a higher acidic nature and generally dissolves too slowly to be effective. This is really only suitable to work in larger swimming pools. Prolonged contact with the spa may cause bleaching of the colour and may even mark it causing a permanent line.

However, there is a form of chlorine that can be used for spa shock treatment (see below). This is sodium DiChlor granular chlorine. It is not excessively alkaline in nature and it is highly dissolvable in granular form.

Spa shock treatment

Shock treatment is the routine of applying a compound to the spa water which oxidises or breaks down the dead organic material left behind from the sanitiser system, as well as non-filterable material such as dirt, soap films, hair spray and perspiration. Allowed to remain in the water, these contaminants provide a food source for bacteria and algae. Regular shock treatments eliminate them and the organics on which bacteria feed.

Regardless of which sanitiser system you use, periodic shocking is essential for clear, clean hot tub water. It will also allow the sanitiser to perform at peak efficiency.

How to test the water

Water testing can be carried out using two methods:

- Using tablets of pH phenol red tablet and DPD tablets to measure bromine levels into a double vial which has colour codes against it, to compare against the colour of the water.
- Using impregnated strips to test pH and bromine levels and comparing them to the readings on the side of the testing jar.

Remember

Read the instructions on the bottle first, as they may vary from brand to brand.

For tablet testing

- Allow the spa to circulate for a minute or two, then take a sample of spa water by dipping the testing vial into the middle of the spa water, but do not fill up to the brim – allow enough space for the lid to go on.
- Into the left side of the phial, drop one pH phenol red tablet, encased within the foil wrapper. Do not touch the tablet, as it will absorb the pH reading from your skin.
- In the right side, add one DPD tablet to measure the bromine levels – again, make no contact with it.
- Replace the rubber cap and give the container a thorough shake to disperse the tablets and then in a good light, compare the readings from the colour chart, and adjust the spa water accordingly.

Remember

Should there be a large abnormal reading of any of the water balance tests, report it immediately to your line manager and do not allow the client to enter the spa – it could be a problem which can be remedied, but you should not put the client at risk.

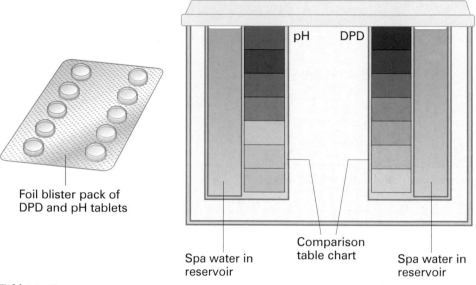

Foil blister pack of DPD and pH tablets

Spa water in reservoir

Comparison table chart

Spa water in reservoir

Tablet testing

For paper strip testing

Follow this simple routine for testing before each spa use, or at least once a week:

- Allow the spa to circulate for a minute or two, then take a sample of spa water in a clean plastic drinking glass – a few millilitres will do.
- Remove a spa test strip from the bottle, and recap tightly.
- Dip the strip in the water just deep enough to wet all test pads, and remove (dip time may vary from brand to brand, so read the instructions).
- Remove excess water by shaking the strip once, briskly, if so indicated in the instructions (procedure may vary by brand).
- Hold strip horizontal, pad side up, for 15 seconds (or as per instructions).
- Make colour comparisons with bottle chart. Adjust the spa water as necessary.

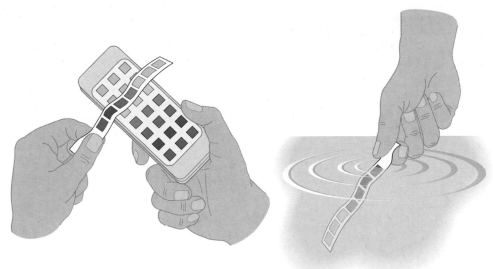

Paper strip testing

Keys to good practice

- Store your test strips at room temperature in a dark, dry location (never outside). The strips themselves must be kept completely dry until ready to use. Cap the bottle tightly, immediately after removing a strip – do not wait until you have finished testing. Prolonged sunlight exposure and heat should also be avoided.
- Watch your fingers – to avoid false readings, never put a wet finger into the test strip container. This will contaminate the unused strips. Be sure to wash your hands before performing the test. Bromine, chlorine or other chemical residues on your hands can interfere with the test results.
- Use fresh strips – discard expired test strips.

Check the expiration date on your bottle. Test strips have a set shelf life. Beyond that date, you cannot be assured of accurate results. False readings mean bad tests, wasted chemicals or equipment damage. Replace expired strips.

Dip the strip to completely cover all the test pads, but do not dip too long in the water. Excessive time will invalidate the test. (Check the instructions.) Also keep in mind that in instances where the amount of bromine or chlorine in the water is quite excessive, it can actually start to bleach out your readings over time. An excessively high level (over 6 parts per million (ppm)) can also result in a false high pH reading. You will have to wait until the bromine or chlorine level comes down to get an accurate test result.

Test results

- If the pH reading is too low, then add the correct additive to bring it up again – usually a powder with pH +. Follow manufacturer's recommendations for use.
- If the pH reading is high, then reduce it to acceptable levels, again following directions for use.
- To adjust the bromine levels, follow instructions by adding another bromine tablet into the flotation basket, or crush one into the filter basket, depending upon the spa instructions.
- Hardness of water will be dependent upon the water supply from the local water authority, and it should offer advice about water softening.

Chemical	Reading
pH	7.2–7.8
Chlorine	2.5–3 ppm
Bromine	2– 4 ppm
Alkalinity	80–160 ppm
Calcium hardness	75–500 ppm

Range of correct readings

Chemical	Function
Sodium carbonate (soda ash)	Raise pH
Sodium bicarbonate	Raise total alkalinity (TA)
Sodium bisulphate (dry acid)	Lower pH to lower TA
Calcium chloride	Raise hardness

Chemicals and their functions

Remember

Spa chemicals are dangerous and must be stored safely in a clean, dry environment. See the COSHH Regulations in, **Professional basics**, page 72, for safe storage guidance and first aid procedures should the chemicals be swallowed or come in contact with the skin.

SPA POOL
A User's Guide

The potential hazards are:

❖ adverse reaction caused by excess heat or overuse, including giddiness and fainting
❖ scalding from water in excess of usual spa temperatures
❖ allergy to chemical used in the spa pool disinfection process
❖ slipping injures caused by wet flooring or from entry or exit from the spa pool
❖ drowning
❖ outlets which if incorrectly designed may cause hair or parts of the body to become trapped against them.

Be aware that:

❖ a spa bath operates at a temperature up to 40°C. Ensure this is comfortable for you
❖ bathing time should not exceed 20 minutes at a time but may be repeated during a session. The warmer the water the less time you should stay
❖ where a spa pool is operated with rest periods you should leave the spa pool during the rest period
❖ some costumes may fade after immersion in the spa pool.

You should not use the steam room if you:

❖ suffer from heart disease or circulatory problems, high or low blood pressure, or from any condition which may affect your reaction to heat
❖ are suffering from infections, skin diseases, sores or wounds
❖ are suffering from an illness causing an inability to perspire
❖ are taking anticoagulants, antihistamines, vasoconstrictors, vasodilators, stimulants, hypnotics, narcotics, tranquillisers or any other medications that make you unsure as to the advisability of using a spa pool
❖ have had a heavy meal within one and a half hours
❖ have consumed alcohol within one and a half hours
❖ are under the age of 8
❖ suffer from any condition that makes you unsure as to the advisability of using a spa pool.

A user's guide to the spa pool

Keys to good practice

Too high a level of bromine in the water will bleach the readings, so you may think that there is not enough bromine to give a reading, and then add more, so exacerbating the problem! If clients were to get into a high bromine spa, their swimming costume could be bleached, and their skin will begin to sting. Fortunately, too much bromine is recognisable by a high smell, a bit like bleach, so use your nose as another form of water testing!

Effects of spa treatment

- Increases the circulation.
- Stimulates the skin and cellular activity.
- Increases general metabolism.
- Raises the body temperature.
- Relaxes muscles through the heat.
- Relieves aches and pains.

Aftercare for the spa

Invite the client to get out of the spa once the water and air jets have been stopped, and provide large towels to wrap the client in order to keep the residue heat in the muscles.

The client should dry off thoroughly, and then get dressed, or relax in a bath robe in the rest area. If the client is going on to have another treatment, such as massage or electrical treatment, time must be allowed for the body temperature to return to normal, and do not give another heat treatment.

Offer the client a large drink of water to replace water lost through perspiration, and ensure the client is in full command of his or her faculties, before attempting to drive or go back to work.

Baths

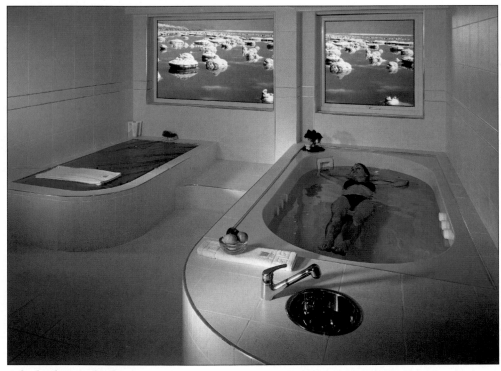

A hydrotherapy bath

Baths are much easier to manage than a spa unit and can also be classed as hydrotherapy. They are a more personal treatment, about the size of a domestic bath, with inlet holes for jets of air or water to be pushed on to the body, giving massage and relaxation. A hydro bath can also provide underwater massage – the massage hose can be hand manipulated by the therapist to target specific areas in order to improve blood and lymph circulation.

Arms

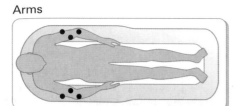

Hips/lower arms

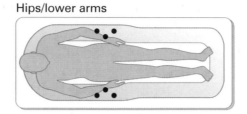

Thighs

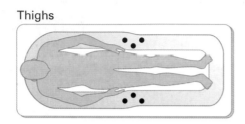

Knees

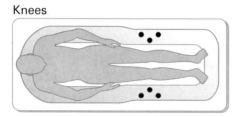

Calves

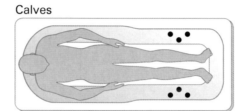

Client being massaged in hydrotherapy bath

The psychological benefits of a hydrotherapy bath

- Reduces stress.
- Soothes irritability.
- Promotes better sleeping patterns.
- Induces mental relaxation.
- Improves concentration through the day.
- Creates a feeling of well being.

The physical benefits of a hydrotherapy bath

- Increases blood and lymph circulation.
- Speeds the removal of metabolic waste.
- Relieves tired and aching muscles.
- Strengthens the immune system.
- Reduces muscular tension.
- Reduces tension headaches.

Foam baths

Foam baths have a warming effect on the body, as the foam generated is an insulator and does not lose its heat as quickly as hot water does. The bath is similar to a domestic bath, but has a plastic duckboard in its base, with tiny holes for the compressed air to be forced through. There is a little hot water in the bath, and most of the bath content is foam in which the client relaxes for up to 15 minutes. Air in the foam traps the heat, there is a rise in body temperature and the client has a very relaxing time – the body is warmed and tissue softened prior to other treatments.

A variety of concentrated foaming agents is available, with aromatherapy essences used for scent. Seaweed and mineral-based foam is also used.

Contra-indications and aftercare are the same as for the spa or steam treatments.

Thalasso therapy

Thalasso therapy is the simultaneous use of sea water and sea air with a preventative or curative purpose, usually under medical supervision, in a site near the sea. The sea water has a three-fold positive effect on health.

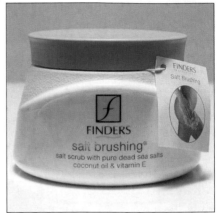

Dead Sea products

1 Effect through the skin. Sea water contains the principal mineral and organic elements needed for cellular life, such as calcium, magnesium, potassium, phosphorous, chlorine and sodium ions.
2 Physical effect. The therapy's stimulating effect is particularly useful in cases where physiotherapy is required, especially through the physical aspect of water motion and its massaging action (only to be taken under medical supervision – not a beauty therapy treatment).
3 Thermal effect. It helps control blood circulation and is both stimulating and restful.

The term 'thalasso' is thought to come from the Greek word *Thalassa* meaning 'sea' and is used to describe any therapeutic treatments involving sea water and seaweed. Many European health spas use thalasso therapy within their treatment packages, for slimming treatments, anti-cellulite and skin rejuvenation. The European Spa Association (ESPA) has strict criteria regarding the term, and how it can be used.

1 Thalasso therapy is an integrated plan for therapy, prevention and health promotion. The plan shall be implemented for defined indications under medical care and with the participation of a qualified expert staff.
2 Therapeutic location immediately by the sea – where the maritime climate has an immediate effect.
3 Sea water shall be used for bathing in natural waters. Suitable sea water that is drawn locally shall be used for inhaling and/or bathing in a bath tub or swimming pool.
4 Marine products should be used such as mud or algae for different applications.
5 Low allergen and clean sea air – the quality of the air must warrant that extended stays in the open air will represent a relieving factor.
6 Associated health promoting measures such as relaxation, change of nutrition and physical exercise shall be included in the plan, to improve overall physical fitness. (ESPA)

If a health spa does not include these criteria, then it is not a thalasso therapy centre.

Sea water is used primarily as it contains at least 60 different minerals and trace elements, most of which are essential to the human organism. These include iodine, iron, copper, zinc, manganese, strontium, molybdenum, boron and a vast range of vitamins, trace elements, minerals and plankton.

Thalasso therapy is a highly effective form of treatment for the human body, since it combines the natural, highly concentrated mineral elements of seaweed and the use of hot water to increase the penetration of these active ingredients through the skin. Hot water dilates pores and blood vessels, making the skin more permeable and therefore more receptive to the active ingredients.

Pools

The bigger health spa club will have a large swimming pool, which needs a lot of water balancing, and uses stronger chemicals than a spa. Swimming pool management is a huge topic and cannot be discussed in detail here. However, a smaller hydro pool is often used as a treatment, and is only 8 feet by 15 feet, but has a powerful pump creating a current which the client has to swim against. This provides resistance to make the muscles work hard and is a stimulating, aerobic exercise. Many physiotherapists use small hydro pools for building up strength in muscles which have atrophied, and need rebuilding.

Water management techniques are exactly the same as for the spa pool – the water is reused, circulated around a heater, with regular chemical checks, and then balanced. The hydro pool is not as high maintenance as a large swimming pool. The pool is also ideal for walking exercises or aqua aerobics.

> ### Keys to good practice
>
> Spa and swimming pool management is governed by the Swimming Pool and Allied Trades Association (SPATA). It can be contacted for advice and guidance on anything from chemical balancing of water to the amount of floor support required for spa installation. SPATA's code of practice is an excellent guide to protecting clients.

Showers

There are three main type of showers used within hydrotherapy:

- the affusion shower
- the shower hydro
- the shower experience.

The affusion shower

This is a relaxing multi-jet shower of warm droplets of water, often seaweed-based or with mineral extracts, which is also infused with aromatic oils. The shower is suspended over a wet table and the water massages the body with varying temperatures and pressures. A lymph drainage massage can also be given.

Most wet tables are moulded of durable ABS plastic, which creates a rounded, silky smooth surface. A trough and drainpipe system surround the central pad which keeps the water draining away when washing off the client. The vinyl-coated foam pad in the middle is easily sanitised and allows the client to be massaged in comfort.

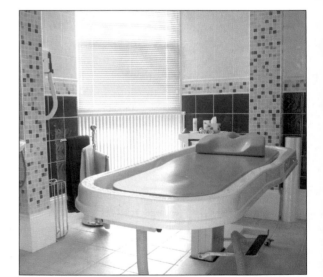

A wet table

The shower hydro

This is automatic water massage, and is usually computer controlled for accuracy of temperature and various methods of application. Specific areas of the body can be targeted by the high-pressured jets, programmed to give precisely timed sequences and differing programmes. These may include wave and back and head massage aimed at specific reflex regions, which are subjected to rapid changes in temperature and pressure.

Kneipp therapy

The use of hot and cold water on the reflex points is based upon Kneipp (pronounced Ka-nipe) therapy. This water therapy system, which was developed in the nineteenth century, is still used in most big spas around the world today. Kniepp therapy employs baths, showers, rinses, wet compresses and water exercises and is used to treat a wide range of ailments from arthritis and rheumatism to sleep disorders and digestive problems.

Kneipp believed that when hot and cold treatments are used alternately, they stimulate the circulation and the temperature receptors within the skin, which improves the health of the tissues in the area. This, combined with regular exercise, water exercise and a high quality diet, led eventually to the development of the health farm and spa experience.

Power jet massage

This is often called a blitz massage or a Scottish douche, and involves the client standing in an open-ended, three-sided, larger shower cubicle, with the therapist at the end of the cubicle with a powerful hose, rather like a fireman's hose! The warm pressurised water can target individual muscle groups, with the client's posture providing a little resistance against the water. The massage is very stimulating and helps both lymphatic drainage and improves the circulation. It is extremely invigorating and sets the whole body tingling through the stimulation of the nerve endings within the skin.

The shower experience

The shower experience has several options ranging from a cold fog mist combined with essential oils, such as a mint essence to enhance a feeling of coolness, especially after a heat treatment, or it can be used with a tropical rain shower massage, with passion fruit essence to invigorate the client before a heat treatment. This is classed as a multi-sensory shower experience with light, sound and scent added.

General showers

After a full consultation, and before the treatment, the client must shower before entering either the sauna, steam unit or spa pool, both for hygiene purposes and to ensure that maximum benefit is gained from the treatment.

Precautions to take when the client showers

There is the risk that the client will fall in the shower or be scalded. To minimise the risk, the following precautions should be taken:

- Explain the use of the shower control to each client before use.
- Make sure that there is a good non-slip mat on the base of the shower cubicle.
- Make sure that clients dry their feet before leaving the shower area.
- Check the thermostatic control on the shower unit frequently.
- If possible, fit the shower with a hand rail. A shower seat could be installed if you have many elderly clients.
- Use disposable paper on the floor where the client stands to dry.
- Once the shower has been used, dry and then wipe with a disinfectant solution.
- Shower gel only is to be provided, due to contamination from common use of soap bars – clients may wish to bring in their own.
- Towels for drying should be placed immediately in plastic bags for washing. Alternatively, clients may bring their own.

Tepidarium

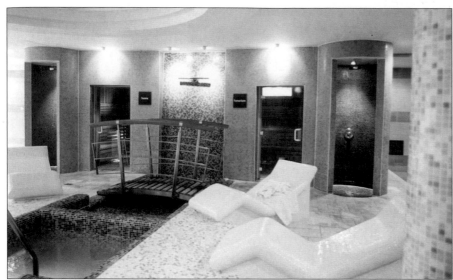

A tepidarium

A stay in the tepidarium, or relaxation room, is protective and stimulating at the same time and clients may stay as long as they wish. The room has an ambient temperature close to that of the body, which induces a healthy fever that strengthens the immune system without overloading the circulatory system.

The tepidarium has a preventive and healing effect and is an ideal way to relieve stress and regenerate the system for young and old alike.

A water feature and a crystal are often used as a focal point in the Tepidarium.

> *Tepidarium*
>
> Ambient temperatures between 42°C and 45°C.
> Dry environment.
> Ideal for regeneration and building up the immune system.
> Has a preventive and healing effect.
> Suggested duration of stay: from 30 minutes, two to three times weekly.

Relaxation room

This should contain comfortable chairs and a small refreshment bar, serving water and fruit squashes to rehydrate the client and allow the body to cool down and relax. The client should always be allowed to cool down for at least half an hour before going back into the reality of the stressful world.

Keys to good practice

Remember to keep the relaxation room well stocked with bottled water, fruit juices and fruit, and treat it just as you would a reception area – keep it tidy and regularly stock check, ordering when a minimum order number has been reached. It may not be the therapists' job to do the ordering, but it is certainly their responsibility to inform the receptionist that stocks are low.

Remember

With all spa equipment used, aftercare should be given. Remember to gain feedback from the client about their impressions and feelings of the treatment, and mark it on the client record card. Explain any possible contra-actions they may experience after the treatment, and what to do if that happens. Make up a suitable treatment plan, and mark it clearly on the record card for future reference, along with a written recommendation for other complimentary treatments. Keep your client record cards up to date, accurate, legible for all to understand and signed by the client.

Knowledge check

1   List ten contra-indications to epilation treatment.

2   List five ways to prevent cross-infection during epilation treatment.

3   What are the benefits of epilation for the client compared with other hair removal methods?

4   Why is it essential to use a magnification lamp during epilation?

5   List four potential risks/hazards within epilation treatment.

6   Give three reasons for your choice of needle within an epilation treatment.

7   List five factors which could affect the client's pain threshold during epilation.

8   What special considerations does a black skin require during epilation?

9   List the benefits of galvanic, diathermy and blend. When would you decide to use each method?

10   Name five epilation aftercare recommendations.

11   Why is hygiene of prime consideration for the wet area?

12   Give ten contra-indications to the wet area.

13   Why is the client's skin type and cultural preferences important to take into consideration?

14   Give three things a new client to the spa may be anxious about.

15   List three conditions where medical approval is required.

16   Give a brief explanation of the term blood shunting.

17   Give four possible contra-indications to treatment.

18   What are the general effects of any heat treatment?

19   State the various types of body wraps available.

20   Give the benefits to be gained from a body wrap.

Resources

Professional associations

Association of Nail Technicians
Alexander House
Forehill
Ely
Cambridgeshire CB7 4AF
Tel: 01353 665577

British Association of Beauty Therapy and Cosmetology
BABTAC House
70 Eastgate Street
Gloucester GL1 1QN
Tel: 01452 421114
www.babtac.com

British Association of Electrolysis
40 Parkfield Road
Ickenham
Middlesex UB10 8LW
Tel: 0870 1280477
Helpline: 01474 325574
www.electrolysis-bae-ltd.co.uk

British Association of Skin Camouflage
c/o Resources for Business
South Park Road
Macclesfield SK11 6FP
Tel: 01625 267880
www.skin-camouflage.net

British Federation of Massage Practitioners
78 Meadow Street
Preston
Lancashire PR1 1TS
Tel: 01772 881063
www.jolanta.co.uk/bfmp.html

British Massage Therapy Council
7 Rymers Lane
Oxford OX4 3JU
Tel: 01865 774123

Federation of Holistic Therapists
3rd Floor
Eastleigh House
Upper Market Street
Eastleigh
Hampshire SO50 9FD
Tel: 023 8048 8900
www.fht.org.uk

Floatation Tank Association
7a Clapham Common
Southside
London SW4 7AA
Tel: 020 7627 4962
www.floatationtankassociation.net

Guild of Professional Beauty Therapists
Guild House
320 Burton Road
Derby DE23 6AF
Tel: 0870 000 4242
www.beauty-guild.com

Hair and Beauty Industry Authority (HABIA)
Fraser House
Nether Hall Road
Doncaster
South Yorkshire DN1 2PH
Tel: 01302 380000
www.habia.org.uk

Hairdressing Council
12 David House
45 High Street
South Norwood
London SE25 6HJ
Tel: 020 8771 6205
www.haircouncil.demon.co.uk

Institute of Electrolysis
PO Box 5187
Milton Keynes MK4 2ZF
Tel: 01908 521511
www.electrolysis.co.uk

International Federation of Aromatherapists
182 Chiswick High Road
London W4 1PP
Tel: 020 8742 2605
www.ifparoma.org

International Nail Association
Guild House
320 Burton Road
Derby DE23 6AF
Tel: 0870 000 4242

Independent Professional Therapists International
PO Box 106
Retford
Nottinghamshire DN22 7WN
Tel: 01777 700383
www.iptiuk.com

Institute of Indian Head Massage
PO Box 1
Windsor
Berkshire SL4 4UZ
Tel: 01753 831 841
www.indianheadmassage.org.uk

Association of Professional Aestheticians of Australia (APAA)
PO Box 96
Robina
Queensland 4226
Australia
Tel: +07 5575 9364
www.apaa.com.au

South African Association of Health and Skin Care Professionals (SAAHSP)
www.cosmeticweb.co.za; www.saahsp.co.uk

Awarding bodies

City and Guilds of London Institute (CGLI)
1 Giltspur Street
London EC1A 9DD
Tel: 020 7294 2800
www.city-and-guilds.co.uk

BTEC
Edexcel
Stewart House
32 Russell Square
London WC1B 5DN
Tel: 0870 240 9800
www.edexcel.org.uk

Confederation of International Beauty Therapy and Cosmetology (CIBTAC)
70 Eastgate Street
Gloucester GL1 1QN
Tel: 01452 421114
www.cibtac.com

International Therapy Examination Council (ITEC)
4 Heathfield Terrace
Chiswick
London W4 4JE
Tel: 020 8994 4141
www.itecworld.co.uk

Qualifications and Curriculum Authority
83 Piccadilly
London W1J 8QA
Tel: 020 7509 5555
www.qca.org.uk

Scottish Qualifications Authority
Hanover House
24 Douglas Street
Glasgow G2 7NQ
Tel: 0141 242 2214
www.sqa.org.uk

Vocational Training Charitable Trust (VTCT)
Unit 11
Brickfield Trading Estate
Brickfield Lane
Chandlers Ford
Dorset SO53 4DR
Tel: 023 8027 1733
www.vtct.org.uk

Australia Council for Private Education and Training (ACPET)
Box Q1076,
QVB PO
New South Wales 1230
Australia
Tel: +61 29299 4555
www.acpet.edu.au

Comité International d'Esthétique et de Cosmétologie (CIDESCO)
Secretariat
Witikonerstrasse 365
8053 Zurich
Switzerland
Tel: +41 1380 0075
www.cidesco.com

Vocational Education and Training Accreditation Board (VETAB)
Level 14
1 Oxford Street
Darlinghurst
New South Wales 2010
Australia
Tel: +61 9244 5335
www.vetab.nsw.gov.au

Business organisations

Association of British Insurers
51 Gresham Street
London EC2V 7HQ
Tel: 020 7600 3333
www.abi.org.uk

ACAS
Brandon House
189 Borough High Street
London SE1 1LW
Tel: 020 7210 3680
www.acas.co.uk

Business Link
To contact your local business link, Tel: 0845 600 9006 or visit www.businesslink.gov.uk

Centre for Accessible Environments
Nutmeg House
60 Gainsford Street
London SE1 2NY
Tel: 020 7357 8182
www.cae.org.uk
Contact the centre for an access audit, a checklist for appraising the accessibility of your premises for people with disabilities.

Consumers' Association
2 Marylebone Road
London NW1 4DF
www.which.net – the Consumers' Association website
www.which.co.uk – the *Which?* magazine website

Data Protection Commissioner
Wycliffe House
Water Lane
Wilmslow
Cheshire SK9 5AF
Tel: 01625 545 745
www.dataprotection.gov.uk

Department of Trade and Industry (DTI)
1 Victoria Street
London SW1H 0ET
Tel: 020 7215 6740
www.dti.gov.uk
A guide to help small businesses may be ordered from the DTI Publications orderline 0870 150 2500.

Health & Safety Executive (HSE)
HSE Information Centre
Broad Lane
Sheffield S3 7HQ
Tel: 08701 545500
www.hse.gov.uk
Contact the HSE for a free leaflet 'Basic advice on first aid at work' (IND(G)215L 1997, published by HSE Books).

The Incident Contact Centre (ICC)
Caerphilly Business Park
Caerphilly CF83 3GG
Tel: 0845 3009923
www.riddor.gov.uk
Holds records on all incidents currently reportable under RIDDOR.

National Association of Citizens Advice Bureaux
Myddelton House
115–123 Pentonville Road
London N1 9LZ
Tel: 020 7833 2181
www.carestandards.org.uk
A voluntary organisation providing impartial, confidential advice on almost any problem.

National Care Standards Commission (NCSC) (England only)
St Nicholas Building
St Nicholas Street
Newcastle-upon-Tyne NE1 1NB
Tel: 0191 233 3600
www.carestandards.org.uk
In **Scotland**, contact the Scottish Commission for the Regulation of Care www.carecommission.com
In **Wales**, contact the Care Standards Inspectorate for Wales www.wales.gov.uk/subisocialpolicycarestandards/index.htm/sponsorship
You must apply for registration with the relevant body if your business offers Class 4 laser treatment and IPL (intensive pulsed light) for non-invasive cosmetic surgery administered by non-medically qualified staff.

The Prince's Trust
Head Office
18 Park Square East
London NW1 4LH
Tel: 0800 842 842
www.princes-trust.org.uk
Helps young people aged 18–30 to set up businesses.

Trading Standards Central
For a local office, visit www.tradingstandards.gov.uk and type in your post code.

Other useful information

- Refer to a directory such as Professional Beauty for comprehensive list of suppliers: www.professionalbeauty.co.uk
- For information on naming a limited company, visit www.companies-house.gov.uk
- When looking for investors in your business a possible source could be National Business Angels Network, 3rd Floor, 40–42 Cannon Street, London EC4N 6JJ, Tel: 020 7329 2929, www.nationalbuangels.co.uk
- For more information on the Disability Discrimination Act 1995, contact the Department of Education and Employment for a series of free booklets, 'Bringing the DDA to life for small shops', the first of which is a hairdressing salon. Tel: 0845 762 2633, www.disability.gov.uk. You can also contact the Disability Rights Commission for advice, www.drc-gb-org
- For advice on fire safety, visit www.firesafe.org.uk
- For cruise liner work, Tel: 020 8909 5074, www.steinerleisure.com
- For a national recruitment agency specialising in placing beauty therapists in a retail environment working for prestigious cosmetic and perfume houses, contact Retail Solutions Recruitment Ltd, 34–35 Eastcastle Street, London W1 8DW, Tel: 020 7436 8484, www.rsr-solutions.co.uk
- For information on gender dysphoria, visit www.beaumontsociety.org.uk (Beaumont Trust) and www.gender.org.uk/gendys (Gendys Network).

- For information about training courses in the audio visual industries, contact Skillset National Training Organisation, 2nd Floor, 103 Dean Street, London W1D 3TH, Tel: 020 7534 5300, www.skillset.org.uk
- For information on full-time courses at colleges, contact Universities and Colleges Admissions Service (UCAS), Rosehill, New Barn Lane, Cheltenham, Gloucestershire GL52 3LZ, Tel: 01242 227788, www.ucas.com

Books

Brown, Loulou, *Careers in the Hairdressing, Beauty and Fitness Industries*, Kogan Page

Taylor, Samantha, *Real Life Guide: The Beauty Industry*, Trotman

Websites

www.educationuk.org

www.educationukscotland.org

www.elemis.com

www.findershealth.com

www.pevonia.com

How to access the Heinemann website

Free web resource

Unit BT30 Provide UV tanning treatments and Unit BT31 Provide self-tanning treatments are available for you to download from our website at www.heinemann.co.uk/vocational, click on: *Hair, Beauty and Holistic Therapies* in the subject list on the left-hand column of the page. From there click on: *Free resources* in the *Resource centre* box in the right hand corner of the page.

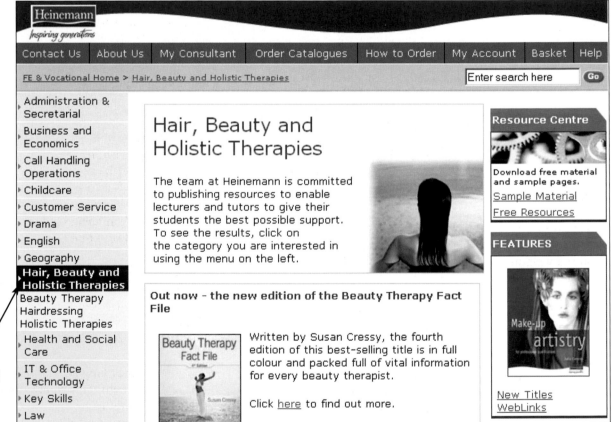

1. Click on: Hair, Beauty and Holistic Therapies

Index

A

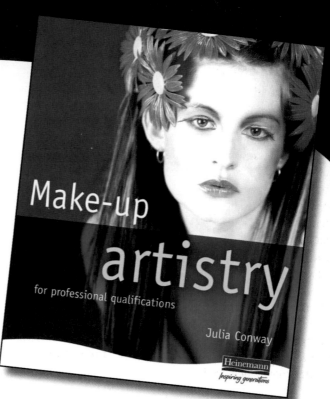
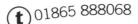 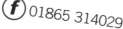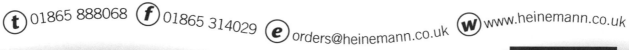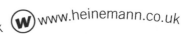
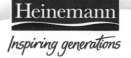

S 666 HAB A

The essential reference tool for both existing practitioners and students

Beauty Therapy Fact File 4th edition

Susan Cressy

The new edition of this best-selling reference book is indispensable to any Beauty Therapy student or practitioner. It has been completely updated and revised in line with the 2004 Beauty Therapy standards.

- The accessible Fact File format allows you to find the information you need quickly and easily.

- The full-colour pages with specially-commissioned photographs and artwork make it visually appealing.

- Includes a new Lifestyle section and a more detailed Spa and Heat Therapy section, making the Fact File bang up-to-date with new developments.

- Written by Susan Cressy, author of a number of highly respected Beauty and Holistics titles.

Beauty Therapy Fact File

4th Edition

Susan Cressy

Heinemann
Inspiring generations

Now in full colour!

Why not order a copy of the Beauty Therapy Fact File today?

Beauty Therapy Fact File
0 435 45142 1

Visit your local bookshop or contact our Customer Services Department for more details:

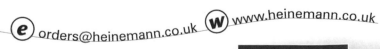

(t) 01865 888068   (f) 01865 314029   (e) orders@heinemann.co.uk   (w) www.heinemann.co.uk

Heinemann
Inspiring generations

H997